HOLISTIC HEALING

for ANXIETY, DEPRESSION, *&* COGNITIVE DECLINE

Brant Cortright, Ph.D.

Published by:

Psyche Media
135 Forrest Ave.
Fairfax, CA 94930

Cover design: Derek Murphy
Copy Editor: Madeline Hopkins

ISBN: 978-0-9861492-2-1 (paperback)

978-0-9861492-3-8 (e-book)

TABLE OF CONTENTS

CHAPTER 1

THE PROBLEM: WHY HAVE MENTAL HEALTH DISORDERS SKYROCKETED IN THE PAST 50 YEARS?

If you feel bad, you're not alone.

Mental health problems have exploded over the last five decades. Childhood rates of depression and anxiety are five to eight times greater than they were in the 1950s and '60s. This isn't due to better diagnosis—the same standardized tests were used then. Plus, now we have sky-high rates of autism, attention deficit disorder (ADD), attention deficit hyperactive disorder (ADHD), eating disorders, and other psychological problems virtually unknown back then. [1, 2]

For adults it's a similar picture. One in eight American adults is currently taking an antidepressant, and one-fourth of those have been taking one for ten years or more. One in four American women age 25–45 is taking an antidepressant. In 2011, the Centers for Disease Control and Prevention reported that the rate of antidepressant use in the United States rose by 400% between 1988 and 2008. Before antidepressants it was estimated that the number of depressed people was 50-100 per million. Now it is estimated to be a *thousand times* greater.[3]

Since each chapter in this book could be a book in itself (and each sentence given a reference), I'll do my best to compress a lot of information into a readable space. Not an easy task considering the volume of information available. In 2016 the American College Health Association surveyed 100,000 college students at 53 U.S.

campuses and found that 84% of the students felt unable to cope, 79% were exhausted, 60% felt very sad, and more 50% were experiencing overwhelming anxiety.[4] College counseling centers are swamped with students seeking relief from anxiety and depression.

Rates of Alzheimer's disease show a similar spike. About 50% of people who reach the age of 85 suffer from Alzheimer's or some other form of dementia. In the past 50 years Alzheimer's rates have gone up more than tenfold, according to the *New York Times*. One in ten seniors 65 or older has Alzheimer's and one in three seniors dies with Alzheimer's or some other dementia. [5] Cognitive decline and mild cognitive impairment, the precursor to Alzheimer's, are seen as part of "normal" aging. But why are rates suddenly rising so quickly?

And it's not just happening with common mental health disorders like anxiety and depression, this explosion is also documented in severe mental disorders such as psychosis and schizophrenia. In his revealing book *Anatomy of an Epidemic*, author Robert Whitaker details the growing mental health crisis in America and the entire developed world. The number of disabled mentally ill has tripled in the last three decades.[6]

Even more alarming: This is all getting worse. According to data from the National Institute of Mental Health, 38% of girls and 26% of boys age 13–17 have an anxiety disorder. I've talked with preschool teachers in despair because a third of their class is on medication. This isn't even grammar school, this is *preschool.*

This crisis has serious physical consequences as well. Research reported in the *New York Times* states, "Americans with depression, bipolar disorder or other serious mental illnesses die 15 to 30 years younger than those without mental illness—a disparity larger than for race, ethnicity, geography or socioeconomic status." [7]

Depression, anxiety, stress, PTSD, ADD and ADHD, addictions, cognitive decline, and other mental health problems are escalating at rates never before seen. More dramatic statistics like these could go on for pages, but probably it's already clear that something is terribly, terribly wrong.

Paradoxically, this is happening when there are more mental services available than ever before. There are more therapists and counselors, more mental health centers, counseling centers, residential treatment centers; more psychiatric medication is being prescribed than at any previous time.

So how can things be getting worse? Why are there more resources available yet a greater need for help ? Why are emotional and mental suffering skyrocketing at this time?

How Did We Get Here?

Why this is happening is considered a mystery. It can't be genetic because the genome takes 50,000—70,000 years to change. Therefore, it must be something in the environment, even if epigenetic changes ensue. But what?

Many causes have been proposed. Some psychiatrists attribute the rise to better diagnosis while others blame drug companies that promote medicating away any kind of emotional pain. Holistic health practitioners see things like environmental pollution, food additives, and sugar as culprits. Some people blame video games, cell phones, or social media. Many therapists point the finger either to more absentee parenting or else to parents who indulge their kids and produce entitled young adults who can't handle failure. Yet none of these alone can explain the enormity of the problem.

All the possible causes have one thing in common: *They all affect the brain.* Moreover, they all degrade the brain in ways that impair healthy emotion regulation.

Why the Brain Is Key

Everyone knows the brain is important, but it's easy to overlook how the brain is responsible for the way you experience life. Everything you experience, you experience through the brain. Every part of you, your body, your emotions and desires, your mental thoughts and images, your dreams and spiritual experiences, your very sense of self, and all of your consciousness is experienced through your brain.

The brain is the master integrator of all the levels we exist on—body, heart, mind, and spirit. The brain shapes everything in life. **The quality of your brain determines the quality of your life.** With a high-quality brain you experience a high quality of life. A low-quality brain yields a low quality of life. A mediocre brain equals a mediocre life.

The health and strength of the self and the brain go together. When the brain weakens, the self weakens. As the brain gets stronger, so does the self. The converse is also true: When the self weakens, the brain weakens. As the self gets stronger, this strengthens the brain.

The physical brain and the psychological sense of self are two levels of one unitary process, two sides of a single coin. Neuroscience and medicine describe the brain; psychology describes the self. Integrating these two languages into a unified whole gives us the most encompassing vision for healing.

Optimal Brain Performance

Optimal brain function means the immense powers and capacities of your brain are available to engage with the world.

A robust, radiant brain shows itself in every area of life. **When your brain functions at peak capacity, life is a joyous adventure.** Not every moment, of course, but with radiant brain health, even life's inevitable suffering can be tolerated without collapse. You meet the world fully, on all planes.

- Physically you have energy, vitality, and an underlying feeling of well-being.
- Your emotion regulation is healthy, so you feel good, enthusiastic, and eager to connect with others and take part in life, able to bounce back after setbacks, energized and joyful.
- Mentally you are focused, able to concentrate and learn, interested and curious about the world.
- Spiritually you are better able to tune in to your inner being, the source of inner peace and love.

You aren't afraid of life or defeated by it. With a robust, radiant brain there comes an expansive sense of self. You don't shrink from life, instead you are ready to pounce on it, like an eager four-year-old, ready to play.

The brain meets the stresses and challenges of living by bringing forth its potentials—your inner talents and abilities. When you actualize your inner self, you creatively develop your capacities in relationships, in school, at work, and at play. Such a robust brain doesn't mean being Einstein or having a high I.Q., it means tapping into the unique genius of *your* brain. Bringing forth *your* potentials carries with it an intrinsic sense of meaning and fulfillment.

It's like paddling downstream on a warm day with the wind to your back. Even a little effort produces big results. But your brain can't reach its highest potentials without the self fulfilling its potentials. The two need to go together.

Actualizing your true nature feels "right" and deeply good, even when things are unpleasant, for you're on the right track to fulfil your deeper self. When bad things happen, as they inescapably do, you aren't as thrown by them and have the resilience to come back quickly.

A robust, radiant brain confers almost total immunity from mental health disorders. Optimal brain health implies that the lower physical systems of the body, like the heart and liver, are healthy also, for if they aren't this usually reduces the brain's operating capacity. Optimal brain health generally means overall radiant health. Radiant health isn't merely the absence of disease, it's a vital state of well-being. There is a healthy glow that feels deeply good and strengthens us to bear the bad times and life's inevitable pain.

A Deficient, Impaired Brain

In contrast, an impaired brain, as in Alzheimer's, Parkinson's, a brain injury or some other form of neurological damage, brings both cognitive and emotional problems. An impaired brain means problems with emotion regulation in some form: interpersonal difficulties, depression, anxiety, stress, chronic anger, shame, hopelessness, or other dysphoric states. It brings cognitive problems such as difficulties with new learning, brain fog, concentration, memory, or executive function.

A low-functioning brain also usually indicates problems in other areas of life, for example physical problems such as compromised immunity, GI disorders, or heart disease; cognitive problems such as difficulties with concentration, memory, or executive function; spiritual difficulties in focusing, meditation, and inner awareness.

Additionally, problems with emotion regulation further diminish the brain. There is measurable cortical decrease with depression, chronic stress and anxiety, isolation, and PTSD. These emotional states actually shrink the brain. [8, 9] The longer a person is depressed, the greater the cortical loss.

When your brain is operating at below capacity, your whole life suffers. Each day is like paddling upstream against the wind in a storm: Much effort produces very little result, and at times you are even pulled backward. The very quality of your sense of self is constructed by your brain.

The Average Brain Today: A Weakened, Fragile Organ

The great majority of people fall midway between these two ends of the spectrum. Only a few percent experience a robust, radiant brain and sense of self. A greater number, perhaps 15–20% of the population, suffer from a deficient or impaired brain due to such things as brain damage or injury, neurological conditions like Alzheimer's disease or Parkinson's, drug or alcohol addiction, or cognitive decline.

For most people who consider themselves healthy, however, "health" is simply the absence of disease, and the average brain today reflects this viewpoint. This so-called health is actually a weakened, fragile condition. It masks a fragility in the stability of the brain and the structures of the self that easily fragment into feeling bad at the slightest pressure. Feelings of inadequacy, shame, anxiety, stress, embarrassment, guilt, and a host of other feelings rush in in a furious attempt to paddle upstream and feel okay once again. The result is anxiety, depression, cognitive decline and an impaired immune system.

Weakened Brain Syndrome

Fragility is a sign the brain isn't operating at an optimal level. This weakness comes from physical and psychological assaults. No one is to blame, for everyone is doing the best they can. The world has innocently stumbled into this state of affairs.

A weakened brain equals a weakened sense of self. With a weakened brain comes a fragile sense of self. Most people don't suffer from low self-esteem, they suffer from fragile self-esteem and the brain weakness that underlies it. An underlying sense of deficiency is the core experience of a weakened brain, often only vaguely felt but periodically breaking through intensely with a strong sense of not feeling okay or shame. The essential wounding of our time is a pervasive feeling of deficiency at the core in the self. It's the outcome of a weakened, fragile brain that physical and/or emotional malnourishment produces.

I have used the phrase "Weakened Brain Syndrome" as the simplest way to describe this phenomenon. A syndrome is a set of signs and symptoms that are correlated together. As with any new diagnostic category, it is through clinical experience that these issues are first noticed, and as is common with other syndromes, current neuroimaging equipment is not yet sensitive enough to measure the difference between a robust and a weakened or toxic brain. The only way to diagnose "Weakened Brain Syndrome" at present is through clinical symptoms.

It may well be that over time a better description of this phenomenon will arise. No matter what it's called, the clinical picture reveals a brain under attack.

A weakened, sub-optimal brain has become the norm. This brain weakness or toxicity has both psychological and physical dimensions. Psychologically the self has fragile self-structures (less emotional resilience), and physically there is reduced brain functionality due to diminished brain capacity, decreased neuroplasticity, and reduced neurogenesis (less neural flexibility).

This fragility indicates a brain on the tipping point, able to swing either way, into greater health or into pain and negativity. The brain's fragility sets a person up for the roster of mental health problems we see today. Such a vulnerable brain may be statistically average or normal, but it's *not* truly, radiantly healthy. From this fragile brain springs depression, anxiety, stress, PTSD, cognitive decline, and the mental health problems of modern living.

But again, why? How did this happen?

The brain is under assault, and it's a "death by a thousand cuts." You don't notice one or two cuts. You don't even notice twenty or thirty. But after one or two hundred, you begin to falter and weaken.

The problem is that since each individual cut isn't noticed, it's hard to say what's wrong. Death by a thousand cuts is invisible. It's utterly baffling why you feel bad. And when people are baffled, they turn to authorities to find out what's wrong. The problem is then compounded when the "authorities" only treat the symptoms but allow the underlying causes to keep festering. This slowly weakens the brain even further, making it increasingly vulnerable to anxiety, depression and cognitive decline.

The brain weakens in two main ways:

1. Neurotoxins that actively damage neurons.
2. Malnourishment so the brain doesn't get enough of what it needs for optimal growth (failure to grow strong).

We live in a highly neurotoxic world, where most brains are raised on the neural equivalent of "junk food" rather than getting genuine nourishment. Neurotoxins and neural "junk food" come in many forms.

It's obvious that nutritional deficiencies and physical neurotoxins hurt the brain. Recent neuroscience research shows that certain psychological influences are also profoundly neurotoxic. Without adequate nourishment at all levels, the brain fails to develop properly and sets the person up for emotional difficulties.

The mental health crisis is a crisis of brain health. As the brain is exposed to neurotoxins—physical ones, emotional ones, as well as mental and spiritual ones—it becomes increasingly vulnerable to depression, anxiety, stress, cognitive decline, and the other mental health problems we see. The self is unstable because the brain is not stable. The converse is also true – a destabilized self weakens the brain. Depression, anxiety, stress, concentration problems, mood swings—all result from a self and brain that are fragile and unsteady.

The answer lies in strengthening the weakened brain and self. When we see how the brain and self are weakened, then we can see how to strengthen them. Let's examine both "neurotoxicity" and "malnourishment" to understand how much damage has been done. These two categories look simple, yet they describe much in modern life and appear in a wide variety of forms.

The good news is that the brain is remarkably resilient. With the right nourishment, it comes back to a remarkable degree and usually can develop into an optimal, peak brain.

How to Heal and Optimize the Brain and Self

As the brain stabilizes, it helps the self to stabilize. As you feel better, you function better, recover faster from stumbles, and operate at higher and higher levels. When this happens:

- Depression recedes and fades away.
- Anxiety and stress reduce as the body relaxes and the brain strengthens.
- Emotion regulation develops and new life choices become possible.
- Memory, learning, and cognitive function increase, which leads to better executive function and feeling more solid inside.
- New depths of inner peace and love and compassion become available.

This book proposes a two-pronged strategy:

1. **Nourish the brain and self to get stronger.**
2. **Minimize what weakens the brain and self.**

Both of these are important, otherwise we'll be spinning our wheels. As long as you continue ingesting neurotoxins, merely adding good things will have only a minor effect. But these two antidotes together reverse the two main causes of the brain's deterioration. The next chapter goes into detail on this two-pronged strategy for developing a radiant, robust brain and self. This is followed by chapters that offer remedies for the disorders addressed by this book.

In identifying what the problems are, it becomes clear how to reverse them. The following discussion is only a cursory survey of these problems, for a thorough examination would require volumes.

The Assault on the Brain: The Rise of Neurotoxins and Malnourishment

A "neurotoxin" is anything that poisons, kills, or debilitates nerve cells (neurons). Since the brain integrates our whole range of experience, it can be poisoned in a variety of ways. Neurotoxic effects also result from lack of nourishment. When the brain fails to obtain necessary nutrients, healthy development fails and brain cell death can occur.

To build and maintain a healthy, robust brain in today's world demands you navigate a daily minefield very, very skillfully. No one sets out to poison their own brain, it just happens growing up in today's world—a world everyone thought was safe but which medical research has recently shown is much more neurotoxic than anyone could have imagined.

Malnourishment: The Other Way to Degrade the Brain

As if the onslaught of neurotoxins wasn't enough, the other factor both mature and developing brains contend with is widespread malnourishment.

There are two key nutrients for the brain:

- physical nutrients (food)
- psychological nutrients

The brain grows through physical food and psychological experience. Both are essential for brain development. **Physical**

food provides the raw material for building neurons and neural connections, but experience, especially emotional experience, shapes how this raw material grows into the developing brain.

The rapidly expanding fields of interpersonal neurobiology, attachment theory and research, developmental neuropsychology, show unambiguously how critical early experience molds the brain as well as how the adult brain's structure and function is molded by ongoing experience. [10, 11, 12] There are also, of course, important forms of mental and even spiritual nourishment for the brain, but overwhelmingly it is early and later emotional experiences that shape how strong and resilient the brain and self are—or how weak and fragile.

Physical and psychological toxins along with physical and psychological forms of malnourishment work together to produce a weakened brain and self.

Physical neurotoxins

We live in a neurotoxic soup. Most people are under the delusion that government regulations keep neurotoxins out of the environment. Sadly, it's not true.

Under the category of neurotoxins, Wikipedia has a list 164 pages long of neurotoxins commonly found in today's environment, and each toxin on the list links to its own Wikipedia page. Of the more than 80,000 chemicals used in industry and whose waste pollutes the air, water, and ground, the Environmental Protection Agency (EPA) in America has no idea how many may be neurotoxic since there are no requirements that safety be proven before using them. Only a small fraction has ever been tested for safety. In many other countries with less regulation the situation is even worse.

Pesticides used on commercial foods are well-documented neurotoxins. Numerous scientific reviews confirm that pesticides which are neurotoxic to insects are also neurotoxic to humans.[13] Dr. David Bellinger, a professor of neurology at Harvard, estimates America has collectively lost 16.9 million I.Q. points due to organophosphates, the most common pesticides used in the U.S. When mercury and lead are added in, he estimates the loss of 41 million I.Q. points.[14]

Glyphosate, the main ingredient of the pesticide Roundup, is the most commonly used organophosphate. It is an antibiotic that kills all-important friendly bacteria in the gut as well as the soil. When the friendly bacteria in the gut are killed off, there are significant mental, emotional, and physical problems. Reduced bacterial biodiversity is linked to mental health problems. [15] Glyphosate stimulates the body to produce zonulin, a molecule that opens up the tight junctions in the intestines that normally protect the body from toxins. When these tight junctions are opened up, toxins flow into the body. These toxins cause the body to mount an inflammatory defense, which soon becomes chronic and further attacks the body and brain.

Zonulin also opens up the tight junctions in the blood-brain barrier allowing toxins to flow into the brain. Further, gliadin, a protein in wheat and gluten, also stimulates zonulin and creates "leaky gut" in everyone who eats it, even though only 1–2% develop celiac disease and only 10–20% of people become gluten sensitive. It's a few short steps from leaky gut and leaky brain to toxic brain.

Eating organic food can reduce this exposure by 70–80%. [14] However, glyphosate is in the dust, groundwater, and rain of 75% of America. It's in commercial meats, which are raised on GMO grains with high glyphosate levels. Almost all corn, cotton, and soy products are GMOs created to tolerate extremely high amounts of glyphosate. Eighty percent of commercial food in the U.S. is contaminated with glyphosate. Currently 600 million pounds are used yearly in the U.S., over 4 billion pounds worldwide.

Many of these chemicals are called developmental neurotoxins because they affect the growing brains of children and babies far more than adults. Testing has shown that American mothers, even those who try to avoid glyphosate, have breast milk with many times the glyphosate levels allowed in European water systems, sometimes 600 times higher.

Since glyphosate is almost everywhere and contaminates so much of the food supply, anyone who eats in restaurants gets exposed. A 2016 study done by researchers at the University of California San Francisco found measurable glyphosate levels in 93% of Americans. Highest levels were in children, where decimating the microbiome is especially harmful since the microbiome affects brain development and permanently alters gene expression.

The Environmental Working Group has published a study of cereal and breakfast bars. They found 43 of 45 conventional cereal products contained glyphosate at potentially dangerous levels, and one in three organic samples had glyphosate, though at lower levels. [16] Ninety percent of cotton grown in the United States is genetically modified, bred to withstand high doses of glyphosate, and glyphosate was detected in 85% of tampons and other cotton hygiene products. [17]

There are more chemical neurotoxins in the environment than ever before. German toxicologist Dr. Richard Straube, found that in the early 2000s, the average person had 20 toxins over the threshold of detection. Now that figure has gone up to over 500. [18]

So just when the tight junctions of the protective blood-brain barrier and intestinal barrier are needed more than ever, the gates have opened, allowing in a flood of neurotoxins. Since the 1980s when glyphosate use exploded, the ensuing leaky gut and leaky blood-brain barrier have resulted in the brain being exposed to levels of neurotoxins that are unprecedented in human history.

Other significant neurotoxins include heavy metals. After plutonium, mercury is the most powerful neurotoxin known. Just a few molecules will instantly destroy brain cells. Everyone alive has some degree of mercury contamination. Common sources of mercury are seafood, dental amalgam fillings, coal-burning factories, and smog.

Some other leading offenders are heavy metals such as lead, cadmium, arsenic, and aluminum. These are present in many home and work environments, including the drinking water of many public water supplies. Smog from auto exhaust, coal-burning factories, and industry produce large amounts of heavy metal pollution.

Chemicals in plastics such as PCBs (polychlorinated biphenyls) and PVC (polyvinyl chloride), and PBA (bisphenol-A) are endocrine disruptors. When these wreak havoc with a person's hormone system, there are emotional, mental, and physical consequences. The lowering of the age of puberty, with six-year-old girls getting their periods and developing breasts, is just the tip of the iceberg, as hormone imbalances have profound effects on mood and how you feel, aside from their well-known carcinogenic properties. Phthalates, found in thermal paper receipts (which you absorb when you touch them), milk containers, and many plastics are also endocrine disruptors that alter levels of hormones and disrupt brain function and mood. [19]

These plastics are not biodegradable but over time reduce in size. They enter the water supply and oceans, and even seemingly clean products become contaminated. Most sea salt, for example, has microparticles of plastic in it. It's estimated that by 2050 there will be more plastic than fish in our oceans by weight. The average person swallows over 68,000 plastic microfibers each year just from the plastic dust landing on plates while eating. [20] The average bottled water contains 325 pieces of microparticles of plastic per liter, another source of endocrine disruptors. [21]

Clothing manufacturers use 20,000 chemicals, many of them carcinogenic and neurotoxic, and produce one-fifth of the world's water pollution. For example, fire retardants in sleepwear, carpeting, and furniture are known endocrine disruptors and neurotoxins.[22, 15] Washing fleece and other synthetic fibers in the washing machine produces microfiber waste water that pollutes waterways, farmlands, and oceans. Of course, this finds its way back into people's bodies, for no one can be hermetically sealed from the environment. We take in what's around us.

Toxic mold from a contaminated house, school, or office can wreak havoc on the brain. The symptoms can look exactly like Alzheimer's or dementia, as well as produce anxiety and depression.

Most indoor air is more polluted than outside air, from outgassing of rugs, upholstery, cooking, and cleaning products. Cosmetics and most skin care products are another key source of endocrine disruptors and heavy metals.

Air pollution in the form of smog produces small particles that are highly neurotoxic. In 2016 the World Health Organization (WHO) reported that 92% of the world's population breathe what it classified as unhealthy air. **Some of the tiniest particles in smog, 2.5 micrometers and smaller, pass through the blood-brain barrier and lodge in the brain.**

Once in the brain these particles act like tiny wrecking balls. They smash into delicate neurons and destroy them, producing a trail of free radical damage, chronic inflammation, and amyloid buildup. When the brain is inflamed and the mitochondria of the neurons have high levels of inflammation, anxiety, depression, and cognitive decline follow.

This is an especially heavy burden on the growing brains of children. Researchers at Cincinnati Children's Hospital showed particular risks to children for mental health disorders from polluted air. Studies linked traffic-related air pollution exposure to increased brain inflammation and generalized anxiety and depression in 12-year olds. [23, 24] Lead author of one study, Cole Brokamp, Ph.D., said in a news release, "This study is the first to show an association between outdoor air pollution levels and increased symptoms of psychiatric disorders, like anxiety and suicidality, in children."

A study in China documented that air pollution affected cognitive performance, especially in older people. [25] Some experts now believe 20–30% of Alzheimer's disease worldwide is due to smog and the tiny particles in the air.

While external environmental neurotoxins are pervasive and require vigilance to avoid them, there are also internal forms of neurotoxins. **Chronic inflammation is one such neurotoxin.** Foods can be classified as pro-inflammatory or anti-inflammatory. The Standard American Diet (SAD) is highly inflammatory and also produces excess free radicals, which are neurotoxic. **Chronic inflammation is a major source of brain deterioration, involved in Alzheimer's and other neurological disorders.** Pesticides contribute to inflammation and make it worse. [26] When things like wheat and glyphosate open up the intestinal and blood-brain barriers, toxins enter, so the body mounts an inflammatory attack that often spirals into autoimmune disorders and diminished mental health.

The mitochondria in cells produce the cells' energy, and when the mitochondria of the brain decay, so does brain function. Inflammation, free radicals, and neurotoxins powerfully diminish mitochondrial function in the brain, directly leading to the mental disorders discussed in this book.

Stress hormones such as glucocorticoids are another internal neurotoxin. Short-term, moderate stress is fine, but chronic or extremely high stress produces high levels of glucocorticoids that kill neurons, especially in the hippocampus. Glucocorticoid excess is implicated in Alzheimer's, cognitive decline, brain shrinkage, anxiety, and depression, reduced immunity, cancer, and heart disease. [8] Chronic stress also raises inflammation levels.

Another source of assault is the microbiome, which consists of the bacteria, viruses, and fungi that line the intestinal walls. They produce chemicals that either help the brain or hurt it, depending upon the type of bacteria present. Poor diet, antibiotics, glyphosate, and other pesticides all damage the microbiome and create health and brain problems that will be detailed later.

Brain injuries such as concussions, hits to the head from car accidents, bike accidents, and athletic injuries not only jar the delicate tissues of the brain but can kill neurons. The brain has the consistency of uncooked tofu or soft butter. When an accident throws this delicate structure against the sharp, bony interior of the skull, the result can be brain damage. A single concussion doubles the chance of Alzheimer's. Recent research into chronic traumatic encephalitis (CTE) in football players shows that continual hits to the head are even more likely than concussion to produce brain damage and dementia.

Electromagnetic fields (EMF) produced by cell phones, computers, and Wi-Fi are damaging to mitochondria by activating voltage-gated calcium channels (VGCC) within the cell. The brain and nervous system are the most vulnerable to EMF exposure with the highest density of VGCCs in the human body. When VGCCs are exposed to EMFs, these channels open up so that about a million calcium ions per second flow through each channel, flooding the cell with calcium, draining magnesium, damaging free radicals, and producing high levels of inflammation. The mitochondria of the brain, heart, and testes are the most vulnerable to EMFs.

Headlines have focused on the more than 50% drop in male sperm count in otherwise healthy young men over the last few decades as one consequence of EMF exposure through laptop use and carrying cell phones in pockets. This decline in fertility rates shows no signs of diminishing. Researcher Martin Pall, Ph.D., has been sounding the alarm for this drop. He says that in animal models early exposure can be reversed but continual exposure results in permanent infertility.

It may be that the rise in anxiety, stress, depression, ADD/ADHD, and autism is the real story, however, as the brain and nervous system have the densest VGCCs in the human body. [27, 28, 29] The brain's mitochondria are extremely sensitive to this disruption. When the neural mitochondria become highly inflamed and oxidized due to the inrush of calcium ions, neural functioning is disrupted and emotion regulation is impaired.

The most comprehensive study of brain development in American youth is the Adolescent Brain Cognitive Development Study, which followed 11,000 children for ten years. Preliminary findings show a premature thinning of the brain cortex in nine- and ten-year-olds who use electronic devices heavily. Thinning of the brain at this developmental stage in youth who use video games, cell phones, TVs, and computers for seven hours a day (not uncommon) has consequences that are not yet known.

When new technologies are introduced into society, there is a lag time before negative consequences become apparent. It often takes 20–30 years before science can establish the toxic health effects of something like tobacco, especially when it's a slow, gradual impact. The introduction of glyphosate and other pesticides, the increase in carbohydrates and sugar and reduction in healthy fat, the use of cell phones and computers, the 80,000 chemicals that have polluted our world—it takes time to comprehend their effects. We are just now understanding some of the potent neurotoxic results such things have.

Physical Malnourishment

The lack of a proper diet produces more brain malnutrition than any other source. If you want to build a beautiful, high-end house, you need to use high-quality building materials, not rotting or inferior wood. It's the same with the brain. To build a robust, radiant brain requires high quality building materials, and the Standard American Diet (SAD) comes nowhere close.

We are just beginning to recover from decades of disastrous dietary policies that have produced the health crisis in the West. This is not the place to go into why these policies came about in the first place. It's a twisted story of junk science exploited by powerful economic forces, governmental acquiescence to industry lobbies, and the revolving door between corporations and government agencies, scientific mob mentality that invalidated opposing views—in other words, many of the usual culprits that influence society.

As a consequence, since the 1960s the medical establishment advocated a diet high in carbohydrates and low in fat. This misguided diet has caused a surge in heart disease, diabetes, obesity, cancer, Alzheimer's, metabolic syndrome, and many chronic diseases, as well as high levels of inflammation, lowered immunity, disordered metabolism, and insulin resistance. No surprise the brain gets hammered also.

Most people in this culture get far too much sugar and too many carbohydrates, too many unhealthy "bad" fats, and too few healthy "good" fats and fiber. The brain is composed of about two-thirds fat, and everyone needs plenty of healthy fat to build a better brain as well as to fuel it. The rise in childhood depression, anxiety, and ADD/ADHD rates began when Americans switched to high carb, low fat diets in the 1960s and beyond. On a low-fat and bad fat, high sugar diet, the growing brain cannot—repeat CANNOT—grow into radiant, optimal health. Plus, there are a number of nutrients that are essential for optimal brain development that very few children or adults get enough of.

Take an average American schoolchild's diet: breakfast of orange juice, a high sugar and carb cereal, low fat milk; lunch of bread, lunch meat, cookies, nonfat milk or fruit juice; dinner of hamburger, French fries, soda, dessert. It's mostly sugar and carbs; high bad fats, low good fats, and little fiber. Such a diet is a setup for a deficient or weakened brain and the mental health problems that follow. More details about this will follow in the next chapter, "The Solution."

Additionally, the average Western diet is highly inflammatory, which inhibits new neuron growth, dampens neuroplasticity, and prevents a fully healthy brain from developing. And a lack of antioxidants means the brain is deficient in antioxidant defenses that protect against the onslaught of free radicals that come with a diet high in sugar, carbs, bad fats, and low in fiber.

Other physical factors that contribute to undernourishing the brain include lack of exercise, especially aerobic exercise. Aerobic exercise (that is, exercise that gets you breathing hard and fast) is perhaps the most powerful way to build up the brain and increase cognitive function—in kids, adults, and seniors. That only a quarter of Americans get enough exercise is another contributor to impaired brain function.

Sleep is another key factor. Most Americans don't get enough sleep for optimal brain health. Most everyone needs seven or eight hours a night. Getting less sleep impairs the brain's self-cleaning process at night performed by the newly discovered glymphatic system. The brain's glymphatic system cleanses the brain's daily buildup of toxins and cellular debris, especially amyloid plaque that figures so prominently in Alzheimer's.

Emotional Neurotoxins

It is probably no surprise to learn that chronic stress, fear, and anxiety are neurotoxic. Chronic or intense stress (such as surviving a military firefight where half the platoon died) can kill neurons and up to one-quarter of the hippocampus can be lost. When trauma happens in childhood, damage to the hippocampus is multiplied, resulting in reduced hippocampal size and vulnerability to future anxiety, fear, stress, and depression. [9]

Childhood maltreatment correlates with lifelong elevated levels of stress and inflammatory hormones. [30] Being bullied either as a child or as an adult, living with intimidation and fear, is neurotoxic. Chronic anger and chronic loneliness also shrink the brain and are neurotoxic. Emotional isolation impairs new brain cell growth and damages brain development. The famous Adverse Childhood Experiences study done by Kaiser and the Centers for Disease Control and Prevention documents the lifelong effects of early stressors. [31] In adults, not only stress but depression can cause the loss of 20% of the hippocampus, with longer periods of depression associated with greater brain cell loss [2]

According to author Joseph Chilton Pierce, expectant mothers who are stressed or anxious give birth to babies with a smaller neocortex (the part that has the higher cognitive functions) and a larger hindbrain (that has the more primitive fight-or-flight survival circuits). Without a well-developed neocortex, there are problems with executive function, emotion regulation, and impulse control, leading to behavior problems, cognitive deficits, and emotional disorders. These babies begin life with significant neural disadvantages. [32]

The emotional life of most adults is rife with emotional neurotoxins—stressful, scary, or anxiety-producing relationships, relationships with emotional or physical bullying or harassment, important relationships where there is emotional coldness, distance, or controlling behavior. On top of this many experience financial stresses, illness, family stresses, worry about politics or the future.

These emotional neurotoxins produce physical neurotoxins that have a profound impact on the brain. Stress also disrupts the tight junctions of the intestines and the blood-brain barrier, allowing in toxins and producing inflammation in the brain and gut.

On the opposite side, as more and more people withdraw from human contact into their cell phones and computers, this lack or diminishing of real, physical relationship creates loneliness, social isolation, and a lack of real intimacy, which in turn produces stress, inflammation, increased interpersonal fear, and anxiety.

Healthy, genuine relationships are necessary to feel good, but with the retreat into screens, this vital emotional nutrient is in shorter supply than ever. The young are the most affected, for the developing sense of self weakens without the crucial ingredient of actual, in-the-flesh emotional relationships.

Stress and negative relationships alter gene expression toward lowered immunity and emotional distress. Stress damages the microbiome, which creates chemicals that lower mood and immunity. This further amplifies feelings of stress, which in turn hurts the microbiome even more. It's a vast interacting system that over time wears away the brain's integrity.

Emotional Malnourishment

Every human being needs high quality emotional contact and lots of it. Almost no one gets nearly enough. The first few years of life are critical for brain development, requiring an emotionally attuned mother or other caregivers to form close, loving attachment bonds. Such a mother is quick to soothe painful feelings and to amplify positive emotions. These relationships get internalized as psychic structure and durable neural pathways. This internal self-structure then allows the person to regulate their emotions—to self-soothe when upset, enjoy pleasure, find love, develop creative work and talents in a meaningful life.

Even as adults, however, we continue to need lots of positive, loving, supportive relationships of all kinds—friends, lover, colleagues, family. The problem is that most people are fed a lot of emotional "junk food," the equivalent of being on an emotional starvation diet, that provides inadequate emotional nutrition. American culture is especially prone to value independence and "the rugged individual," and an overemphasis on this results in isolation, loneliness, and a massive deficiency in quality relationships. (Some other cultures err on the opposite side and have too much contact that is stifling, engulfing, or enmeshed, which also prevents optimal development.)

Western culture has seen a gradual fraying of the relationship bonds that create a healthy brain and self. As divorce levels have risen and family structures have collapsed; as economic crises have increased stress levels along with drug abuse and alcoholism; and as cell phones and electronic media have exploded, the quality of human contact has eroded in the last several decades.

An emotionally attuned, loving, empathic mother or caregiver is rare to start with. Throw in financial stresses, relationship stresses, work stresses, cell phones, the internet, social media, and you get many mothers with a distracted brain.

In experiments with monkeys, researchers found that a distracted, stressed mother monkey produced offspring that developed lifelong anxiety, high levels of stress hormones, depression-proneness, and susceptibility to a variety of health concerns including heart disease and cancer. [8] The experimenters didn't even include cell phones or the internet. With the human brain so sensitive to early social interactions, how could children raised with distracted caregivers not have some weakness in their brain and self-structures as a result?

Parenting and actual relationships have taken a major hit with cell phones, computers, social media, and the internet. Restaurants are filled with silent families, each member looking at their cell phone rather than talking to each other. The heartbreaking scene of a mother focused on her cell phone, ignoring her crying baby in the stroller who's reaching out its arms for her is all too commonplace. Computer tablets have become virtual nannies and babysitters. Two-year-olds prefer interacting with an iPad to interacting with people, but encouraging this deprives the child of what it needs most.

Surveys show a third of people who text prefer texting to talking with an actual person. Most people check their cell phones 150 times a day (once every six minutes). Teens spend 8–11 hours a day on a screen. Ninety percent of 18- to 29-year-olds sleep with their cell phones. Video games and cell phones are viewed by many as addictions rivaling heroin. Many teenagers and 20-somethings seem more attached to their cell phones than their families.

When cell phones substitute for in-person, face-to-face interaction, essential emotional nutrients are lost. A world of virtual relationships creates a virtual sense of self, along with the ghost-like sense of not feeling entirely solid or firm.

So-called screenagers, who spend eight to eleven hours a day in front of screens, suffer incalculable harm. And when a two- or four-year-old's babysitter is a tablet, the consequences for the solidity of the self are even greater.

Our sense of self is molded by the quality of early emotional relationships that we internalize. Inadequate emotional nourishment produces a shaky sense of self. As this continues into adolescence and adulthood, the problem only worsens. Combined with inadequate nutrition, the brain's emotional malnourishment produces a fragile, unstable self that is highly vulnerable to stress, anxiety, depression, and all the rest.

Mental Neurotoxins

Pessimistic attitudes create chronic stress as the person is always bracing for the worst. Catastrophizing leads to anxiety and paralyzing fear, producing stress hormones and increasing inflammation; in other words, more neurotoxins. Optimists live 19% longer than pessimists.

Critical self-talk is a kind of mental autoimmune disorder, and it's reached epidemic proportions. When the self attacks itself, this negative, critical self-talk produces stress hormones and shame. The feeling of shame is so difficult to bear because it directly undermines our sense of self and makes us feel unworthy, not okay, unlovable.

Shame produces inflammation. [33] The "average" brain of the average person in the U.S. today is highly vulnerable to shame. The fragile brain that produces the fragile self easily fragments in challenging situations or when self-esteem is threatened (e.g., calling yourself a "loser" or "stupid" or feeling rejected). When the self fragments in the face of an assault like this, shame and inflammation result.

Lack of mental stimulation, deadening routine, or overstimulation and mental overwhelm all slow natural brain growth to a crawl, shrink the brain and create a neural environment that readily fragments.

Mental Malnourishment

The brain thrives on stimulation of all kinds. Cognitive stimulation in school, college, and throughout adult life are crucial for developing the brain. Lifelong learning after graduation is essential to prevent cognitive decline and to stay sharp. Computers and the internet are amazing tools to stimulate the mind and provide access to information in an instant. But technology is a double-edged sword.

One downside is that attention spans are decreasing at an alarming rate. A recent study put the average adult attention span now at five seconds. Clearly this limits how much real comprehension there is. And as wonderful as entertainment is, when so much screen time is devoted to computer games, movies and TV, music and sports, and so on, this mental "junk food" simultaneously starves the brain with empty mental calories and over activates it with a constant barrage of stimulation. The mental "hangover" is a weary mental numbness. The more overstimulation there is, the greater the mental numbness that follows.

Standardized testing shows that college entrance exam average scores have been falling for several decades, with record low levels reported in the last five years. Weakened Brain Syndrome (WBS) shows itself in many different ways and lowering cognitive function is yet one more symptom.

Spiritual Neurotoxins

Spiritual neurotoxins include frightening or shaming belief systems that threaten eternal punishment if the person isn't perfect or doesn't conform to rigidly prescribed behavior. Lack of meaning is another form, and lack of meaning produces changes in gene expression and stress hormones similar to chronic adversity. [34] The spiritual importance of meaning can hardly be overstated, for meaning is neuroprotective. When something is meaningful, it allows a person to endure even the greatest suffering, as *Man's Search for Meaning*, Viktor Frankl's classic work, demonstrates. [35]

Spiritual Malnourishment

As organized religion has declined in the West, there have been two different reactions to this. On the one hand, some people awaken to spiritualty and become seekers who imbibe the wisdom of several different spiritual traditions. On the other hand, many others lose sight of spirituality entirely in an increasing secularization. They adopt completely materialistic values bereft of a spiritual orientation. This creates an existential or spiritual void.

Such a spiritual void unmoors a person and makes the outer world the measure of all things. This outward, superficial orientation is profoundly disturbing, for there is no peace to be found there. The outer world is a field of constant flux and change. Peace is not to be found outwardly, only inwardly. But if there is never any inward focus, if life is a continual outward distraction, the necessary inner journey is never taken.

Although some can create a sense of meaning in life without an explicitly spiritual orientation, for many people such a spiritual void casts them adrift. Feeling lost in a meaningless universe without a larger sense of significance, self-gratification becomes the primary life impulse. Sensory pleasures are the only momentary relief from the stresses, existential fears, and anxieties that overshadow living. A spiritual anomie results, and, devoid of the renewal provided by inner peace, love, and joy, the ongoing stress can weaken the brain and immune system, and open the door to despair, existential anxiety, addictions, and other emotional disorders.

A Perfect Storm

Make no mistake about it: **The brain is under attack on multiple fronts.**

Never in evolutionary history has the brain been exposed to such a vast quantity of neurotoxins. Just at the time when the brain needs its protective blood-brain barrier the most, it has never been so vulnerable due to disruptions in the tight junctions that create a leaky gut and leaky brain, letting in more of these neurotoxins than ever.

A single neurotoxin is bad enough. A whole mix of physical neurotoxins together can wreak havoc on the brain, especially the growing brain of a child. Throw in emotional and other neurotoxins, and you've got a highly toxic stew. Then combine this toxic stew with malnourishment on all levels, particularly on the body level with deficient diet and emotionally with inadequate emotional sustenance, and the resulting brain weakness is far more vulnerable to the neurotoxic environment.

One additional problem is that most people don't even realize their brain is weakened and compromised. For example, many Alzheimer's patients don't realize how much they are cognitively impaired—because the very instrument that registers the problem is itself damaged. It's similar with a weakened brain. And since the slippage happens slowly, it all gets normalized and the person believes everything is fine. Only afterward, when your brain begins functioning on a higher level, do you realize how diminished you were.

Remember, glyphosate has been found in 93% of Americans. That's 93% of the population that has some degree of leaky brain/toxic brain, and that's just one neurotoxin out of hundreds. Multiply this by some number (10, 20, 100—we don't even know how many) and the result is the average brain today—weakened, poisoned, compromised.

Most everyone suffers from some degree of impaired brain function, but very few know it. Often only when symptoms such as anxiety, depression, or cognitive decline appear does the person realize something is wrong.

The burden of this neurotoxicity and malnourishment falls disproportionately on the young. When emotion regulation structures fail to develop optimally, we see the result in soaring anxiety and depression rates. On the other side of the age spectrum, older people notice the burden with memory problems and premature cognitive decline.

It's a perfect storm of countless neurotoxins colliding with early and continuous forms of malnourishment.

To give an overly simple illustration of this perfect storm and its multiple moving parts, consider how problems with early attachment relationships affect the brain. It's well understood in developmental psychology that myriad attachment difficulties lead to problems in internalizing strong emotion regulation structures. The lack of these internal structures increases stress hormones, which interfere with brain development. Additionally, cortisol and other glucocorticoid stress hormones kill off high numbers of good bacteria in the intestinal lining, allow an overgrowth of damaging bacteria, and disrupt the tight junctions that normally keep out damaging contaminants.

When the intestinal barrier is breached, harmful bacteria, viruses, proteins, and other toxins leak into the system. This also disrupts the tight junctions in the blood-brain barrier, so some of these same toxins enter the brain and disrupt neural functioning.

Now add in several courses of antibiotics and a diet that includes pesticides such as glyphosate, phthalates, and other neurotoxins that far more powerfully disrupt the membrane lining of the gut and blood brain barrier. What should be a protective barrier becomes a sieve. The brain's balance is thrown off even more as greater numbers of toxins enter and damage the highly sensitive neurons and the brain's microbiome and upset the hormonal and neurotransmitter balance. Emotion regulation is further eroded. This makes it harder to establish healthy relationships, leading to further stress hormones, anxiety, and other symptoms, in a progressive descent.

Anxiety, depression, and negativity are natural feelings when the brain is under sustained, daily assault. How could such a person *not* see the world as dangerous, dark, and hard to navigate? The brain senses *something* is terribly wrong or dangerous in the world, but it doesn't know what.

When the threat isn't clear, danger becomes global or else the brain fixes on something, anything, so it can make sense of these feelings. Real dangers are amplified, and the brain goes on high alert, hypervigilant. The world is dangerous because the brain is getting battered. Only when the brain is healthy and strong does the world become safe again.

The emotional pain this creates can either look like a psychological problem that needs therapy, or a biological illness that needs medication.

It's not just a double whammy, it's a double, double whammy: Physical neurotoxins together with psychological neurotoxins in combination with physical malnourishment together with psychological malnourishment. This quadruple whammy turns into a vicious downward spiral where neurotoxins and malnourishment reinforce one another. Significant malnourishment enfeebles the brain, rendering it more vulnerable to neurotoxic attacks and less able to recoup later. Neurotoxins further enfeeble the brain, rendering it more damaged by further malnourishment.

As the brain declines, all aspects of life erode. Emotion regulation is a central function of the brain, and it's often the first to go. No wonder we have an epidemic on our hands. The brain throws up all these symptoms to get our attention. Symptoms are the brain's way of saying, "Something is wrong! Pay attention here! Something is terribly, terribly wrong!"

Why Medication Is Rarely the Answer

Modern medicine has produced breakthroughs to improve the health of our species. Better sanitation, antibiotics, fixing broken bones, curing of many illnesses that previously were fatal—it's a tribute to science and medical discovery how much longer people live, from an average lifespan of 47 in 1900 to 77 in 2000. But the picture is far from an unbroken march toward perfect health nirvana.

While medicine has greatly curtailed the leading causes of death from infectious disease—tuberculosis, pneumonia, and diarrhea—there remain many diseases that medicine cannot cure or even treat. Chronic diseases are now the leading cause of death. Heart disease, cancer, stroke, type 2 diabetes, and Alzheimer's lead the list. According to the CDC, in 2012 half of all Americans had at least one chronic disease.

One critique of modern medicine is that its reductionistic thinking works well for broken legs or diseases with a single infectious agent that can be treated with a drug, but it is ill-equipped to deal with diseases that have multiple dietary and lifestyle causes—hence the current epidemic of chronic illness.

One important distinction is between cure and symptom relief. An antibiotic may cure a bacterial infection forever, but giving painkillers to someone with a painful infection must not be confused with curing the disease.

Much of modern medicine has become the treatment of symptoms rather than the discovery of cure. While symptom relief can be helpful to a suffering person, such medications always come with side effects, which often lead to additional medications to manage the side effects.

For many diseases, the medical-pharmaceutical complex has developed into a subscription model of taking symptom-relieving drugs for years or a lifetime. There are many factors that contribute to this, from the complexity of diseases to the quest for higher profits driving the search for solutions. While a subscription model may be better for business, for everyone else it's obviously preferable to find a cure and remove the suffering permanently.

It's the same story when it comes to the mental health field. Psychiatric drugs are necessary and very helpful at times. But there is a large shadow side to this medication which is rarely acknowledged. In most cases these drugs only reduce or mask the symptoms. They don't "cure" emotional or mental disorders.

The widely used benzodiazepine anti-anxiety drugs are depressants. They slow down the central nervous system, slow metabolism, and lower blood pressure. Taking a depressant lowers anxiety and can provide much needed relief. But these drugs also impair a person's presence and ability to think; they slow reaction time and dull aliveness. This medication temporarily reduces or masks anxiety. It does not cure anxiety.

Antidepressants increase certain neurotransmitters and change mood (although they are effective less than 50% of the time). For some people they are important and clearly helpful, and after a few months or years of improved functioning and getting their emotional needs met, they can then stop without slipping back into depression. For most patients, however, this is not the case. No drug company will claim antidepressants "cure" depression, instead they temporarily reduce the symptoms of depression. For some patients the brain adapts to the antidepressant, makes fewer neurotransmitter receptors, and with long-term use the antidepressant induces chronic depression. [36]

Alzheimer's drugs are almost completely ineffective and only postpone a worsening of symptoms by a few months. ADD and ADHD medication provides the nervous system with a temporary boost that masks the symptoms of these disorders but does not cure it.

The side effects of psychiatric medications are often so severe that patients stop taking the drugs. For example, more than half of patients taking antidepressants lose their sex drive, have erectile dysfunction, or inability to orgasm (and if all this isn't depressing, what is?). Other common side effects include: weight gain, sleep disturbance, daytime drowsiness, nausea, headaches or migraines, blurred vision, increased depression, constipation or diarrhea.

The False Analogy of Insulin

The psychiatric field likes to compare the use of psychiatric medications to the use of insulin by those with type 1 diabetes. A type 1 diabetic can't make insulin. Providing the patient with insulin may not cure the disease, but it manages it quite effectively and allows the person to lead a relatively normal existence, even though the person needs to take insulin for life.

As the parent of a type 1 diabetic son, I can't express how grateful I am for modern medicine's discovery of insulin and its life-giving consequences. However, as a psychologist I can't help but notice the false equivalence this analogy draws.

Insulin is what the body requires to metabolize glucose, the single hormone the body needs for this function. But when it comes to the brain, it's a whole different story.

For example, take the serotonin deficiency theory of depression. This has been highly marketable due to its simplicity. The idea is that lack of serotonin causes depression, and adding serotonin, just like insulin, will fix the depression. So appealing was this idea that it has become a 16 billion dollar a year industry, even though research has now shown this model to be incorrect.

First of all, there is no serotonin deficiency in depression. Chapter 4, "Holistic Healing of Depression," goes into greater detail on the research behind the myth of the "serotonin deficiency theory of depression." Most studies show depressed patients have normal levels of serotonin. Some studies indicate patients have higher than normal levels, a few show lower levels, but most show normal levels. [37] How can adding more of something there is no deficiency of be compared to supplying the body with missing insulin?

Secondly, there are over 100 known neurotransmitters, and more than 20 are involved in mood regulation. Additionally, there are dozens of other biochemicals that regulate mood, such as hormones, growth factors, enzymes, transcription factors, and protein families.

The complexity of a brain that produces human consciousness is unfathomable. With multiple redundancies, various feedback loops and backup systems, the neural conversation between all these elements that contribute to how we feel is an order of complexity far beyond our current understanding.

To increase a single chemical or say that anxiety or depression is "because" of too much or too little of one or two chemicals is a hopelessly simplistic, outdated view of the brain.

An increase in a single brain chemical changes the whole intricate balance of neural communication. Replacing one missing hormone (insulin) that has specific actions is not comparable with the psychiatric situation of boosting one chemical that is not deficient (serotonin) among dozens and dozens of other neurotransmitters, hormones, enzymes, transcription factors, etc. that are in continuous, multifaceted communication, mutual feedback and interactive mutual self-regulation. It's like comparing apples to refrigerators.

Third, the serotonin deficiency theory of depression has given way to one in which neurogenic factors are key. Chapter 4 details how antidepressants' effectiveness comes by increasing the rate of neurogenesis and neuroplasticity, not by adding serotonin to the brain's soup. Even when antidepressants do "work," it's through an entirely different mechanism than adding serotonin to the system. The insulin analogy breaks down before it can take off.

Antidepressants are the best case. When it comes to anti-anxiety drugs the analogy is more untenable still. The widely prescribed anti-anxiety agents, the benzodiazepines, do not exist in nature or the body. This class of synthetic chemicals bludgeons the mind, dulls the senses, slows reaction time, confuses thinking, interferes with memory, reduces presence, is addicting, and causes brain damage. [38]

In cases of extreme anxiety or crisis, benzodiazepines can certainly be helpful. They act like a sledgehammer on the GABA system to reduce neural excitability. In the right amount they provide symptom relief even while reducing presence and cognitive ability with only slight "zombification." Much more common are higher doses of Xanax or Klonopin or Ativan or Valium that amplify this zombification effect. Since the brain is dulled, the person usually doesn't realize how powerfully numbed they are until they get off the medication.

Even worse, it's being given to children whose brains are still developing. It is not yet known to what degree brain damage will be seen in adults who were prescribed benzodiazepines as children.

The comparison of benzodiazepines to insulin is a mistake, which in logic is called a category error. A category error is very bad science, but because it sounds plausible on the surface, it's become "successful." Modern psychiatry, with its potent medications, has been compared to trying to do brain surgery with a blunt axe.

Yes, you'll affect the brain and how the person feels. But there is significant collateral damage.

Some symptoms may be reduced for some people, yet clubbing the brain with such powerful chemicals bring changes that are only beginning to be understood. For instance, taking an SSRI antidepressant (which temporarily boosts serotonin in the brain) causes the brain to downregulate serotonin production, so that an increasing dependence on the drug is created. This makes it all the more difficult to stop taking the medication later on. That they "work" by reducing and suppressing symptoms (though generally only slightly better than a placebo) confounds the situation further by mimicking success.

Psychiatric medications do not cure emotional disorders, they dampen symptoms. The brain of someone with anxiety does not have a shortage of Xanax, nor is a depressed brain short on Prozac. Someone with ADD/ADHD is not suffering from a lack of Adderall or amphetamine. These are all synthetic drugs that do not appear anywhere in nature. To heal the brain, we need to look beyond patentable, synthetic medications that beat the brain into muffling symptoms. We must understand how the brain grows and heals (see Chapter 2, "The Solution").

Psychiatrist Peter Breggin, M.D., author of *Talking Back to Prozac* and *Medication Madness,* said in response to being asked what people don't know about psychiatric medication, "They don't know that all psychiatric drugs are neurotoxins. They don't know that they aren't correcting biochemical imbalances, they are causing biochemical imbalances." [39]

Faulty reasoning with false analogies is poor science, even though it may be genius marketing for pharmaceutical companies. Is this what Western healthcare and psychiatry have come to: turning children and the population into zombies? Is this really the best we can do? There must be a better way.

The Importance of Painful Symptoms

Pain is a signal that something is wrong. A painful toothache signals the need to go to the dentist to fix a cavity. Once you make a dental appointment and set in motion the process to fix it, the pain is no longer necessary. Then you can take a painkiller until the dentist fixes the cause by filling the cavity. But if all you do is take painkillers, the problem will get worse, the decay will increase.

The massive suppression of the pain of mental disorders in America and the developed world is akin to taking painkillers without fixing the cavity. No doubt about it, mental disorders will multiply when the underlying problem isn't fixed. Freud called this "the return of the repressed." Emerging needs and feelings don't just go away. The psyche expresses its needs continually, and whatever we push down will come back up until this information is integrated.

For example, a patient came to me complaining about still feeling depressed and anxious despite having been on an antidepressant for many years. When I asked about his life he reported a stressful job and marriage. In probing further, it came out that he'd been having an affair for the past six years; he was involved in some shady and illegal dealings through his work; and he felt guilty about not spending time with his kids. How could he not be anxious and depressed? His life was massively out of alignment with his deeper values and self.

Most anyone would be anxious and depressed in circumstances like this. Such feelings are beneficial signals that things are off. Numbing the pain with an antidepressant only enables a bad situation to become worse. His anxiety and depression didn't go away until he straightened out his marriage, his job, and his relationship with his kids, and came into alignment with his own deeper sense of internal integrity. He needed to feel and understand what his pain was telling him. Instead of taking antidepressants he could just as well have been using alcohol or heroin. Far too often, that's what psychiatric medications have become—legal drugs that suppress symptoms.

This is one reason why rates of mental disorders have increased so much. Although temporary pain relief may appear to help in the short run, over the long run the world gets worse when we suppress symptoms, not better. The current solution? More and newer medication or higher doses. And of course, more of the same thing results in more of the same poor results. Sticking our collective heads in the sand isn't working.

Has Psychiatry Become Part of the Problem?

As modern psychiatry has morphed into bio-psychiatry over the past 50 years, the field has increasingly become an extension of the pharmaceutical industry. At first, beginning in the 1960s and '70s, psychiatric education in the bio-psychiatry model was influenced by the large drug companies. Then in the '80s and '90s educational materials were paid for and developed by drug companies. Now the training of psychiatrists is almost entirely organized and controlled by the drug industry mentality.

When psychiatry is controlled by the pharmaceutical mindset, an unhealthy mutual dependence arises. The pharmaceutical industry makes vast sums of money from patentable drugs. Natural brain nutrients like omega-3s or curcumin, which can't be patented, are ignored. Psychiatrists make their living by writing prescriptions for patented drugs. No one needs to see a psychiatrist for fish oil or curcumin. So Big Pharma and psychiatry are joined together in a professional embrace of mutual financial dependence.

Any challenge to this psychiatric-pharmaceutical industrial complex threatens the livelihood of both, and dissenting voices and research are dismissed. But sooner or later the larger truth will win out, I believe, even when powerful financial resources are arrayed against it.

For the great majority of psychiatrists, treatment equals prescribing drugs. Conventional psychiatry has become the marketing arm of the pharmaceutical industry, pushing ever more powerful, mind-altering drugs.

The massive introduction of powerful brain drugs is dulling the population, numbing the aliveness of countless millions, and squashing the symptoms we should be listening to. It's no wonder zombie movies and TV shows are so popular—they symbolize what's happening now, the dulling and numbing of great masses of people.

Surprisingly, the majority of antidepressants and anti-anxiety drugs are not prescribed by psychiatrists but by primary care physicians. Most anyone can walk into a doctor's office and walk out with prescription for an antidepressant or tranquilizer. Primary care doctors who have almost no real training in psychiatry prescribe these drugs like candy.

There isn't real evil here, just well-intended physicians who want to relieve suffering. Most have no idea how medications can increase suffering in the long term. It's the same with psychiatrists and employees of pharmaceutical companies. Nearly all the people I know in these fields are well-meaning individuals who believe they are helping to relieve suffering. No one should be demonized. They are just trying to help people with the only tools they have. When all you have is a hammer (prescribing brain-altering drugs), everything looks like a nail (brain imbalances that need drugs).

It is also important to note some exceptions; a small percentage also do psychotherapy. Similarly, not all medication is negative; sometimes it is helpful to relieve anxiety or give a sleeping pill to suppress the symptom and provide a bridge to better functioning.

To add another layer of complexity to this picture, sometimes a round of antidepressants results in the person functioning better and tapering off. Sometimes medication does work as advertised. And to confuse the situation further, most conditions do improve without treatment, so when the person feels better, it appears that the medication "worked."

Psychiatric medication is not all bad or all good. It's a more complex picture. Sometimes medication works just fine with minimal problems. However, I believe they are overprescribed most of the time, and worsen the problem in the long run, but a more nuanced view sees both the good they offer as well as the destructive effects they have overall.

To the degree that psychiatry uses medication to relieve intense, acute distress or to contain out-of-control symptoms, psychiatry is helpful. The degree to which medication becomes chronic and simply suppresses symptoms is the degree to which psychiatry has become part of the problem. Unfortunately, the great majority of the time, psychiatry results in symptom suppression and therefore contributes to the problem.

Psychology Has Only Half a Solution

Psychotherapy is effective in many cases, but why isn't it more effective? For some it is life-changing and powerfully transformative.

For others it is ineffective. For many more it is much less effective than it could be.

By its near exclusive emphasis on psychological factors, psychotherapy has mapped the psyche but ignored the physical foundation of brain health. With a weakened brain, a weakened, fragmentation-prone self follows naturally. Healing the self may help the brain but does not heal it.

De-Mystifying the Perfect Storm

When psychiatric medications that should contribute to the solution actually are part of the problem, this mystifies the perfect storm even further. To solve this problem means de-mystifying it by naming the contributing factors. So, we have this quadruple whammy of 1) physical and psychological neurotoxins together with 2) physical and psychological malnourishment shrouded by a 3) mystifying process of treatment that worsens the problem by suppressing its symptoms but is languaged as "correcting a biochemical imbalance." It's a complex picture where insidious forces interact to produce an epidemic that's growing relentlessly.

We know many ways to heal the self. But are there natural ways to heal the brain without the side effects of psychiatric medications? Yes. Are they used? No. Therefore, this book. The strategy of symptom suppression versus true brain healing is the larger issue. Which would you choose?

The Problem of Specialization and the Fragmentation of Knowledge

Specialization has produced enormous benefits as knowledge in all fields has multiplied exponentially. But a downside is that specialists think within their own narrow domain and increasingly only talk to others in that same sphere of expertise. They can become insulated from new, emerging paradigms and knowledge outside that area.

Specialization, especially in medicine, treats different parts separately and loses track of the whole. I had a friend who had massive pain in his heart area. He went to a gastroenterologist clutching his chest in the belief it might be heartburn from acid reflux. His chest pain was so great he could barely get through the exam. After the doctor told him there was nothing wrong with his esophagus or stomach, that he'd be fine and shouldn't worry, he was unable leave the office for hours due to intense pains in his chest. He died that night of a heart attack. Even without medical training, who besides a specialist wouldn't have considered that this man clutching his heart was having a heart attack?

We know a great deal about how to heal the brain. Psychiatry, in one of medicine's great ironies, generally leads in the opposite direction, weakening instead of healing the brain. The medical field, with a few notable exceptions, is remarkably ignorant on the role of diet and nutrition.

Early in the 20th century, as science was making breakthrough discoveries with antibiotics and new drugs, medical schools made a fateful decision. Medical schools decided to specifically exclude nutrition from medical education and instead focus upon pharmaceutical medications. The mold was set so medical and psychiatric education became centered upon prescribing drugs.

The result is that the great majority of physicians have never had even a single course in nutrition, at most they've had an hour-long lecture. This decision by medical schools to exclude nutrition was bad enough for regular medicine; for psychiatry it was a disaster.

It's a shame. A medical education could be excellent preparation to understand the connection between food and mood, and how to strengthen the brain. Instead, psychiatric education dismisses nutrition in favor of prescription medications that often make the whole problem more damaging. As a consequence, conventional medicine and psychiatry lack the conceptual tools with which to understand, diagnose, and truly heal this present brain crisis.

The field of psychology has been torn by internecine wars between different schools. Cognitive therapists put down psychoanalysts; Jungians fight with Freudians; somatic therapists make fun of talk therapy; each school striving for its own supremacy. There is some movement toward a blending of best practices and theoretical integration, but much too little.

The specialized training each school of psychotherapy requires develops a cult-like adherence in its trainees to one particular school's approach as the best way to heal the self. "If it worked for me, it should work for everyone" is a common belief.

A theoretical one-up mentality plagues much of modern psychotherapy. This results in a Tower of Babel situation, where the various schools of psychotherapy become silos that rarely talk to therapists outside their particular silo. This muddies the waters even further.

Integration, Not Further Fragmentation

To heal the fragmentation of knowledge brought about by specialization requires breadth and width, not merely depth in a particular field. Psychiatry has been focused on the level of effect but ignores the level of cause. Psychotherapy addresses only half of the problem. Meanwhile the multiple factors that weaken the brain and self go unaddressed, and they deteriorate further.

The usual debate between psychology and bio-psychiatry frames the issue in terms of a chicken and egg problem: Which came first? Do biological problems cause depression and anxiety or do psychological problems and unskillful living cause biological effects? But this creates a false dichotomy that doesn't exist. We are psychophysical beings. The chicken and egg evolved together. It's both/and rather than either/or.

On the one hand, as psychology has increasingly specialized, its focus on psychotherapy disregards the body and brain; lip service is paid to the physical with an occasional referral to a psychiatrist for medication. On the other hand, as bio-psychiatry has been captured by the drug mindset, its focus on medication disregards the psyche; lip service is paid to the psychological with an occasional referral to a psychotherapist for therapy. Going in opposite directions is exacerbating the problem, not solving it.

Dickens was right when he wrote, "It was the best of times, it was the worst of times." We know more about brain health, and we have more resources to support the healing and growth of the brain and self into radiant vitality than at any other period in history.

At the same time, our environment is vastly more polluted with neurotoxins, and there is greater malnourishment and mystification than ever. It's never been a better or worse time for the brain.

The knowledge we need is there but not in conventional psychiatry or psychology alone. The fields of holistic health, nutritional science, functional and integrative medicine, depth psychology, interpersonal neurobiology, transpersonal psychology, attachment theory, and developmental neuroscience provide the missing pieces. They only need to be put together into a new, meaningful whole. Although more information waits to be discovered, we already know a great deal about how to heal the brain and self.

This approach can be called holistic therapy, integral or integrative psychotherapy, functional psychology, for as yet there is no standard name for this emerging field. To heal the mind-body split, psychotherapy must fully integrate the brain, just as psychiatry must give more than a tip of the hat to psychology.

Yet out of this specialization and fragmentation come the outlines of a new resolution. Perhaps this fragmenting separation was even necessary to create the conditions for a larger dialectic; thesis and antithesis producing a greater synthesis. The more both sides pull apart, the more an integrating wholeness comes into view.

CHAPTER 2

THE SOLUTION:
HEAL AND STRENGTHEN THE BRAIN AND SELF

True healing requires a holistic, whole brain approach. The goal is to strengthen the weakened brain and self so they grow into radiant health. As the brain gets stronger and stabilizes, the self becomes stronger and more stable. And as the self stabilizes it steadies the brain. The person starts to feel good, then better and better.

The brain grows from two directions: physical and psychological.

No matter what age, all brains need both *physical* and *psychological* nutrients to thrive. Optimal food and other physical factors build a vibrant, radiant brain. And everyone needs *psychological* nutrients to create strong, coherent self-structures and neural pathways that can regulate emotion, find love, joy, meaningful work and intimacy, and meet the challenges of life.

Not getting enough of either physical or psychological nourishment weakens the brain and creates fragile self-structures, paving the way for anxiety, depression, cognitive decline, and other problems.

With proper food the brain can grow, and with psychological nutrients a strong, coherent self can grow. The growing self doesn't need perfect parents (otherwise we're all lost). Simply a "good enough" mother, father, or caregiver will do.

Similarly, even with the best *psychological* nurturing, without proper *physical* nourishment, the structures of the self and neural pathways that support this will be frail and weak. We need both physical and psychological nutrients.

Nourish the brain on all levels, holistically, to create a vital brain and self. This is the fundamental principle on which this book is based. The flip side to nourishing the brain is detoxifying and avoiding further neurotoxins.

The following chapters will go into this in more detail, but this chapter notes that there are some common brain problems in depression, anxiety, and cognitive decline. Common neural mechanisms in these three disorders include a central role of the hippocampus and hippocampal atrophy, lower levels of BDNF (brain-derived neurotrophic factor), and neurogenic slowing, which reduces the rate of neurogenesis and neuroplasticity.

Since the psychological causes, however, are so very different for these three problems, they will be examined in the following chapters rather than here. This chapter focuses on the physical side of the plan to heal, strengthen, and stabilize the brain. The following chapters will carefully examine the psychological aspects of each disorder and then tweak the basic physical plan in this chapter to precisely match each disorder.

The Holistic Approach

The discovery of holism marks an important corrective to the reductionist, atomistic approach of conventional medicine. Traditional medicine views the body and brain as a machine. When a part is broken, fix it or replace it, either with a pill (e.g., an antibiotic) or a new part (e.g., a hip replacement). This modern medical approach has achieved spectacular success with things like broken bones or bacterial diseases.

However, when it comes to the current epidemic of chronic diseases and mental health crises, such fragmentary thinking is quite limiting, for it ignores the interrelated nature of the body, brain, and self. We exist on different levels: an inner soul or spirit and an outer body, heart, mind. All four levels, or subsystems, are interrelated, and they all come together in the brain. Nothing in the brain exists independently from everything else. The brain exists in a complex network of interactive, interdependent relationships.

A central pillar of the holistic view is that the organism has a natural tendency toward health and growth. The intelligence of our human organism is vast, far greater than the intellect. Holism is the understanding that our organism reacts as an organized whole to every experience. You can't deal with one part without affecting the whole.

When a person loses a limb, this affects the balance of the whole body as well as affecting the rest of the person. When someone loses sight, the other senses heighten to compensate and there are also emotional, mental, and spiritual effects. Although we exist as a multilayered body, heart, mind, and spirit, these form a single whole. The brain integrates these multiple channels to produce a unitary experience of your "self" and consciousness. It is to this greater whole that holism constantly points.

Holistic thinking rather than fragmentary thinking is needed to address the systemic nature of the present epidemics, both physical and psychological. Unfortunately, as noted in the previous chapter, a limitation of many holistic or integrative health practitioners is that while they focus on the wholeness of the body, they only give a tip of the hat to the rest of our being—heart, mind, and spirit. Conversely, while many depth psychotherapists focus on the heart, mind, and spirit, they minimize the body and brain. A truly holistic approach integrates all four levels, for neurotoxins and malnourishment come in all forms.

When we intervene on all levels, they work together synergistically. The body-heart-mind-spirit organism reacts as an organized whole to being nourished or poisoned. Conversely, physical healing supports psychological healing just as psychological healing supports physical healing.

Radiant Brain Health

The resilience of the human brain is extraordinary. Even after being beaten down, poisoned, or starved, with proper nourishment and care, the brain can come roaring back into vibrant health.

We haven't known how to revitalize the brain until now.

Only in the past decade or two has research uncovered these revolutionary findings:

- The brain is being poisoned and malnourished from multiple directions.
- We now know what many of these physical and psychological neurotoxins are.
- It's clear how neurotoxins shrink the hippocampus, resulting in anxiety, stress, depression, and cognitive decline.
- The brain not only rewires itself (neuroplasticity or synaptogenesis) but regenerates itself (neurogenesis).
- The rates of neurogenesis and synaptogenesis are the most important biomarkers for brain health and general well-being.
- The rate of making new brain cells (neurogenesis) and new connections (synaptogenesis) can be increased, probably by five times or more, with profound effects on the brain, the self, and quality of life.
- We understand the optimal diet to stimulate brain growth and repair.
- We know the optimal psychological nutrients to stimulate the brain and self.

Much of this research is so new that most doctors, nutritionists, and health practitioners, those who were educated in outdated models of the brain, are not aware of these findings.

The Neurogenic Revolution

The discovery of neuroplasticity over 50 years ago marked an important shift in how the brain is viewed. The brain is continuously making new connections among neurons, rewiring itself to adapt to an ever-changing environment. With the discovery that synapses between neurons make new connections with other neurons, a process known as synaptogenesis, medical science realized the brain was more resilient than previously thought.

Then in the late 1990s researchers discovered that not only does the brain make new connections, it actually makes new brain cells throughout our lifetime, a process called "neurogenesis." Before this it was considered settled fact that the brain stops growing new brain cells in our early twenties, and after this there is only a gradual die-off of neurons.

The discovery that the brain grows new brain cells throughout our entire lifespan changed the entire field of neuroscience and upended decades of medical doctrine about the brain. At first, this discovery of neurogenesis was merely a change in understanding about the brain. But within 10 years it became clear that the rate of neurogenesis and synaptogenesis is one of the most important, if not the most important, indicators of brain health as well as emotional and cognitive health.

Fred Gage, Ph.D., the neuroscientist who first confirmed that neurogenesis occurs throughout the human lifespan, found he could increase the rate of neurogenesis in mice by five times through an "enriched environment," which had healthy food, running wheels for exercise, lots of friendly mice to play and mate with, and a complex, changing environment. It was kind of like the mouse equivalent of a holistic treatment.

He found that, while certain things like aerobic exercise strongly increased neurogenesis, the brain pruned about half of these new neurons fairly quickly *unless* the brain was engaged in multiple other ways. Then there was a very high survival rate together with accelerated neurogenesis. That is, he found that all the factors of diet, exercise, emotional and mental stimulation acted synergistically to produce and maintain a high rate of neurogenesis.

It may be too much to call these "super mice," but they had strong cognitive and emotional advantages over their peers with normal neurogenesis rates. [25]They were smarter, learned faster, were more courageous and social, and appeared protected against stress, anxiety, and depression.

As the neuroscience studies rolled in, it became clear that increasing your neurogenic capacity results in improved learning, better memory, improved mood and emotion regulation as well as enhancing overall *presence.* [1] You are more *there,* more present.

Movement Is Life, Stasis Is Death

Healing the brain and self involves increasing the brain's neurogenic capacity. This means increasing the rate of neurogenesis and neuroplasticity in order to bring more movement and life to a sluggish, weakened brain.

The brain isn't a static "thing," it's a living, ever-moving *process*. Don't think of the brain as a computer. It's not a static, dead machine. Rather, the brain is a living, growing organ in constant movement. The brain is closer to a slow-moving amoeba or jellyfish than a circuit board. The brain is ever moving, in continual flux.

The rate of the brain's movement determines how you feel and how well you think. A slow, sluggish brain shows itself in anxiety, stress, depression, brain fog, and cognitive decline.

Neurogenesis and neuroplasticity are reduced in people with chronic anxiety, depression, and cognitive decline—and when chronic there is measurable brain shrinkage. Even gene expression is altered. In depressed patients, the most disrupted genes are those for brain growth factors such as BDNF and fibroblast growth factor-2, which also play a key role in resilience. [2]

If you suffer from brain fog, memory problems, or cognitive decline, this can indicate reduced neurogenic capacity. The hippocampus is not keeping up with the need for enhanced cognition and creating new memories. The brain's neurogenic rate has declined and with it, cognitive performance.

Every experience, every thought, feeling, sensation, and desire changes the brain. Reading these words is changing your brain right now. The brain is exquisitely sensitive and responsive to its inner and outer environment, continuously adjusting to this ever-changing movement of internal and external events.

New connections, new neural pathways, and new brain cells are continuously forming. Both physical food and psychological food (experience) stimulate brain growth.

At the same time the brain is building up, it's tearing down (pruning) unused connections. Unused neural connections and debris are cleared out every day (and especially every night when we sleep), while new neural pathways are laid down with every experience. At the molecular level all the cells of the brain are replaced and rebuilt every seven years. Not just in children, adult and senior brains are also in constant motion, building up and tearing down all the time, continually remodeling. The brain is always "under construction."

Common Factors in Anxiety, Depression, and Cognitive Decline

This chapter details some of the neural mechanisms that anxiety, depression, and cognitive decline all have in common. Inflammation, insulin resistance, poor gut health, sleep disturbances, and various neurotoxins lie behind many of these symptoms. There is one brain system, however, that has emerged as key to brain health or illness—the hippocampus.

The brain is an enormously complex structure, with different regions and subsystems. The hippocampus is a central structure in brain health, for it's the lynchpin of memory, new learning, cognition, and emotion regulation: It's where neurogenesis takes place and where neural death often first occurs. Alzheimer's, for example, massively attacks the hippocampus.

In Praise of the Hippocampus

Why has Mother Nature endowed this part of our brains for continuous growth? Why is the hippocampus chosen for this gift of the fountain of youth? Perhaps nature has selected the hippocampus for this distinction because it's so central to so many functions: body, heart, mind, and spirit.

The hippocampus (actually there are two hippocampi, one in the right hemisphere and one in the left, though it's usually referred to in the singular) looks like a crescent moon or curved silkworm. It has two ends, the temporal (or ventral) and septal (or dorsal).

The septal end is involved with memory, new learning, and cognition. The hippocampus processes new memories; it doesn't store them. That is, it aggregates their different features and organizes them into coherent memories that provide the person with a sense of continuity in time and space. This is why, as Alzheimer's attacks the hippocampus, new memories fail to form and memory falls apart.

When memory fails, it takes executive function and the higher cognitive processes along with it. As Alzheimer's progresses the person seems to slip away, for memory is the foundation on which the self is built. When the hippocampus shrinks and neurogenic capacity declines, memory goes and the self begins to dissolve.

The temporal end is involved with emotion regulation, especially of stress, anxiety, and depression, as well as spatial relations and the body. This side of the hippocampus connects with other brain systems in the limbic system that process emotion, including the amygdala. Not only poor diet but things like chronic or high stress, anxiety, and depression actually kill neurons in the hippocampus.

Certain meditation practices appear to increase neurogenesis along the entire length of the hippocampus, which underscores its importance.

The Aftermath of Neurogenic Slowing

So much of the current neurotoxic environment slows down neuroplasticity and neurogenesis. This neurogenic slowing reduces a person's capacity for change and adaptability. Neurogenic slowing brings in its wake anxiety, depression, and cognitive decline, depending upon a person's genetic, physical, and psychological vulnerabilities and age. Neurogenic slowing is one of the most insidious features of the current world, affecting most people to some degree.

A neurotoxic environment can impair different brain regions, but often the hippocampus is first. Neurogenic slowing is both the canary in the coal mine and the toxic gases the canary warns of. It's both a preliminary signal or rumbling of impending trouble as well as, when sustained, a cause of reduced brain capacity that brings the host of psychological problems that the program in this book seeks to reverse.

To jump-start change involves increasing your neurogenic rate until you reach your neurogenic potential. Once reached, the goal is to maintain your neurogenic stride so you are capable of rapid change and mental/emotional resilience. When neurogenesis and neuroplasticity increase there are dramatic changes: We see cognitive enhancement and rapid learning, robust emotional resilience, and protection against depression, anxiety, and stress. [1] Remember, neurogenic capacity can be increased by at least fivefold, probably more. [3]

What Is Mental Health?

As a psychology professor at the graduate level for over three decades, I came to see how poorly most mental health professionals understand what mental health is. At one conference I attended, someone asked this question to an audience of over 500: "Who has had even a single class in mental health during their training?" Not one hand went up. "Who learned about mental illness and psychopathology?" Every hand rose. It is paradoxical that the field of mental health is so exclusively focused on pathology and has hardly begun to map out the higher possibilities of the psyche.

Mental health is on a continuum ranging from severe psychopathology to the "normal neurosis" of everyday life and extending up into higher ranges first envisioned by Abraham Maslow and humanistic psychology that have been called "flourishing."

The level of "normal neurosis" that the vast majority of people function at is fine for getting by in everyday life. However, it pales in comparison with the joy, creativity, and enhanced functioning that is the hallmark of those self-actualizing individuals at "the farther reaches of human nature." [4]

Therapy and personal growth and healing open the doors to these higher realms of flourishing. Unfortunately, too few people do the inner work needed for such transformation. Because the average brain is so weakened, therapy is not as effective as it is when the brain is strong and glowing. The field of mental health at present is more of a promise than an accomplished fact.

This book extends flourishing into the physical level of brain health. Just as there are higher possibilities psychologically, so there are much higher possibilities for brain health. This book is about healing from the disorders of anxiety, depression, and cognitive decline. But its goal is much greater than this. It points the way to levels of human flourishing that surpass the current levels of weakened brains and simply existing. Psychological flourishing and radiant brain health go together, complete each other, find their highest fulfillment when brain and self are raised to their greatest possibilities.

We want the brightest, most luminous brain and self to express the whole range of our powers and abilities:

- to think clearly, lucidly, creatively
- to feel fully, deeply, richly
- to experience deep intimacy, love, and connection with others
- to enjoy our senses and bodily life and take in the immense beauty of the natural world
- to spiritually open within to our loving center of peace

This is possible for almost everyone. With proper nourishment, the brain and self naturally thrive and strengthen. Clearly, there are some people, such as those with advanced Alzheimer's or severe brain damage, whose brains are already so compromised that full repair is not possible, though even here healing can occur. But for the great majority of people who simply operate well below capacity, so much more is possible.

When the brain gets stronger, the self operates at a higher level, especially in terms of emotion regulation, cognition, and creativity. Concurrently, when the structures of the self become more cohesive, there is greater coherence and efficiency within the brain, and this in turn allows its potentials to emerge more fully. Physical and psychological nutrients work together to strengthen the brain and stabilize the self. This is holistic healing of the brain and the self.

It's worth repeating that each individual needs a unique combination of physical and psychological (that is somatic, emotional, mental, and spiritual) cleansing and repair. Some people move into a higher level purely through diet; some move purely through psychotherapy; for some both are needed. While both are optimal for most people, in practice healing on one side or the other may suffice.

Have You Reached Your Neurogenic Potential?

Is your brain growing? Is your self growing? The two go together. The idea is to repair, rejuvenate, and renew your neurogenic capacity. When your neurogenic rate is high, the brain is moving, growing, renewing. The result is you feel good, clear, and sharp.

Falling short of your neurogenic potential means you don't function as well as you could. The first part of this dietary plan heals and strengthens the brain so you reach your neurogenic potential. You start feeling good and performing at a higher level.

Can You Maintain Your Neurogenic Stride?

The second part of the Healthy Brain Diet begins once your neurogenic rate has reached its optimal level. After you've hit your neurogenic stride, then the Maintenance Phase of this plan begins. The Maintenance Phase is designed to keep your brain performing at a peak level throughout your lifespan.

A Note on the Nature of Evidence

While brain imaging technology has come a long way, it still only gives very partial, limited information about what is happening in the brain. For this reason, much of what neuroscience knows about the brain has been learned from animals, especially mammals, which share the same brain systems as humans. The fundamental architecture of the brain is identical in all mammals: the triadic brain system of reptilian brain stem, mammalian emotional limbic system, and neocortex. It's the size of these brain systems that vary by species. In humans the neocortex accounts for 30% of the brain, whereas in monkeys the neocortex is only 12%, and in dogs it's 4%. However, the basic structures are the same across species.

Mammals such as monkeys, dogs, mice, and humans also share the same neurotransmitters. Antidepressant drugs such as SSRIs (selective serotonin reuptake inhibitors), SNRIs (serotonin-norepinephrine reuptake inhibitors), and NDRIs (norepinephrine-dopamine reuptake inhibitors), work in the same way in all mammalian species. Stress and depression show similar neural effects in humans, mice, and monkeys.

Measuring the rate of neuroplasticity and neurogenesis is a scientific feat that has only recently been achieved through brain imaging that looks at blood flow, BDNF levels, glucose utilization, and increased brain volume. These are key markers of neurogenesis and neuroplasticity. Neurogenesis can currently be inferred in these ways but can only be confirmed on autopsy. This is another reason animal studies have been crucial in learning about this.

While most of the studies in this book are done with humans, some are done with animals. It takes science time to confirm the results in humans. Inevitably, as science moves forward, some of the information in this book will be modified and refined.

Scientific progress is not a straight upward line. Rather it moves ahead in waves, and conventional medical practice lags about 20–30 years behind the latest research. While there is a great deal of recent evidence in nutritional science on the effectiveness of supplements, for example, many physicians have not kept abreast of these findings and disparage nutrition as a road to health, relying exclusively on drugs instead.

The alternative, to wait 20, 30, 50 years for absolute confirmation, is a choice some will make. In addition, it often takes a few months to feel better as the brain heals, so some people don't take supplements because there is no immediate effect. Yet everything in this book is backed up by scientific research. For those who want to make use of the best available data and to make their own choices about their health, please continue reading.

Part 1 of the Plan: Diet and the Body

This plan is in two parts. The first part (this chapter) details the physical side of regenerating the brain against depression, anxiety, and cognitive decline, since these share many common brain pathways. The focus here is on diet, sleep, exercise, and detoxification.

The second part (the following chapters) details the psychological side to heal and strengthen the self, which are different for each disorder. The chapters on each disorder further tweak the dietary recommendations to emphasize specific nutrients and supplements shown to be helpful.

DIET

"Let food be your medicine, and let medicine be your food."
Hippocrates

Most of this section is devoted to diet, the single most powerful physical influence on the brain. Most people eat too much that's harmful to the brain and not enough of what nourishes it. The result is a malnourished, weakened brain.

To build a better brain, it's crucial to understand how the brain evolved. Then it becomes clear what the brain really needs, as opposed to what it currently gets or craves or is readily available.

The human brain is the crown jewel of evolution, the product of 200 million years of beta testing since the mammalian brain first emerged. The modern human brain is the product of further testing as the first humans arose 200,000 years ago from a diet of mostly fat, moderate protein, and some carbohydrate mixed in with a great deal of fiber. Our genetic programming was never designed for either the massive amounts of sugar and carbohydrates, or the low fat, oxidized fat, and low fiber most people consume, not to mention the pesticides, synthetic chemicals, and processing much food undergoes.

Further, since access to food was variable, human DNA evolved in feast or famine cycles, that is, periods of no food (what we now call fasting) were interspersed with periods of plenty. Regular eating didn't happen until agriculture was invented, about 10,000 years ago, the mere blink of an eye in genetic time.

What's good for the brain tends to be good for the rest of the body. For example, foods that are good for the heart and cardiovascular system also help the brain because 20% of the body's blood goes to the brain through a rich supply of blood vessels. When the heart and blood vessels work well, so does the brain. Things like chronic inflammation that damage the heart and blood vessels also damage the brain.

A general dietary principle is: If it's good for the brain, it's good for the body. When we build a healthy brain, a healthy body comes with it.

Healthy Brain Diet

These are general guidelines for a diet that nourishes the brain. Each person needs to experiment with how to customize this diet to your individual needs. There is no "one size fits all" approach when it comes to eating. Each body and brain is unique, with different genetic strengths and vulnerabilities, a unique environment and microbiome, a different history with unique mineral, metabolic, and other deficiencies. For example, an estimated 80% of Americans have some degree of insulin resistance and would do well to cut down on carbohydrates, but the 20% who don't may be able to eat larger amounts of sugar and carbohydrates, at least until they, too, develop insulin resistance and then need to curtail their carbohydrate intake.

What your body needs will depend on your unique metabolism and what you can tolerate. The body is highly adaptive, so what you need when you're 20 may be very different from what's best when you're 40 or 60. It's a continual process of adaptation.

All discussions of diet need to acknowledge that nutritional knowledge is a moving target. We know more than ever before, but there is still so much that is unknown that we need to approach this area with a great deal of humility. Dietary fads come and go as science becomes more precise in its understanding. For 50 years fat was "bad"; now we know this ignored differences between oxidized and non-oxidized fat as well as failed to distinguish between unhealthy trans fats and other very healthy fats. Inevitably, ten years from now, as science marches forward, current understandings will be honed by new discoveries.

Four Pillars of the Healthy Brain Diet

Eating according to these principles brings about an epigenetic shift to express those genes that support brain, mitochondrial health, and healthy aging. A discussion follows that unpacks each principle:

1. neurogenic
2. ketogenic
3. anti-inflammatory
4. gut friendly (prebiotic, probiotic, tight junction supporting)

Neurogenic: Stimulates Brain Growth through Increasing the Rates of Neurogenesis and Neuroplasticity

As new research on neurogenesis and neuroplasticity rolled in, it became clear that a person's rate of neurogenesis and neuroplasticity are key to the quality of life. Research has tied the rate of neurogenesis and neuroplasticity to everything from mood regulation to executive function. [1]

Low rates of neurogenesis and neuroplasticity are associated with problems in emotion regulation, leading to anxiety, stress, depression, hopelessness. Cognitive decline, memory deficits, and learning problems are also tied to a low rate of neurogenesis and neuroplasticity.

As mentioned in the previous chapter, there is now convincing evidence that the "serotonin deficiency theory" of depression is a myth. Chapter 4, "Holistic Healing for Depression," goes into the research that undermines the myth of serotonin deficiency in greater detail. For now, it's important to understand that the rate of neurogenesis and synaptogenesis are reduced in depression and anxiety.

The majority of studies show serotonin levels are normal in depressed patients, so serotonin levels are not a biomarker for depression, nor are antidepressants addressing a "serotonin deficiency." Recent research shows it's not the increase in serotonin that affects depression but the increase in neurogenesis and neuroplasticity. On the other hand, lower levels of BDNF (or brain-derived neurotrophic factor, which stimulates neurogenesis and neuroplasticity) *is* a marker for depression. [5]

High rates of neurogenesis are associated with healthy emotion regulation and positive feelings of joy, peace, fulfillment, and love. Cognitive benefits also accrue: rapid learning, increased executive function, cognitive enhancement, and increased problem solving. [1]

When the brain is producing new neurons at a high level, neuroplasticity is high. Neuroplasticity refers both to the process of making new connections among existing brain cells (synaptogenesis) as well as neurogenesis. The human ability to change and evolve, to creatively adapt to new situations, to learn new things, and respond freshly to life, requires neurogenesis and synaptogenesis operate at peak capacity. A high degree of neurogenesis and neuroplasticity are hallmarks of a healthy brain.

Brain Food

To build a strong, resilient, radiantly healthy brain means, first and foremost, increasing the brain's rate of growth, neurogenesis, and synaptogenesis through a neurogenic diet. It's essential to stimulate the brain's natural growth, its rebuilding and strengthening capacities, by increasing neurogenesis and neuroplasticity. Neurogenic foods do this in part by increasing levels of brain-derived neurotrophic factor (BDNF), a substance made by the body which is like miracle-grow for the brain.

A variety of chemical messengers stimulates neural growth, collectively they are known as "neurotrophins." They include:

- Brain-derived neurotrophic factor (BDNF), the most important neurotrophin, has a powerful effect on increasing neurogenesis and neuroplasticity

- Nerve growth factor (NGF), works with sensory neurons and sympathetic neurons as well as pain receptors
- Neurotrophin-3 (NT-3), which stimulates sensory neurons
- Neurotrophin-4 (NT-4), which is not well understood
- IGF-1, which helps neuron survival and regulates insulin

The most widely studied neurotrophin is BDNF. It acts like fertilizer for new brain cells and new neural connections. It appears to be the main signal for turning on neurogenesis and neuroplasticity. There are things that lower BDNF, such as certain foods, inflammation, chronic stress and anxiety, physical assaults, and emotional and sensory deprivation.

Conversely, there are things that increase BDNF, such as certain nutrients, emotional states of well-being, mental stimulation, and spiritual practices. The key is to increase BDNF levels naturally and safely, by aligning with the brain's own systems.

When BDNF levels are artificially increased by injecting BDNF directly into the body, it has the opposite effect and strongly inhibits cognition, memory, neurogenesis, and neuroplasticity. There is an astounding network of safety mechanisms in the brain that simply cannot be overridden. Attempting to do so does violence to the brain's interconnected, complex protective systems and throws off its homeostatic balance.

The key is to work *with* the brain to heal and strengthen it. Naturally raising BDNF levels increases rates of neurogenesis and synaptogenesis and corrects the neurogenic sluggishness involved in cognitive decline, depression, and anxiety. In the words of the Greek physician Hippocrates, "Natural forces within us are the true healers of disease."

These new neural circuits will help to solidify these changes and protect against future emotional assaults. There are a number of nutrients that dramatically increase the rate of neurogenesis and neuroplasticity. A more comprehensive discussion of these can be found in my previous book, but this list includes nutrients newly discovered to be effective in the last few years.

The Value of Supplements

The depletion of the soil over the past century has drastically reduced the amount of nutrients in food. Pesticides that have killed beneficial bacteria in the soil that are needed for plants to absorb nutrients, topsoil erosion, soil depletion and other modern farming methods produces vegetables that lack the nutrients that were in them decades ago.

Additionally, while it may be possible to get the minimum amount of nutrients to avoid disease through diet alone, it is not possible to obtain higher amounts of many nutrients that are needed for healing without concentrating certain factors through supplementation. Some people are prejudiced against supplementation. I would suggest openness to the thousands of studies that show supplements to be helpful.

While conflicting studies often make headlines, the great majority of studies show the following nutrients are highly beneficial to brain function. This list is meant to be inclusive so you can pick and choose what fits for you. This list may seem daunting, so only take what seems right for you. Some people will begin with a few, others will want to jump in. You don't need to try to do everything. At the end of this chapter, I'll suggest an easy way to start.

Neurogenic Nutrients:

Omega-3 fatty acids. The single most important nutrient for your brain is the complex of fatty acids called omega-3s. Of the three omega-3 fatty acids (ALA, DHA, and EPA), the most important is DHA. Sixty percent of the brain is fat, and one-third to one-half of this is DHA. DHA is the fundamental building block of the brain. EPA is also important for its anti-inflammatory effects. Omega-3s have been shown to dramatically increase neurogenesis and BDNF levels.

Neuroscience researcher Sandrine Thuret, Ph.D., of London's Kings College, showed a 40% increase in neurogenesis by adding omega-3s as reported in *Science Daily* in 2007. Other studies have shown equally impressive gains in neurogenesis, elevated BDNF levels, increase in brain size, and neuroprotective benefits from omega-3s. [6, 7, 8]

In the ongoing tearing down, repairing, and rebuilding of our brains' cellular structures, we want to consume high-quality fats in order to continuously rebuild our brains with the best fats possible, beginning with omega-3s. Unfortunately, it's estimated that 95% of the American population is deficient in omega-3s. A diet high in unhealthy or "bad" fats slows down neurogenesis and creates inflammation, but a diet high in healthy or "good" omega-3s reduces inflammation and raises neurogenesis to a higher level. [9, 10]

Omega-3s work in a number of ways besides increasing neurogenesis. They build up bigger, more functional brains by increasing neurite growth, enhancing neuronal cell transmission, increasing neurotransmitter release, and protecting against inflammation and oxidation. [7, 11, 12]

DHA is the single most important nutrient for the brain. Of the 60% of the brain that's composed of fat, a third to a half of it is DHA. Some evolutionary biology thinkers link the growth of the human brain over the last few million years to access to DHA through fish and meat.

Researchers raised monkeys on two diets, one low in DHA and the other high in DHA. Then they looked at their brains. The monkeys on the low DHA diet had very simple, undifferentiated brains with limited neural networks. The monkeys on the high DHA diets, in contrast, had brains that were highly complex, richly differentiated, with well-organized neural networks, almost like those of human beings. [13, 14] When it comes to the brain, complexity is good.

Omega-3 is critical to maintain high levels of brain and cognitive function. Higher omega-3 levels in the diet are associated with larger brain volume in the regions involved in executive function and emotion regulation. Omega-3 supplemented adults had lower anxiety and were more able to take risks without increased impulsiveness. Bigger and more functional brains result when taking more omega-3s. Lower omega-3 intake is associated with impaired learning and memory; higher risk of Alzheimer's, ADD, and ADHD; and cognitive decline. Higher intake is tied to reduced risk of cognitive decline and Alzheimer's, as well as providing protection against other risk factors for cognitive decline such as diabetes and heart disease. [15, 16, 17]

Getting a plentiful supply of DHA is the single most important thing you can do for your brain. Omega-3s are important for healing traumatic brain injury (TBI), and neurologist Michael Lewis, M.D., who worked in Iraq with many TBI patients, uses high doses (18 grams daily) for two weeks, then returns to three or more grams daily. [18, 19] "If you have a brick wall and it gets damaged, wouldn't you want to use bricks to repair it?" asked Dr. Lewis, founder of the Brain Health Education and Research Institute. "By using [omega-3 fatty acids] in substantial doses, you provide the foundation for the brain to repair itself." [20]

Further, omega-3s have been shown to be as or more effective than prescription SSRI antidepressant medication in treating depression. Joseph R. Hibbeln, M.D., from the National Institute on Alcohol Abuse and Alcoholism (NIAAA) said in an interview, "The strongest evidence was found for managing major depressive symptoms, with the effect of omega-3s being at least as great, if not greater than, antidepressant medications." [11, 21] This makes sense because, as noted in an earlier chapter, depression is linked to decreased neurogenesis and increasing neurogenesis helps alleviate depression.

Low levels of omega-3s are linked to lower IQs in children, higher rates of cognitive decline, Alzheimer's, and other cognitive impairments such as ADHD and dyslexia. [22, 23]

A report in the January 22, 2014, issue of the journal *Neurology* reveals lower brain volume and smaller hippocampus size in older adults is associated with lower omega-3 levels. Lead author James Pottala, Ph.D., concluded, "This study adds to the growing literature suggesting that higher omega-3 fatty acid tissue levels, which can be achieved by dietary changes, may hold promise for delaying cognitive aging and/or dementia."

Omega-3s are found in abundance in cold water fish, including wild Alaskan salmon, coho and sockeye salmon, black cod, sablefish, sardines, and herring. It is possible to obtain one of the essential fatty acids (ALA) from flax oil, and the body can convert this to the other two critical fatty acids (EPA and DHA), but this conversion is extremely inefficient. According to the Pauling Institute at Oregon State University, a mere 8% is converted to EPA and 0–4% is converted to DHA in healthy young men.

Some people do not manage even this minimal conversion rate, and the process deteriorates with age. This is why fish oil is recommended as the best source for omega-3s, although new sources from algae have recently appeared for vegetarians. Vegans and vegetarians have significantly lower levels of DHA in their bodies, which is a cause for concern. Supplementing with flax oil alone has shown increased EPA levels but not increased levels of the more important DHA. [24] The newer, supplemental algae sources have, however, been shown to increase DHA levels.

When obtaining fish oil in capsule form, it is preferable to buy molecularly distilled products, to ensure that no mercury or other heavy metal contamination is present. Look for equal amounts of DHA and EPA. While this is an expensive supplement, remember, there is no better financial investment than your own brain. Many capsules are 1,000 mg (1 gram), and although the U.S. government recommends at least 3 grams daily, most people can use 3–4 grams daily. The ratio of EPA to DHA ideally is 1:1, however, if you have high inflammatory levels (based on high-sensitivity C-RP blood test, over .5 for men or 1.0 for women, more on this test later), then a 2:1 ratio is preferable to bring down the inflammation quickly.

Green tea. Green tea contains polyphenols, the most powerful of which is epigallocatechin gallate (EGCG), a type of catechin. Green tea's polyphenols have been shown to increase neurogenesis, BDNF levels, and to have strong health benefits ranging from cancer prevention to fat loss, plus cardiovascular benefits, immunity improvement, and glucose reduction. [25-28] ECGC and green tea's other polyphenols not only increase neurogenesis but, like blueberries and omega-3s, exert powerful anti-inflammatory as well as antioxidant effects. Green tea has clear cognitive benefits and improves working memory, which is one of the most difficult cognitive functions to increase. [29]

It's important to remember that although green tea has less caffeine than regular tea, usually half or a third as much, this amount is still stimulating. It seems less stimulating because it also contains L-theanine, one of the polyphenols present in green tea that produces relaxation and also increases BDNF levels. Some people like and want caffeine stimulation while others do not. For those who are sensitive to caffeine or want to avoid it, caffeine-free green tea extracts are available.

Optimal range is the equivalent of about 8-10 cups of green tea daily but not the equivalent amount of caffeine. Look for decaffeinated extracts standardized to at least 40% polyphenols, or even better, 98% polyphenols with 75% catechins and 45% ECGC. Standard doses are 300–725 mg once daily. More than this can, in rare cases, be toxic to the liver. Higher amounts with caffeine should be monitored for overstimulation. Additionally, caffeine, even in low doses, decreases neurogenesis, so eliminating or reducing caffeine is advised. [30, 31]

Curcumin. Curcumin provides the yellow color in the curry spice turmeric. It has strong neurogenic effects, as well as being a powerful anti-inflammatory and antioxidant compound. Aging populations who consume curcumin show better cognitive performance. [32, 33] It reduces beta-amyloid and plaque formation in aging humans and has high potential as part of an anti-Alzheimer's strategy. It has also shown strong antidepressant effects, which naturally follow from decreasing inflammation and increasing neurogenesis. [34]

Here again, like so many things, more is not necessarily better. Too little and there is no effect, but extremely high doses, on the other hand, appear to be toxic to cells. [32] Some people report feeling an analgesic numbness with too much. Just the right, moderate amount bestows highly beneficial effects on the brain, BDNF levels, and neurogenesis. Typical amounts are 200–1,200 mg daily, so experiment to see what's right for you.

Because it is poorly absorbed, there are several ways to enhance this. One is to make smaller particles (submicron dispersion technology). Another is to add piperine (a pepper extract) or phospholipids such as eggs or lecithin to enhance bioavailability. Research has shown not only increased absorption but also additional antidepressant effects when these are added. Piperine or lecithin can be added to a curcumin or turmeric supplement for little additional cost. Most good supplement companies already enhance assimilation in one of these ways.

Blueberries. Blueberries have a wide range of brain-enhancing effects. Numerous studies show adding blueberries to the daily diet of mice increases neurogenesis significantly. [35-37] Further, blueberries seem to protect against cognitive decline, inflammation, oxidation (free radical damage), radiation, and glycation. [38-52] It would be hard to find something with such broad and powerful brain and cognitive-enhancing effects. Consuming about a cup a day is the equivalent human portion that animal studies have suggested.

Blueberries are packed with polyphenols, especially flavonoids called "anthocyanins" that stimulate neurogenesis. More specifically the anthocyanin dye, which causes the dark blue color, crosses the blood-brain barrier to stimulate neurogenesis. This anthocyanin dye is also present in black currants, blackberries, and bilberries, though these have not been studied as extensively.

Blueberries have been shown to reverse cognitive decline in both humans and animals. Mice bred to develop Alzheimer's showed improvements in memory when fed blueberries, and two neuroprotective chemicals were higher in these mice. Humans with cognitive decline showed improvements after consuming blueberries daily. Aside from increasing neurogenesis, blueberries allow better communication among neurons, something called "signal transduction," and they also protect against brain injury, stroke, certain neurotoxins, excitotoxicity, and so may help with Parkinson's, MS, and other neurodegenerative diseases as well. [53]

Studies have shown that blueberry extracts are as effective as fresh blueberries. In most animal studies it's the extract that is used. This makes daily blueberry intake possible for those who don't have access to fresh blueberries. Although blueberries are a low sugar fruit, they still do contain sugars, which this diet seeks to minimize. Blueberry extracts are preferable due to their lack of sugar. Look for extracts with the highest amount of anthocyanin content. Some are available at 25%.

Hesperidin. This flavonoid is found widely in fruits and vegetables and has been shown to increase the rate of neurogenesis by 25–41%. With most nutrients we don't yet know if the neurogenesis increase is due to a greater rate of neuron birth or survival. With hesperidin we do know. It comes via an increase in the survival rate of neural progenitor cells. Thus, like an "enriched environment," it functions to keep alive the newborn neurons rather than having them die off early on. [54] Since the brain prunes new brain cells and can eliminate half of them rather quickly, this nutrient is important to ensure that newly formed brain cells survive at a high rate.

Regular hesperidin is difficult for the body to assimilate, but a form of hesperidin called methyl chalcone is much more bioavailable and well worth the slight extra cost. Dosage is 500 mg, 1–2 times daily.

Ginkgo biloba. This has been hailed as a memory booster for some years now. While some studies failed to show improvements in patients with dementia, other studies have confirmed cognitive and memory improvements. Research shows it does increase neurogenesis, raise BDNF levels, enhance cognitive function, as well as reducing amyloid beta plaque in Alzheimer's. [55, 56] Recommended dose is usually given as 120 mg per day of standardized extract.

Luteolin. This compound from peanuts has strong anti-inflammatory and antidepressant effects on the brain as well as increases neurogenesis and BDNF. [57-59] The usual amount in many formulations is too small to have much effect, so 50–200 mg daily is recommended.

Taurine. This amino acid has recently been shown to have a strong effect on neurogenesis; 1,000 mg (1 gram), 1–2 times daily.

Rosmarinic acid. This comes from oregano or basil. It does triple duty as a compound that is neurogenic, anti-inflammatory, and antioxidant. It's sold most commonly under the brand name Origanox; 500–1,000 mg (1 gram), 1–2 times daily. A new source of rosmarinic acid has recently come on the market in the form of spearmint tea developed by Neumentix.

Quercetin. This flavonoid is widely found in many fruits and vegetables. It increases neurogenesis and BDNF levels, and it has anti-inflammatory, antioxidant, and other beneficial health effects. Standard dose is 500 mg, 1–2 times daily. [55]

Apigenin. This is a little-known compound present in many fruits and vegetables such as grapefruit, celery, and parsley. It has been shown to induce neurogenesis. [60] Standard dose is 50 mg, 1–2 times daily.

Vitamin E. In large doses vitamin E promotes neurogenesis. Paradoxically, vitamin E deficiency also promotes neurogenesis. [61] This makes sense given that mild or acute stress can promote neurogenesis, while stronger or chronic stress slows neurogenesis. Vitamin E has many other health benefits for heart health, cancer, eye health, and as a general antioxidant, so it is a helpful vitamin to consider including in your diet. Much research has found that the gamma form is more potent and preferable when choosing a supplement, with effective doses range from 200–400 i.u. per day.

Piperine. This extract from pepper appears with many supplements because of its ability to increase absorption of such things as curcumin. It also increases neurogenesis and BDNF levels in higher amounts. Standard dose is 95% extract, 10 mg, 1–2 times daily.

DHEA and pregnenolone. Pregnenolone is a precursor to DHEA, which in turn is a precursor to testosterone, estrogen and other androgens. Both are called "youth hormones" because levels decline with age. In large amounts they increase neurogenesis and may be neuroprotective against Alzheimer's. [62, 63] Usual doses are lower, 10–100 mg daily.

Huperzine A. This is an extract from a Chinese herb that has neuroprotective effects, shows promise as an Alzheimer's treatment by increasing a neurotransmitter involved in memory (acetylcholine), and it increases neurogenesis and BDNF levels. [64] Usual doses are 200–800 mcg daily.

Baicalin. This extract from Chinese skullcap is a polyphenol that is neuroprotective, reduces amyloid in mice, is anti-inflammatory, and promotes neurogenesis. [65] Depending upon the concentration, usual doses of Chinese skullcap extract are 100–400 mg, 1–2 times daily.

Icariin. This flavonoid from the Asian plant commonly known as horny goat weed increases BDNF levels, stimulates neurogenesis, is neuroprotective, has anti-amyloid and anti-inflammatory properties, and has both anti-stress and antidepressant effects. In aging rats it improves cognitive function. [66] Depending upon the strength of the extract, 300–500 mg, 1–2 times daily.

Ginseng extract. Ginseng has been shown to increase neurogenesis, protect the brain from injury and stroke, enhance memory, and have antidepressant effects. [67-69] The biologically active saponins include different ginsenosides, which have been studied extensively for decades. This herb causes some people to feel overstimulated. Just because it may be good for you doesn't mean it's right for you. As with all information in this book, each person must make his or her own determination.

Tryptophan and 5-HTP. Tryptophan and 5-HTP are chemical precursors to serotonin, and increased serotonin levels appear to upregulate neurogenesis. [70] As noted earlier it seems that increased neurogenesis rather than serotonin leads to antidepressant effects. Tryptophan can also be used as a sleep aid in larger amounts (2.5 grams before bed), as can 5-HTP (200–400 mg before bed). Doses for tryptophan are usually 500–1,000 mg; for 5-HTP usually 50–200 mg, 1–2 times daily.

Whole soy foods such as tofu, edamame, soy milk, soy nuts as well as soy isoflavone extracts containing daidzein and genistein. Soy has been shown to be neuroprotective. Key extracts, particularly daidzein and genistein, have been shown to increase neurogenesis. [71] It is believed that the isoflavones present in soy mimic estrogen, and estrogen has also been shown to increase neurogenesis. This is true for naturally occurring estrogen, but not for non-bioidentical hormones such as Premarin, which decrease neurogenesis. [72, 73]

Because of the increase in estrogenic compounds from soy intake, men should exercise caution with soy and soy extracts. Some males have reported decreased sex drive with soy or soy extract use. Testosterone, like estrogen, has been shown to promote neurogenesis, and it appears that both male and female sex hormones are equally neurogenic.

Rhodiola. This herbal adaptogen from Siberia has alkaloids that stimulate neurogenesis. Because it is stimulating, it is best taken in the morning rather than the evening, and sensitive individuals may want to avoid it. Standard dose is 200–700 mg, 1–2 times daily.

Melatonin. This hormone secreted by the pineal gland has long been known to have health benefits. The body secretes melatonin at night, when it's dark and we're asleep. Levels drop as we age, as does neurogenesis and, conversely, sleep disturbances increase. Melatonin increases neurogenesis and helps regulate it. [74-76] It also increases the immune system's capacity and has anti-cancer effects. Melatonin can be used as a sleep aid at night.

Some research suggests the body adapts to taking melatonin regularly and downregulates its own production in response. Hence, pulsing melatonin usage, that is, cycling in and out of using it, is advised. With dosage there is wide individual variation. The lower range is .2 or .3 mg up to 10 mg per night. This is a vivid example of how everybody needs to individualize their own dosages and nutrients.

Mulberry. This plant has long been used in traditional Oriental medicine, and it has been shown to stimulate neurogenesis. Standardized extract is 500 mg daily.

Red sage aka danshen aka salvia. This plant also has a long history in traditional Oriental medicine, especially for stroke recovery. It has been shown to have a strong effect in increasing neurogenesis. [77] Available as a 60% extract, 1,000 mg (1 gram), 1–2 times daily is usually recommended.

Bacopa. The adaptogenic herb increases neurogenesis and has strong antioxidant properties. It is neuroprotective and has antidepressant and anti-anxiety effects. [78] Different extracts require different dosages. Twenty percent bacosides would suggest 200–800 mg daily, spread out over 1–3 doses. Some people should not take it before sleep, although others find it helpful for sleep. Experiment and see.

Goji berry aka wolfberry. This tasty dried berry from the Himalayas has long been known for its powerful antioxidant properties, but it has now been confirmed that it possesses strong neurogenesis-stimulating effects as well as enhancing sexual performance. The pro-sexual effects are believed to be related to the increase in neurogenesis. [79] As with any dried fruit, be aware of the high sugar content. Available as dried berries, a juice, or as a 60% standardized extract 500 mg, 1–2 times daily.

Grape seed extract. This compound, which is beneficial for the heart and circulatory system, has been shown to increase neurogenesis. [80] Available as an extract standardized to 90%

polyphenols, 100 mg, 1–2 times daily. Some people find this stimulating.

St. John's wort. This herb has been demonstrated to be effective in depression. Some studies show it to be more effective than SSRIs for mild to moderate depression, and it has fewer side effects. It is used more widely in Europe than the United States, where it is a prescription medication. It increases neurogenesis and BDNF levels. [81, 82] Standardized extract 300–1,800 mg, 1–3 times daily.

Ketone bodies. Beta-hydroxybutyrate is the main ketone body produced when consuming a ketogenic diet. This has been shown to increase the rate of neurogenesis and neuroplasticity, BDNF levels, as well as stimulating autophagy. In a ketogenic diet, your body produces this naturally, but you can also purchase exogenous ketones to boost ketone levels.

Berberine. This yellow extract has strong anti-inflammatory and glucose-regulating properties as well as increasing BDNF and neurogenesis. It also has been shown to have antidepressant effects. Standard doses are 400 mg, 1–2 times daily.

Lithium. This mineral is used in the treatment of bi-polar disorder in large amounts and has shown neuroprotective benefits from the brain shrinkage caused by the disorder. It increases BDNF levels in the brain. It can also be taken in small (e.g., 2–30 mg) amounts, but some people find it makes them relaxed or sleepy. For anxiety reduction this can be just what's needed, but otherwise watch the effects on your consciousness if you decide to experiment with this. More recent recommendations are micro doses of 300 mcg per day which does not seem to produce noticeable effects.

Additional Nutrients that Increase BDNF and Other Neural Growth Factors

BDNF is the major, but not only, neurotrophic factor in increasing brain cell growth, but its presence does not ensure that neurogenesis is occurring. These nutrients are neurogenic in that they increase BDNF, neuroplasticity, and probably neurogenesis, but further research is needed to confirm their increase in neurogenesis.

Magnesium-L-threonate. Brain levels of magnesium are correlated with cognitive performance. Most people are deficient in magnesium, even those who take supplemental magnesium, since it only passes the blood-brain barrier in limited amounts. A new form of magnesium developed at the Massachusetts Institute of Technology (MIT) called magnesium-L-threonate has been shown to significantly increase magnesium levels in the brain, boost cognitive performance, increase BDNF levels, and prevent Alzheimer's cognitive decline in mice. [83-84] Usual dose is 2,000 mg daily (three capsules), but many people need more. Some people need up to 12 capsules to reach the desired magnesium blood levels. Experimentation is necessary to find what your body needs. As a sleep aid, people report taking 3 or more at dinner.

L-carnosine and beta-alanine. Beta-alanine is an amino acid precursor to L-carnosine, which is a powerful anti-glycating, anti-inflammatory, heavy metal chelating, and antioxidant agent. It increases BDNF levels and may have anti-anxiety and antidepressant effects as well. Carnosine has the additional properties of strongly reducing beta amyloid plaque in the brain (a key feature of Alzheimer's) as well as rescuing mitochondrial age-related dysfunctions. [85] Usual dose is 1,000 mg (1 gram) of beta-alanine or 500 mg of L-carnosine, 1–2 times daily.

Vitamin D. It is known both as the "sunshine vitamin" and the "happiness vitamin," but vitamin D deficiency is still widespread. It is an antioxidant, anti-inflammatory, and neuroprotective. Vitamin D increases BDNF levels and has been shown to help with depression, even forms of depression not linked to seasonal affective disorder (SAD). It is very difficult to get enough from diet alone unless you spend a lot of time in the sun. Blood tests can show your level, with ideal ranges between 60–100 ng/mL. According to a recent study in *Anticancer Research,* it requires almost 10,000 i.u. daily to get a majority (97%) of the population to reach 40 ng/mL. [86]

Magnolol. This is an extract derived from magnolia bark and has been used in Chinese medicine to treat depression. It increases BDNF levels and may be protective against the amyloid beta plaque in Alzheimer's. [87] It also appears to reduce the stress hormone cortisol, and since cortisol levels increase with time, this compound or other strategies for reducing cortisol are helpful in aging. Reducing cortisol in itself upregulates neurogenesis. It comes as an extract of 90%, 200 mg and as a patented product called Relora. Take 1–2 times daily.

Alpha lipoic acid (ALA). This antioxidant also increases BDNF levels. This nutrient is stimulating for some people, so exercise caution with dosage level. Usual dosage ranges are 50–300 mg, 1–2 times daily.

Ashwagandha. This is an Indian herb long praised for its regenerative powers. It increases dendrite growth and has demonstrated anti-anxiety, antidepressant, neuroprotective, and cognitive-enhancing effects. [88] Studies suggest it increases neurogenesis, and while definitive experiments have not yet been carried out to confirm this, we do know BDNF levels are increased. Doses depend on the concentration of the particular extract, but 5–8% extracts are commonly taken 1–2 times daily.

Resveratrol. The research has been mixed on this compound. Because it mimics some of the effects of caloric restriction, some researchers have assumed it would therefore promote neurogenesis. Studies show conflicting results, however; some show neurogenesis is inhibited, others show neurogenesis is promoted. The initial enthusiasm over resveratrol's health benefits has given way to more limited expectations, with greater benefits for overweight or ill subjects. Some people feel spacey taking resveratrol at higher doses, so you need to find out for yourself. Doses vary from 20–400 mg daily.

Cocoa flavonoids and chocolate. While there have been numerous claims made that chocolate and the flavonoids found in cocoa increase neurogenesis, at the time of this publication it has not been shown to be true, although BDNF levels are increased. [89] While some studies have failed to show any cognitive effects, two studies did show cognitive improvements and several have shown mood improvements. [90, 91] The flavonoids in cocoa demonstrate health benefits for the heart and vascular system, and this may in turn help brain function. One drawback is that cocoa comes with the stimulant theobromine, a close relative of caffeine, which probably impairs neurogenesis along similar pathways that caffeine does.

Milk thistle extract. This herb, also known as silymarin, is widely used for its beneficial effects on the liver. It also is neuroprotective. Although it does not appear to increase BDNF, it does increase NGF (nerve growth factor) and promote neurite growth. [92] Usual doses are 300 mg, 1–2 times daily.

Lion's mane. Like silymarin above, this mushroom also does not increase BDNF but it does increase NGF. It has not yet been shown, contrary to much of the hype on the Web, to increase neurogenesis, but it does increase neurite growth and synaptogenesis; 300–3,000 mg daily.

Pantethine. This is a precursor to the vitamin B5, but its action is believed to occur along other pathways. It increases BDNF, has antidepressant effects, and can be stimulating. [93] Usual doses are 50–500 mg daily.

Phosphatidylserine. This compound is produced by the brain to build new brain cells. Levels decrease as we age, and it is available as a supplement in the United States (in Europe it is by prescription only). It is effective in enhancing memory in older adults, has shown antidepressant effects, and it increases BDNF levels. [94, 95] Doses range from 100 mg daily for memory enhancement to 300 mg for antidepressant effects. In higher doses it can be stimulating, which may contribute to its antidepressant effects, though some people find it has an opposite anti-anxiety effect.

Cinnamon. This flavorful spice upregulates BDNF as well as another neurotrophin (NT-3), but taking pure cinnamon can be toxic. [96] It's better to take a cinnamon extract that has removed the toxins. Doses vary depending upon the extract.

Nutrients that Decrease Neurogenesis and Should Be Avoided or Minimized

Along with eating nutrients that are neurogenic, the complement to this is avoiding or minimizing things that decrease neurogenesis. These include:

- high amounts of food (overeating)
- foods high in sugar, carbohydrates, and unhealthy fats

- inflammatory foods (deep-fried foods, processed foods, common cooking oils like safflower, soy, sunflower, corn, and cottonseed), trans fats, refined grains, sugar, conventional, feedlot-raised meat, eggs, dairy
- alcohol is neurotoxic and slows neurogenesis even in small amounts
- caffeine (Sorry, but even the smallest biologically active amounts of caffeine have been shown to inhibit neurogenesis. Plus, it's a vasoconstrictor, which makes blood vessels smaller. You want more blood to your brain, not less.)
- deficiencies in vitamins A, B-1, and B-9 (thiamine and folic acid)

A summary of all the neurogenic foods in this chapter is listed in Appendix A

Ketogenic: Metabolically Flexible to Burn Fat, Not Just Glucose

Before jumping into the ketogenic part of the Healthy Brain Diet, some nutritional context is in order. It's important to first understand the three major food groups, called macronutrients. Macronutrients consist of fat, protein, and carbohydrates. All calories come in one of these three forms. The ketogenic diet changes the ratio of fat, protein, and carbohydrates that most people consume, shifting it from mostly carbs to mostly healthy fats.

Fat

The first guideline is to eat plenty of healthy fats. Remember, the brain is composed of 60% fat. It needs a constant supply of healthy fats to build, maintain, and remodel itself. It also uses fat for energy more efficiently than glucose.

But wait, isn't fat supposed to be "bad" rather than good?

Fats made up 50–80% of our ancestors' diet for millions of years. Humans are superbly adapted to thrive on mostly fat. Your brain needs lots of good, healthy fats, both to power the brain as well as supply the raw material to grow a healthy brain—every day, for the brain is rebuilding and remodeling itself continually.

In the 1960s Americans got 45% of their calories from fat, 13% of the population was obese, and less than 1% had type 2 diabetes. Since the 1960s, fat has been demonized as carbohydrates took over the food pyramid. Now, with the great majority of calories coming from carbohydrates and a minority from fat, two-thirds of Americans are overweight, 34% are obese, and 12–14% have type 2 diabetes, according to the *Journal of the American Medical Association.* As noted in the previous chapter, childhood rates of anxiety and depression are now five to eight times what they were in the 1960s.

This is a worldwide phenomenon. The *New England Journal of Medicine* reported on June 12, 2017, that one-third of the world is overweight, even countries with low income. This amounts to 2.2 billion people, with the U.S. leading the way in childhood obesity.

Poor diet, usually in the form of too much sugar, carbohydrates and unhealthy fats together with not enough healthy fats are now identified as the key driver of obesity, diabetes, heart disease, metabolic syndrome, inflammatory diseases, and Alzheimer's.

This information is finally getting into the popular culture more, so this discussion will only present a condensed summary. For more complete information please see my previous book, *The Neurogenesis Diet and Lifestyle*, and other excellent books on this: *Grain Brain* and *Brain Maker* by David Perlmutter, M.D.; *Eat Fat, Get Thin* by Mark Hyman, M.D.; *Headstrong* and *Super Human* by Dave Asprey; *Fat for Fuel* by Joseph Mercola, M.D.; and *Why We Get Fat* by Gary Taubes.

Healthy and Unhealthy Fats

The best diets for the brain get 50–80% of calories from healthy fat.

What makes a fat healthy or unhealthy? To simplify a complex topic, it depends on three things: *the type of fat, the amount of that type, and how it's prepared.*

The type of fat is important. These are the four types of fats (called fatty acids):

1. saturated fats (meat, dairy, palm and coconut oil)
2. monounsaturated fats (olive oil, avocados, nuts)
3. polyunsaturated fats: omega-3s (fish) and omega-6s (vegetable oils)
4. trans fats

We need the first three, none of the last. Trans fats' dangers are well catalogued by now. They are highly inflammatory, lead to heart disease, diabetes, and all manner of metabolic problems. The FDA banned trans fats by 2018, but small amounts will still appear in foods, mainly processed foods with half a gram or less, but it all adds up. It's wise to stay away from processed foods.

The *amount* of each type of fat is important. Saturated fat is the most stable form of fat. The myelin sheath that protects neurons is made of saturated fat and helps neural impulses travel better. Saturated fat makes up tissues and cell membranes that hold cells together. Main sources of saturated fat are meat and dairy, cocoa butter, coconut and palm oils.

We need a certain amount of saturated fat, but the jury is still out on how much. Until recently saturated fat was seen by the medical profession as "bad" because of the belief it raised cholesterol levels. But current science has overturned this. The liver makes most of the body's cholesterol, and dietary sugar and excess carbohydrates are the major culprits that increase cholesterol for most people [97] Saturated fat has a role when going overboard, but these days lack of saturated fat is more often the problem.

Standard medical practice usually lags about 20 years behind science. Much of the medical profession is still fat phobic. One symptom of this fat phobia is excessive use of statin drugs to lower cholesterol. One in four adults, including half of all senior men and a third of senior women, is on a statin with largely unintended consequences, particularly for the brain. Cholesterol has been demonized for decades, but more current thinking shows it to be critical for optimal brain function (as well as for thousands of metabolic processes like making hormones and vitamin D from sunlight).

The brain needs cholesterol for learning and memory, which is why it's so rich in cholesterol. Twenty-five percent of the body's cholesterol is in the brain, and when statins lower cholesterol levels, they often lower cognitive function, sometimes triggering transient global amnesia. The well-known Framingham Heart Study did cognitive testing on 2,000 men and women. Those with the highest levels of cholesterol had higher cognitive function, whereas those with the lowest levels had the greatest cognitive decline and lower scores on executive function, attention, and reasoning. [98] Seniors with the highest cholesterol levels lived the longest.

Researchers now see that cholesterol-reducing medications inhibit neurotransmitter production, leading to impaired memory and other cognitive functions. [99] Higher cholesterol levels reduce the risk for dementia, contrary to prevailing medical opinion. [100] MIT researcher Stephanie Senoff, Ph.D., links rising Alzheimer's rates to both low fat diets and statin drug use, and predicts a coming tidal wave of Alzheimer's from the widespread overuse of statins. [101]

Newer research has shown the fallacy in early studies which created the current prejudice against fats. These poorly done early studies failed to see that it's not cholesterol but *oxidized* cholesterol which creates the problem. Consuming oxidized cholesterol and fats is the real problem, as we'll examine in more detail soon. Eating cholesterol (e.g., eggs) does not raise your cholesterol levels since about 80% of the body's cholesterol is produced by the liver. The myth that eating fat causes heart disease is, according to Gerald Mann, M.D., of the *New England Journal of Medicine,* "the biggest scam in the history of medicine." [102]

Saturated fat is no longer seen as "the bad guy" it once was, but how much a person can safely consume may vary. This is an example of a moving target in nutrition. Conventional guidelines run about 10%, but since how saturated fat reacts in the body depends upon how much carbohydrate and sugar are consumed, [97] other authorities put no upper limit on it if a person is low carb. Recent studies have challenged this, noting high LDL and high very low density particle numbers in some but not most ketogenic dieters, while other studies have found the opposite.

The question of how much eating saturated fat raises blood levels is not settled science, since it depends upon the rest of the diet, genetics, the biome, and other unknowns, for example rare genetic conditions can predispose someone to high cholesterol levels. Perhaps for now it's best to have a moderate limit on saturated fat, 10–20% of calories, although many people do fine on more. Since large individual differences exist, a fasting lipid panel testing is helpful to see what works for you (discussed later in this section on diet).

Monounsaturated fats are healthy in any amount. They are good for the heart and cardiovascular system, which is why the Mediterranean diet is recommended to reduce heart disease. Olives and olive oil, avocados, some fish, and many kinds of nuts like macadamias, pecans, cashews, and almonds are high in monounsaturated fats. Freedom to eat these is not license, however, as going overboard with calories will increase weight at some point.

Polyunsaturated fats (omega-3s and omega-6s) are needed by the body, but the *amount* is all important. Omega-3s are anti-inflammatory and necessary to help keep inflammation levels low. Fish oil is the main source of omega-3s, along with algae-derived extracts.

As discussed earlier, omega-3s are fundamental building blocks of the brain and are anti-inflammatory and drive anti-inflammatory gene expression.

Omega-6 is inflammatory and necessary for the body to mount an inflammatory defense against infection or injury. But too much omega-6 creates a general inflammatory response that is extremely unhealthy for the body and brain. Excess dietary omega-6 can lead to chronic inflammation, and the promotion of vegetable oils in cooking has led to exactly this.

Historically the ratio of anti-inflammatory omega-3 to omega-6 was 1:1 or 1:2 (some authorities say as much as 1:4), but modern diets are closer to 1:20 or 1:30 or even 1:50, which leads to high inflammation levels. Most people consume far too much omega-6. All vegetable oils should be banned from the kitchen, with the exception of olive oil and avocado oil. Most everyone would benefit from more omega-3s and far fewer omega-6s.

How fat is prepared is critical. Heat, oxygen, and light oxidize fat, especially polyunsaturated fats, the most unstable of all fats. Vegetable oils oxidize readily, even with low heat. This is one reason to avoid cooking with vegetable oils (the other is that they are full of omega-6's). Better to also avoid canola oil, which is monounsaturated but 90% is GMO, and it's exposed in processing to high temperatures, bleaching, deodorizing, and caustic refining.

When oxidized fats and cholesterol (e.g., from cooking meats at high temperature or cooking with vegetable oil) are eaten and absorbed into the blood, they oxidize the cholesterol and fats in the blood, which creates inflammation and paves the way for heart disease, inflammation, cognitive decline, and a host of other ravages. [103, 104]

All oxidized fats, including french fries, onion rings, and all deep-fried foods, should be avoided, for the high amounts of inflammation they produce "chew up" the inside of the blood vessels. Best to cook with coconut oil, butter, ghee, or lard, as these do not oxidize at high temperatures.

Unhealthy fats are everywhere, so vigilance is needed to avoid them. **Unhealthy fats to avoid:**

- margarine
- fried foods, especially anything deep-fried (french fries, tempura, buffalo wings, potato chips, calamari, corn dogs, fish and chips, spring rolls, falafel, onion rings, donuts)
- burned, charred, blackened meat, fish, chicken
- vegetable oils (safflower, soy, corn, cotton seed, peanut)
- cooking with vegetable oils (even olive oil)
- eggs cooked at high temperature
- processed foods

Yes, these things taste good, but then so does arsenic when it's well-prepared. Just because you're used to eating slow poisons doesn't make them non-toxic, nor does avoiding them condemn you to asceticism. There are plenty of healthy, delicious alternatives, as explored in a later section.

Low to Moderate Carbohydrates

Excess sugar and carbohydrates are overwhelming a body that was never made for such quantities. Sugar and carbohydrates are rare in the wild. As humanity spread out of Africa about 100,000 years ago, there was occasional access to some fruit, and the added fat it created may have been helpful in getting through the winter. Further, most carbohydrates in the wild come with great amounts of fiber, which moderates how quickly the sugar pours into the system.

Insulin allows cells to utilize glucose and is the hormone that drives eating and fat storage. Excess carbohydrate gets converted into excess fat. Type 1 diabetes is an autoimmune disorder where the body kills its own insulin-producing islet cells, so insulin must be injected. Type 2 diabetes is when continuous sugar and carbohydrates (all of which convert to glucose or blood sugar) overpower the body's needs and the cells of the body become insensitive to insulin (insulin resistance), so the body must make more insulin to meet the rising glucose levels. Higher insulin levels damage almost every organ in the body, the brain in particular.

When insulin levels are high over years, the brain deteriorates, along with eyes, kidneys, nerves, and other organs. Ninety percent of diabetics are type 2, which has become an epidemic, with one out of three people expected to develop it and most Americans already insulin resistant or on a prediabetic trajectory. Alzheimer's appears to involve a problem with glucose metabolism and is being called type 3 diabetes. [105, 97]

Because of a high sugar and carbohydrate diet, an estimated 80% of the American population has insulin resistance, the first step toward diabetes. Higher insulin levels also mean higher glucose levels, which cause cellular damage through a process called glycation, the cross-linking of proteins. The browning of a chicken on a rotisserie is due to glycation as the sugars in the meat cross-link the proteins. Glycation produces advanced glycation end-products (AGEs); these are one of the main drivers of aging, disease, and brain deterioration. Just eating foods high in AGEs increases glycation (such as meats cooked at high temperatures) and accelerates oxidation and brain stress. [106, 3]

Cognitive decline and high blood sugar levels track perfectly. The higher your blood sugar and insulin, the faster will be your rate of cognitive decline. [105] Drinking sugared soda in childhood is linked in mice to aggressive behavior as adults, as well as higher inflammation levels. [107] Insulin resistance and the higher blood glucose that comes with it produce the three main drivers of brain dysfunction: glycation, inflammation, and oxidation. [105]

Insulin resistance is increasingly referred to as "carbohydrate intolerance," because excess carbohydrates (which, remember, the body converts to sugar) exceed the body's capacity to process glucose. The most effective way to reduce insulin resistance is by cutting down on carbohydrates. Standard medical practice when people are lactose intolerant is to avoid lactose. Gluten intolerance is best treated by staying away from gluten. The same logic applies here: Reduce carbohydrates to recover from carbohydrate intolerance.

Insulin spikes that occur with sugar are particularly harmful. Although all net carbohydrate gets converted to sugar (net carbohydrate is carbs minus fiber, which the body doesn't metabolize), the surge of glucose and insulin that follow a sugary soda or dessert inflict extra heavy damage. Eating complex carbohydrates (foods with fiber or starch) is preferable to simple sugar because the glucose enters the system more slowly. Again, what each person's body can tolerate is an individual matter.

Cutting down on carbohydrates, especially sugar, in a carbohydrate obsessed society is hard at first, but soon after making the change it becomes second nature, habitual and easy. Carbohydrates lurk everywhere, tempting you in the form of sugar, pastries, bread, potatoes, rice, most cereals, desserts, soda, fruits, and fruit juices. Healthy sweet alternatives are stevia extract and monk fruit extract, which have zero sugar, carbs, or calories.

One of the most important blood tests to get as part of a yearly physical exam is called the hemoglobin A1c (HemA1c). It's a snapshot of blood glucose levels over the past three months. Although conventional medicine considers anything below 5.8 to be "normal," beware. "Normal" is not "healthy." Cognitive decline accelerates for every .1 increase over 5.2. Lowering your HemA1c is one of the most important things you can do for the health of your brain.

If you are relatively young and blood testing shows no insulin resistance, then consuming sugar and carbohydrates may be fine. But understand that almost everyone sooner or later develops insulin resistance with a high carb diet, and at that point carb reduction becomes important. Most people with type 2 diabetes are undiagnosed. Most with prediabetes similarly go undiagnosed. Although it takes years of high blood sugars to damage the brain and body, it is nevertheless occurring silently, relentlessly, and will inevitably undermine your brain and sense of well-being. The sooner you catch this, the better.

Moderate Protein

Protein abounds in the developed world. Most people get too much rather than too little protein. Protein builds muscle, tissues, cartilage, skin, blood, and enzymes. You need to get a minimum amount to replace the muscle that breaks down during the day.

Protein builds up the body in large part by stimulating the mTOR pathway. mTOR, which stands for the mechanistic (previously mammalian) target of rapamycin, is a metabolic pathway that promotes cell growth, including, unfortunately, cancer.

The body has two modes that need to be balanced: growth and repair. The body needs to balance the growth of new tissue and the repair of damaged tissue. Every day brings new damage to bodily tissues (including neurons) that need to be repaired. If the body is only in growth mode, this repair doesn't happen very efficiently. If the growth cycle could perfectly equalize the damage-repair cycle, the body would never age. But over the years the repair capacity diminishes and aging inevitably sets in. Nevertheless, you want the repair cycle to be as good as possible for as long as possible.

mTOR slows down the repair cycle and pushes the body into growth mode. Too much growth leads both to cancer, which is growth run amok, and to neurodegeneration. [108] The body needs to repair the brain daily, in an ongoing way. It's a delicate balance: Too much growth stimulates cancer and neurodegeneration, while not enough growth means loss of muscle mass.

It turns out that mTOR is tied to protein and insulin levels. Evolutionarily, when food was scarce the body shifted into repair mode; when food was plentiful (high protein, glucose and insulin) the body moved into growth mode. High insulin levels activate mTOR. Excess protein gets turned into glucose in the liver via gluconeogenesis, which in turn raises insulin and then can be stored as fat. The body uses those high glucose levels to power new growth (including growth of cancer cells that require glucose for fuel).

Many experts who are tuned in to the mTOR pathway recommend a daily protein intake of about a half gram of protein for every pound of lean body weight. For a 130-pound person with 20% fat, 80% of 130 = 104 lbs. of lean body weight, or 50 grams of protein per day. For a 160-pound person with 20% fat, 80% of 160 = 128 lbs. of lean body weight, or 64 grams of protein daily. Most people consume 100 grams daily, almost double this amount, which can promote cancer, raise blood sugar, and over time degrade brain function.

The easiest and most effective way to lower mTOR is to reduce protein to the minimal amount needed to maintain muscle mass. A person's activity level, weight, and age are the chief variables. If you are pregnant, older, or very active physically, you need about 25% more protein whereas if you are sedentary you may do better on a half gram of protein for each pound of lean body weight.

Older adults need both more strength training and protein to protect against muscle loss. Sarcopenia, or loss of muscle mass, is very common in older adults and a key indicator of mortality risk. Higher protein intake in your 60s and older will mitigate against frailty and losing muscular strength. As with everything dietary, you need to experiment to find out what's right for you.

Shifting your brain out of degeneration and into repair and regeneration mode is an important element to feeling good. Having one "protein fast day" per week, when you eat significantly less protein, is a good way to stimulate your body's repair mode, as is intermittent fasting.

With this macronutrient context, the stage is set to understand a ketogenic diet.

Using Fat for Energy in Ketogenic and Low Carb Diets

The brain is an energy hog. Although the brain is just 2% of the body's weight, it uses 25% of the body's oxygen and nutrients and 60% of its glucose in the resting state. [109]

Although almost everyone in the world uses only glucose for energy, glucose is a "dirty" fuel. It produces by-products that damage the body in the forms of inflammation, oxidation, free radicals, glycation, and it is not energy efficient.

The cleanest, most efficient source of energy for the brain is fat, in the form of ketone bodies. Ketone bodies (specifically beta-hydroxybutyrate, acetoacetate, and acetone) are created in the liver as an alternative energy source to glucose. When the brain has a choice, it preferentially utilizes ketones for energy rather than glucose.

Ketones burn cleanly and sharply reduce oxidation and inflammation. [110] Harvard ketone researcher Dr. Richard Veech calculates that the heart works at 28% higher capacity with ketones compared to glucose. [111] Because of the similarity between the heart and the brain's mitochondria, it is believed the brain's metabolism, efficiency, and energy improve by about this amount as well—a rather astonishing figure. Having your brain operate at 28% greater efficiency is like taking your six-cylinder car that's been chugging along on three or four cylinders for a turbo-charged tune-up. Optimal brain health means your brain is firing on all six cylinders, not just a few.

When your brain is powered by ketones, there's a sense that it's operating on a higher level: You feel more clear, there's greater calm and peace, more emotional resilience so you're less likely to be thrown into emotional turmoil. The enhanced brain metabolism of ketosis (using ketones for energy) has a powerful effect on emotion regulation and general well-being. In short, your brain works better in ketosis.

The word that ketone researchers are using to describe the effects of being in ketosis on the brain is "neuroprotective." A diet that allows the brain to utilize ketones is called "ketogenic," and such a diet is used medically to successfully treat epilepsy. Ketogenic diets are also being used with Alzheimer's disease, Parkinson's disease, multiple sclerosis (MS), and cognitive decline—most anything that affects the brain and nervous system. Since cancer cells only use glucose for fuel and cannot use ketones, it's also being tested as an adjunct to cancer medications as a metabolic treatment to starve tumors.

The evolution of the human brain occurred with the help of ketosis. For hundreds of millions of years the evolving brain alternated between cycles of feast and fast. Before the recent development of agriculture, pre-human ancestors and hunter-gatherer societies had periods of scarcity. The body and brain adapted to periods of no food by burning fat stores for energy rather than glucose. Everyone, even those who are thin, has enough fat to power the body for about two months without eating. In contrast, the liver's glycogen stores run out after about 12–14 hours.

There needs to be a balance between the body's two modes of growth and repair (feast and famine). Periods of not eating (fasting) allow the body to shift into repair mode itself instead of continual growth mode. Utilizing fat stores for energy helps the body's repairing and restoring capacity.

When the body has a steady supply of carbohydrates (which eventually get turned into glucose), it loses its ability to burn fat. Ninety-five percent of people are sugar burners exclusively. To become keto adapted, or a "fat adapted" fat burner, usually takes two to four months of ketogenic, low carb eating. This can be jump-started by fasting for a few days. After becoming keto adapted, the body burns fat in the form of ketones for fuel.

The increase in metabolic efficiency is well documented. When a person is in ketosis inflammation goes down significantly, mitochondrial efficiency increases, and the number of mitochondria goes up, which leads to more energy, oxidation is greatly reduced, and free radicals decrease, while insulin sensitivity goes up. It is used to treat type 2 diabetes for this reason. [110, 112]

What do fasting, aerobic exercise, and caloric restriction have in common? They all increase neurogenesis and produce ketones.

[113, 114] The ketone beta-hydroxybutyrate stimulates the expression of BDNF, which increases neurogenesis. A ketogenic diet is also neurogenic.

The effects of being in ketosis are profound. There is a stabilization of the brain, the self, emotions, and mood that comes with ketosis. It is well understood now that anxiety, stress, and depression are alleviated by increased neurogenesis and BDNF levels. Cognitive benefits also accrue. [114]

What I've found in my clinical practice is that a ketogenic diet seems to be highly healing for the brain and allows many to feel better very quickly. Even in anxiety-provoking situations, the person reports feeling much less anxious, as if the feelings of anxiety have less power and the person is sustained by a quiet hum of positive feeling.

It's similar with depression. Being in ketosis for a few months is perhaps the strongest anti-depressant diet there is (although it can be enhanced further as explained in the chapter on depression). Within a month or two, some depressed clients have reported a remarkable lifting of their depression. Studies are now underway to explore this further. ADD and ADHD as well as cognitive decline and even Alzheimer's have been improved with a ketogenic diet. Again, anything involving the brain (and all mental disorders clearly involve the brain) may be helped with the greater neural efficiency of ketosis.

Anyone interested in learning more about ketosis should explore some of the research in this rapidly expanding field. Jeff Volek, Ph.D., and Stephen Phinney, M.D., Ph.D., are two researchers who've spent decades investigating ketogenic diets. Their book, *The Art and Science of Low Carbohydrate Living,* is a bible in this field. Jimmy Moore's *Keto Clarity* is a good starter book. Dominic D'Agostino, Ph.D., is a university researcher with many informative YouTube video interviews.

Brain benefits of a ketogenic diet include:

- increased neurogenesis, neuroplasticity, and BDNF production
- improved insulin signaling and lowering of blood glucose levels
- reduced inflammation

- reduced oxidative stress
- improved mitochondrial functioning and mitochondrial biogenesis
- balancing glutamate (excitatory) and GABA (calming)

So, if a ketogenic diet is so wonderful, why doesn't everybody do it? For one thing, few people have heard of it, although it's becoming better known. Secondly, it's challenging to eat this way because it involves eating very few carbohydrates. A ketogenic diet is very high fat, moderate protein, and low carb. Many people find it difficult to give up carbohydrates, at least initially.

We live in a carb-addicted world. Go to any grocery store and most of the food on display is various forms of sugar and carbs. A ketogenic diet means, for most people, eating no more than 20–30 grams of carbs a day (although some people can consume up to 50 grams). It's a radical shift in how most people eat. It's hard at first, but after you make the switch, it becomes easy and natural.

There are other ways to enter ketosis: caloric restriction, fasting, intermittent fasting, and exogenous (outside) ketone consumption. Caloric restriction involves continuous undereating while providing all essential nutrients. The chief drawback is continuous hunger, not an enjoyable way to live. Almost no one can do it, so not much time needs to be spent on it.

Fasting puts a person into ketosis quickly, within two or three days. If you are not keto adapted, you may feel sick as your body detoxes and begins self-repair, but by day three the hunger goes away and not eating is no longer a problem. Your body rapidly adapts to fat burning when there are no food sources. Most people report feeling very good from day three on as ketone levels soar. If you are already keto adapted, fasting doesn't bring about the cleansing reaction and is much easier to do. Fasting is gaining in popularity, and *The Complete Guide to Fasting* by Jason Fung, M.D., is an excellent resource.

Intermittent fasting is becoming the most widely used form of fasting, for it combines the main benefits of fasting without being too depriving. Since glycogen stores in the liver are used up in about 14–16 hours, by not eating for 14–18 hours each day the body begins to burn fat for energy and enters into the fasting state. Intermittent fasting means restricting meals to a four- or six- or eight-hour window each day. Thus, if your last meal is at six p.m., not eating again until ten a.m. the next morning or noon will give sixteen hours of fasting. This allows your body to burn fat for energy and raise ketone levels in the process. It is probably the most painless method of increasing fat metabolism. There are many variations: eating in a four-hour window, eating once a day, not eating every other day. Each person needs to discover what works best.

Once you become keto adapted, the experience of hunger changes dramatically. For someone who is a sugar burner, hunger pangs increase after several hours and soon make a person feel kind of crazy and frantic for food. But when your body can use its own fat for energy, this intense, out-of-your-mind desperation for food doesn't happen. You feel hunger, but it's not a big deal. It's easy to forget to eat, since you are powered by ketones all the time. Eating becomes a choice, not a compulsion.

Another option that makes ketosis more accessible is consuming exogenous ketones. Dietary ketones are referred to as exogenous (or external) ketones as opposed to endogenous ketones (ketones the body makes internally). Exogenous ketones can take the form of MCT oil (from coconut oil) or actual ketone bodies. The marketplace for exogenous ketones is fast expanding, and they are now available in many forms.

Coconut oil has seven different fatty acids. The two most powerful for ketone production are caprylic acid and capric acid, which together comprise just 15% of coconut oil. Better MCT oils contain these two only, but cheaper forms of MCT oil also include lauric acid, which accounts for 50% of coconut oil, is good for you, but doesn't convert to ketones. Pure caprylic acid (known as C-8) is also commercially available, the purest and rarest form of MCT that converts to ketones most readily.

MCT oil is hard on the digestive system, so most people can only do a tablespoon or less of MCT oil without developing diarrhea. A person can build up over time, however, to be able to ingest higher amounts (a few tablespoons) without the intestinal distress. Powdered forms of MCT oil are more easily tolerated.

Is there a difference between exogenous and endogenous ketones in terms of brain heath? Producing your own ketones generally feels better, but there is clearly a boost in brain function either way since the brain prefers ketones and selectively metabolizes ketones over glucose. Recent research showed that in a rat model exogenous ketones raised blood ketone levels and reduced anxiety [115] The full metabolic effects of a ketogenic diet are not possible with using only exogenous ketones but nevertheless, many of the benefits are.

Utilizing exogenous ketones, however, does not mean a person is keto adapted or metabolically flexible, merely that the body is using the external ketones that were ingested. Achieving metabolic flexibility means going off carbohydrates for long enough that your body adapts through going ketogenic.

There really is no way to describe how good it feels to be in ketosis. The only way to really know is to try being ketotic for a few months to see how it feels. Then you can decide how you want to power your brain. The ideal is to be metabolically flexible so your brain can run on ketones and glucose. To become keto adapted takes a few days of fasting or two months or so of ketogenic eating with careful monitoring.

Here again is an area where individual differences in metabolism show themselves. Some people do great on a ketogenic diet for years on end. Some people, after improving blood glucose levels and insulin sensitivity, experience a rebound of insulin resistance after a period of time and need to cycle out of ketosis periodically (one or two days a week or a week every month or two). Some people will not stay in ketosis for long but periodically cycle in, say through intermittent fasting. Some will use exogenous ketones and forego adopting a ketogenic diet.

Each person must find his or her own unique way. Since the body continually adapts to its present environment, mixing it up through cycling or pulsing (by intermittent fasting, for example, or cycling keto) is increasingly being seen as a way to keep the body flexible.

When a person is metabolically flexible and able to metabolize fat for energy, this has an immediate impact on mood. In the heightened energy efficient state of ketosis, the brain works at peak levels. Aside from being neurogenic, ketosis is a high-performance state that powerfully improves emotion regulation. A quiet feeling of well-being infuses the system and stabilizes the sense of self. It provides a kind of emotional ballast that keeps emotions, especially anxiety, stress, and depression, from capsizing the self. It may not solve all problems, but it creates a state that is emotionally robust and resilient, and problem-solving flows more easily.

It helps cognitive decline by giving the brain a better fuel source than glucose, and since most people with Alzheimer's and cognitive decline have a problem with glucose metabolism, there is an immediate improvement in cognitive function for many.

Keto Foods

Medical researcher Stephen Phinney, M.D., Ph.D., coined the term "nutritional ketosis" to describe the ketone level in the blood that is necessary to reap the health benefits of ketosis. Entering nutritional ketosis means having blood ketones that range from 0.5 to 5.0 mmol/L. Blood testing is the gold standard for measuring ketone levels, although breath monitors are also available. Only by testing can you know if you are truly in nutritional ketosis. Most people I've worked with start out eliminating a great many carbs and believe they have gotten into ketosis, only to test and discover that they fall short. Once you know you either are or aren't, you can tweak your diet accordingly and fully enter nutritional ketosis.

Until recently, the only real choice was a meter with expensive test strips, but newer models are now on the market with much cheaper strips. Once you've gotten into steady, reliable ketosis and know what it feels like, testing is rarely necessary.

The adjustment period to regain your ability to use fat for energy rather than just glucose requires a little time. For most people it takes a month to mostly adapt and two or three months to fully adapt. Some people experience a mild "keto flu" during the first week or so of adjustment, but if you take supplemental electrolytes, particularly potassium (300–800 mg), magnesium (200–400 mg preferably in the form of magnesium glycinate, as other forms can cause loose bowels), and salt (1/4–1/2 tsp) these effects can be eliminated or much reduced.

The carbohydrates that need to be stopped in order to enter ketosis include the usual suspects such as: sugar, wheat, starchy vegetables (like corn, beets, peas, yams), most dairy (which has high amounts of lactose or milk sugar), most fruits and all fruit juices, ketchup, soft drinks, dried fruit and trail mix, energy bars, granola.

Instead, a ketogenic diet consists of non-starchy, high-fiber vegetables and low-sugar fruit that provide the bulk of food. These include:

asparagus
avocados
bell peppers
berries
bok choy
broccoli
brussels sprouts
cabbage
cauliflower
celery
chard
collards
cucumbers
eggplant
grapefruit
green beans
jicama
kale
leeks
lemons
limes
mushrooms
onions
parsley
radishes
salad greens

scallions
spinach
sprouts
summer squash
tomatoes (except cherry tomatoes, which can have excess carbs)
zucchini

The bulk of calories, however, come from healthy fats. These include:

almond milk
avocado oil
butter (organic and grass-fed or pastured)
cheese (except blue cheese)
coconut
coconut milk
coconut oil
pastured eggs
extra-virgin olive oil
ghee (grass-fed)
grass-fed meat
MCT oil (medium-chain triglycerides)
nuts and nut butters (especially macadamia, almonds, pecans)
olives
pastured, organic chicken
seeds (pumpkin, sunflower, flax, chia, sesame)
sour cream (organic, grass-fed)
wild-caught, low-mercury fish

Calories also come from protein, such as

eggs (pastured, organic)
grass-fed cheese
grass-fed, organic meats
greek yogurt
nuts
pastured, organic chicken
wild-caught, low-mercury fish

As you can see, this is quite a wide range of foods to enjoy. It's hardly a severe restriction on what to eat, rather permission to eat well and enjoy. Fats provide satiety, no need to feel hungry!

The internet is now full of keto-friendly, healthy desserts that are sweetened with stevia and/or monk fruit, so that a sweet tooth can be happily indulged.

A summary for easy reference in is Appendix A.

Anti-inflammatory

Inflammation is behind most chronic diseases today: cancer, heart disease, diabetes, arthritis, Crohn's disease, inflammatory bowel disease, lupus, eczema, lung issues including asthma, even bone health. Inflammation is also at the root of virtually all neurodegenerative diseases, such as Alzheimer's and other dementias, Parkinson's, multiple sclerosis (MS), and cognitive decline.

What's emerged more recently is how mental health issues involve inflammation. Depression, anger disorder (chronic anger), and aggressive behavior, stress, anxiety, ADD/ADHD, bipolar, schizophrenia, and other emotional disorders are directly tied to inflammation. [105, 116, 117]

The distinction between acute inflammation and chronic inflammation is crucial to understand. Acute inflammation is an important immune response to infection or injury. As the body mounts an inflammatory defense, blood flow increases and signaling proteins called "cytokines" are released to attack the invader or heal the injury. Ideally the infection or wound heals, inflammation recedes, and the body returns to normal. This is one reason the body needs omega-6s, to help the body's inflammatory capacity.

Chronic inflammation occurs when the body's inflammatory response doesn't turn off and the body turns on itself to destroy its own cells. Instead of attacking an outside invader, the body's inflammatory cytokines turn on their own tissues, devastating normal cells. Chronic inflammation develops in a number of ways: a proinflammatory diet (like the SAD), food sensitivities, leaky gut (which virtually everyone has to some degree), chronic infection, toxicity, and simply normal aging.

Because chronic inflammation is not noticed by the person, it is called "the silent killer." As inflammation levels rise in aging, it accelerates the aging process and is known as "inflammaging." Quenching the fires of inflammation and keeping levels low is essential for brain health, physical health, and emotional health. Chronic inflammation in the brain creates brain fog and other impairments in cognition and emotion regulation.

Neurons are the most complex cells in the body, and these crown jewels need a high degree of protection. The body's defense systems are finely tuned to spot an invader and keep it out by way of the blood-brain barrier, a kind of safe house within the body's already formidable defenses.

When an injury like traumatic brain injury (TBI) or a foreign agent like a virus or bacteria affects the brain, cytokines are released and a type of glial cell called microglia mounts an immediate healing defense. However, when inflammation becomes chronic, the microglia and inflammatory cytokines turn on the brain's own cells and attack neurons.

Ever wonder why you don't think as well when you have a stuffy nose? That's because the high levels of inflammation are both healing your body and interfering with your brain. High levels of inflammation impair neurons' mitochondria and lower cognition as well as emotional resilience.

As discussed earlier, chronic inflammation is the single greatest threat to the brain. Neurons are particularly vulnerable to inflammation, which rapidly increases brain shrinkage. With the blood-brain barrier now more compromised than ever before (through things like glyphosate, gluten, stress, antibiotics, and poor diet), more and more neurotoxins are able to intrude past the blood-brain barrier. When these intruders set off inflammatory responses, inflammation levels rise. With ongoing intruders, inflammation is higher and more sustained than ever before in history. Brain inflammation has become rampant.

This would be very depressing if nothing could be done. But in fact, there is a great deal that can be done to lower inflammation. Eating an anti-inflammatory diet is vital for brain health. Here again, it's a twofold strategy: Avoid pro-inflammatory foods (e.g., deep-fried foods, vegetable oils, sugar), and consume anti-inflammatory foods and supplements (e.g., olive oil, vegetables, turmeric). A list of these foods is given at the end of this section.

It is also important to determine if there is a chronic infection that needs to be addressed. One common issue is gingivitis (gum disease). Bleeding gums and low-level gum disease are a risk factor in both heart disease and cognitive decline due to the general inflammatory response the body mounts to fight it. Lyme disease, herpes, CMV, and other infections need to be dealt with to lower inflammation levels.

Oxidation is the third main assault on brain health, after inflammation and glycation. Oxidation is when an oxygen molecule combines with an element and changes it. Rust is oxidized iron; an apple slice gets brown as it oxidizes; fire burning a log is oxidation. In the body osteoarthritis is oxidation of a joint; cardiovascular disease is oxidation of the vascular tree. Oxidation degrades the entire system but the brain is particularly susceptible to oxidative damage.

Most people are familiar with the term "free radicals." Free radicals (technically called "reactive oxygen species" or ROS) are molecules that rapidly cause oxidation. Free radicals damage all parts of the cell: the proteins, lipids, mitochondria, as well as causing genetic damage to DNA. Neurons, being the most complex cells in the body, are the most sensitive to oxidative stress. When free radicals enter the brain, all hell breaks loose.

The body protects itself from free radicals with antioxidant defenses. Certain vitamins, such as C and E, and amino acids such as cysteine are necessary so the body can manufacture its own antioxidants. Eating a diet high in antioxidants (such as polyphenols in berries, green tea, and dark chocolate) helps insure that the body's defenses aren't overwhelmed by oxidative stress.

The high toxic load that comes from pollution and the stresses of modern living mean that oxidative stress is high—again, higher than at any time in history. Combine this with the reduced effectiveness of the blood-brain barrier and you have a brain subjected to more free radicals than humans have ever been.

One example of how oxidation affects the brain is through the small particles in smog that are so tiny they cross the blood-brain barrier. These minute particles (smaller than 2.5 micrometers) not only damage neurons by themselves but set off a free radical cascade that damages and weakens the brain. Cerebral shrinkage and cognitive decline are also tied to this small particle load. Dementia rates for women living near a busy freeway were double those of women in less polluted areas. [118]

Oxidation seldom acts alone. Oxidation and inflammation usually act together to inflame and oxidize the brain. The small smog particles in the example above not only produce massive amounts of free radicals but a highly inflammatory response. Free radicals almost always evoke an inflammatory cascade that enhances pro-inflammatory gene expression. Oxidation and inflammation are tightly linked. It is currently believed that this is why some antioxidant clinical trials have not been successful as they failed to include anti-inflammatory agents or use antioxidants that also had anti-inflammatory properties. [119] Glycation acts with both oxidation and inflammation to damage neurons. [3]

Colorful fruits and vegetables tend to be the highest in antioxidants. This is why everyone is encouraged to eat a rainbow of foods—a variety of colors from reds and yellows to blues and purples (blueberries, blackberries, spinach, red bell peppers, pecans, green leafy vegetables). Blues, purples, and dark reds are best, and a more complete list is given at the end of this section.

Anti-Inflammatory Foods

An anti-inflammatory diet means avoiding foods that are pro-inflammatory and including some of the foods and herbs listed below. Pro-inflammatory foods to avoid are: deep-fried foods; over-cooked, burned, or charred meats; bad fats; excess carbohydrates; and, of course, sugar.

Foods that decrease inflammation are worth inviting into your daily diet, depending upon the degree of chronic inflammation in your body.

Anti-inflammatories:

apigenin (50 mg, 1–2 times daily)
benfotiamine (a form of B-1 or thiamine, 150–600 mg daily)
berberine (400 mg, 1–2 times daily)
borage oil or evening primrose oil (1 gram, 1–2 times daily, contains GLA)
boswellia extract (100 mg daily, or more if in pain)
black cumin seed oil (500 mg, 1–2 times daily)
blueberries and blueberry extract (highly anti-inflammatory)
carnosine (500–1,000 mg, 1–2 times daily)
cat's claw (500 mg, 1–3 times daily)
Chinese skullcap (baicalin, 4:1 concentrate, 400 mg, 1–2 times daily)
curcumin (highly anti-inflammatory, amount depends upon the form)
fisetin (100 mg daily)
ginger (daily as an extract, amount depends on concentration)
green tea extract (98% catechins, decaffeinated, 500–1,000 mg daily)
nettle root extract (500 mg, 1–2 times daily)
omega-3 fatty acids (3–4 grams daily)
P 5 P (most bioavailable form of B-6, 50–100 mg, 1–2 times daily)
piperine (pepper extract, 10 mg, 1–2 times daily)
pycnogenol (maritime pine bark extract, 50–100 mg daily)
rosmarinic acid (500–1,000 mg, 1–2 times daily, extract most available as Origanox)
sulforaphane (from broccoli sprouts extract, best with myrosinase) dosage depends upon extraction process
tart cherry extract (500 mg, 1–2 times daily)

How much of these anti-inflammatory nutrients to consume daily? It depends upon the degree to which inflammation is an issue for you. To get an initial idea of what you need, there are a number of standard blood tests that are very helpful to meet your brain's unique metabolic needs. Although everyone should be ketogenic and neurogenic, the amount of anti-inflammatory nutrients needed depends on blood tests, especially hs-CRP (high-sensitivity C-reactive protein).

There are a few antioxidants that are essential for your body to produce its own antioxidant defenses. There are also quite a number of anti-inflammatory herbs and nutrients that lower inflammation without the deleterious side effects of nonsteroidal anti-inflammatory drugs (NSAIDS).

Anti-Inflammatory Antioxidants:

vitamin A
vitamin C
vitamin E (especially in the form of gamma tocopherol)
lipoic acid
cysteine or NAC (precursors to glutathione)
ubiquinol (Co-Q10)

A summary of these are included in the full Healthy Brain Diet summary in Appendix A.

Gut Friendly: Probiotic, Prebiotic (High Fiber), Tight Junction Supporting

The more science learns about intestinal health and the microbiome, the more significant it appears to be for the brain and emotional health. The intestinal tract is so rich in neurons, it is called the "enteric nervous system," and sometimes referred to as the "second brain." It's the only organ with its own independent nervous system, connected to the brain via the vagus nerve. It has an enormous role in how we feel.

The microbiome consists of those friendly bacteria that line the mucous membrane of the intestinal tract. While initial estimates had gut bacteria outnumbering the body's cells by ten to one, more recent studies have revised this. Researchers now believe that the cells in the human body and the microbiome are close to equal. The microbiome number ranges from 30 to 50 trillion, and the number of cells in the body is about 40 trillion, each living in a mutually beneficial relationship. [120]

These bacteria produce vast amounts of chemicals that are essential for us to thrive. Some of these chemicals fight diseases like cancer and are central to the body's immune system. Others regulate mood, protect against fear, stress, and depression, and are essential for emotional resilience.

The microbiome produces more than 30 neurotransmitters, including dopamine, GABA, epinephrine, BDNF, acetylcholine, and melatonin. Ninety percent of the body's serotonin is produced by the digestive system. The microbiome has a profound effect on both physical and emotional health.

The diversity of different bacteria is central to gut health. In any ecosystem, the greater the diversity and complexity of organisms, the healthier and more robust the system. Reducing the number of diverse species in an ecosystem puts that ecosystem at risk of collapse.

Indigenous populations never exposed to antibiotics have 20,000–30,000 different strains of gut bacteria. In contrast, most people in the developed world have only 10,000 different strains or less, sometimes just 500 or 1,000 (especially those with serious illnesses like cancer). This severely reduced microbiome is a major health hazard since it severely compromises the body's ability to protect itself and make the nutrients and neurotransmitters it needs.

Four important points about gut bacteria:

1. The gut microbiome strongly influences mood and feelings.
2. Seventy percent of the immune system is in the gut.
3. Problems with the intestinal wall and tight junctions are virtually universal, leading to widespread leaky gut and leaky brain, which let in toxins, increase inflammation, and weaken brain function.
4. The above points dynamically interact: How you feel has a powerful effect on the immune system and affects the microbiome as well as gut and blood-brain barrier permeability.

The microbiome's production of neurotransmitters, hormones, neuropeptides, and proteins such as BDNF (brain-derived neurotrophic factor, the key protein that stimulates neurogenesis and neuroplasticity) have a major effect on how you feel. Anxiety, stress, depression, and cognitive decline are disorders linked to gut bacteria.

Researchers took two groups of mice, one group genetically bred to be anxious and timid, the other strain known for their courageous exploratory behavior. They then transplanted the microbiome of each group into the other group. The results were startling. The courageous mice suddenly became meek and anxious; the timid, anxious mice became fearless explorers. [121] It appears that the microbiome alters gene expression related to anxiety, fear, and courage. In other words, the microbiome trumps genetics by turning important epigenetic switches on or off. The epigenetic effects of the microbiome are only beginning to be explored.

Experiments with human beings bear this out. Introducing two strains of bacteria (*Lactobacillus helveticus* and *Bifidobacterium longum*) to 55 participants with mild anxiety or depression for 30 days resulted in a 50% reduction in depression scores and a 55% improvement in anxiety scores. [122, 123]

The gut bacteria had this impact through different pathways: by reducing inflammatory signaling molecules and downregulating the genetic expression of cytokines; by reducing cortisol, adrenaline, and other glucocorticoid stress hormones; by increasing levels of BDNF and doublecortin (a protein marker of new brain cell formation); by increasing GABA and GABA receptors; and by increasing vagal tone. [124] In these ways and others not yet understood, such as epigenetic expression, your mood and feelings are powerfully affected by your gut bacteria.

The intestinal walls are where the body absorbs nourishment from food and keeps out toxins. The integrity of the intestinal membrane is key. When this membrane is too porous it allows toxins, food pieces, bacteria, viruses, molds, and other proteins to enter the body. Acute inflammation, high levels of cytokines, and free radicals result as the body tries to fend off the invasion. If the immune system is working well, these invaders are neutralized.

However, when the immune system is overwhelmed by the sheer mass of invaders from overly porous membranes (e.g., leaky gut) that continuously flood the body, then inflammation becomes chronic as the immune system's defense spreads to attack the body's own cells. Chronic inflammation and high levels of oxidation move from the intestinal tract (which continues to be inflamed) to the brain and rest of the body. Health deteriorates. Cognition deteriorates. Mood deteriorates, with collateral damage to the brain, heart, and other organs.

Anyone who lives in the developed world is exposed to things that kill off the microbiome. A single course of antibiotics generally wipes out about two-thirds of gut bacteria. When it starts to grow back, the good bacteria are often overwhelmed by the growth of harmful bacteria and the balance in the gut can be permanently upset. Many courses of antibiotics over years devastate the microbiome. Even doing probiotics religiously afterward only adds in 5 to 30 strains, but the goal is to get from a sparse 1,000–10,000 to a healthy 20,000–30,000. How to do this is detailed soon.

Antibiotics are also given to cattle, chicken, and pigs to fatten them up. Eating commercial meat contains a residue of antibiotics that also kill bacteria in the gut (as well as adding to weight, just like in cattle). Glyphosate, a pesticide that is also an antibiotic, has this same effect of wiping out bacteria in the gut (and contributing to obesity).

The microbiome, just like the brain, is affected by both physical factors and psychological factors. A person's emotional state, including stress, anxiety, fear, trauma, depression, all increase stress hormones and inflammation, damage the microbiome, and increase the permeability of the intestinal membrane. The result is leaky gut. Leaky gut then exacerbates intestinal disorders by letting in toxins, increasing inflammation and oxidation, interfering with microbiota, and further increasing the feelings of anxiety, stress, fear, depression—which makes the gut even more leaky and porous, and on it goes.

It's a vicious cycle. The gut's immune system is influenced by negative emotions as well as negative relationships and becomes leaky (as does the blood-brain barrier). This leaky gut (and brain) with its reduced immunity causes a host of downstream metabolic changes, such as chronic inflammation, that increase negative emotions and make relationships more difficult, which makes the gut leakier still, etc., in a downward spiral. It is important to remember that all systems interact: Emotions and relationships affect the immune system, microbiome and gut permeability, which impact emotions and relationships, which further negatively affect the gut.

An overly porous, leaky gut is caused by problems with the tight junctions. Tight junctions, as explained earlier, are the one-cell thick membranes that maintain the boundary between the outside and inside of the intestinal wall. When tight junctions are operating well, they allow nutrients in and keep out toxins, molds, bacteria, viruses, and food particles. However, when tight junctions are porous and leaky, they let in the very toxins they were designed to keep out.

Tight junctions are also key to the integrity of the blood-brain barrier: They keep out harmful pathogens and let in what nourishes and protects the brain.

One of the greatest threats to the brain and emotional health (as well as to the body and physical health) is disruption of a person's tight junctions. As noted earlier, virtually everyone in the developed world has some damage to their tight junctions, so a leaky gut and leaky brain are nearly universal.

With a leaky gut and brain come a toxic gut and toxic brain. Remember, in *everyone* (not just the gluten-sensitive) gluten stimulates the release of zonulin, which opens up the gates of the tight junctions in the intestines and at the blood-brain barrier. And the pesticide glyphosate, which is present in almost everyone's diet, strongly stimulates the release of zonulin, which further disrupts the tight junctions' gates in the gut and the brain, accelerates this toxic inflow to the brain of poisons, bacteria, molds, and inflammation. Compromised brain health is an inevitable result.

The gut microbiome has been dubbed "the third brain," as it powerfully influences mood and behavior. Aside from the microbiome's production of neurotransmitters and peptides and other chemicals that influence both the first brain and the second brain (the enteric nervous system), the gut's microbiome seems to have a "mind of its own." There is evidence the microbiome exerts an influence over behavior and mood, even shaping the choice of foods a person makes.

Recent discoveries by Canadian researchers show that the brain has its own microbiome. [9] If the enteric nervous system is the "second brain," and the intestinal microbiome is the "third brain," then this is the "fourth brain." It was long believed that the brain is a sterile environment that keeps out noxious bacteria, proteins, and toxins via the blood-brain barrier. This is the case with all other animals and mammals, except, it turns out, for primates. Alone among animal species, only primates have brains that are populated by microbiota. Some researchers have theorized that the growth of the large brain in primates is even due to their microbiota.

This research is so new that the full implications aren't known. It is very difficult to study this, for it involves invasive procedures to access the brain's environment, so routine testing of the brain's microbiome is not possible. It's clear that some of the same difficulties encountered in the intestinal microbiome apply here. Antibiotics that ravage the microbiome population and ecosystem also affect the brain, and tight junction disruptions (due to glyphosate, gluten, anxiety and stress, toxic bacterial overgrowth, etc.) that let in neurotoxic proteins, viruses, damaging bacteria, and other particles such as small smog particles damage both the gut as well as the brain and mood.

The existence of a third and fourth "brain" with our gut and brain microbiome is a new finding that raises more questions than answers. If our microbiome, both gut and brain, influence the first and second "brains," what does this mean for free will? Are we doing something because we want to or because the brain's or gut's microbiota influence us to do it? Of course, all four "brains" get integrated by the brain itself into a single consciousness.

Just as we have different parts to ourselves (subpersonalities) that contribute different feelings and motivations to an integrated sense of self, so the brain integrates these various voices or influences into a unified whole. This research, however, opens up the question of what this unified whole that is one's "self" actually is, for some of this appears to be nonhuman in nature.

Although the number of human cells and the number of microbiota are about equal, the nonhuman DNA of our microbiome outnumbers our human DNA by 100 to 1. Their DNA influences the epigenetic expression of our DNA. So, what is human and what is nonhuman? What is "me" and what is "not me"? And how can this be influenced toward greater mental health?

The near universality of these conditions—decimated, shrunken microbiome in gut and brain; leaky gut, leaky brain—leads to a toxic gut and toxic brain that sustain chronic inflammation. The mental health effects are so wide-ranging and powerful they can hardly be overstated, ranging from anxiety, brain fog, cognitive decline, memory problems, difficulty concentrating and ADD/ADHD, depression, addictions, greater vulnerability to trauma and PTSD, stress, Alzheimer's and other neurodegenerative diseases. Restoring an optimal microbiome environment and tight junction integrity in the brain is paramount. Otherwise it's like trying to fill a sieve with water.

But what are the best practices to regenerate the gut and brain microbiome? Since brain health is so closely linked to gut health, how can the integrity of the tight junctions in the gut and the blood-brain barrier be restored? How can brain inflammation be reduced? And how can the gut-brain axis become optimally healthy going forward?

Here again it's the same dual strategy:

1. Eat and drink what nourishes the microbiome and tight junctions.
2. Avoid or minimize what is harmful.

In terms of what to actually do, this means, first, to heal the intestinal barrier (tight junctions); second, repopulate the microbiome with healthy, plentiful strains of bacteria; and third, provide a nourishing intestinal environment in which the microbiome can thrive.

To heal the intestinal barrier and rejuvenate the tight junctions so they do their job of keeping out the bad stuff and letting in the good, several things are helpful.

If you are lectin sensitive, avoiding lectin-rich foods can heal the intestinal barrier. Omega-3s are helpful, together with fermented foods. Avoiding alcohol and medications that disrupt the tight junctions also is important, including proton pump inhibitors and NSAIDs, such as ibuprofen. [125]

Additionally, several types of probiotics have been shown to increase the integrity of the tight junctions. *Lactobacillus plantarum* and *Lactobacillus reuteri* reduce gut wall permeability, according to Swedish researchers. [126] Bacillus spore strains increase tight junction integrity, and spores have greater survival rates through the harsh stomach acid that can kill many probiotics. [127]

In animal and cell studies the following bacterial strains have helped heal a leaky intestinal membrane. [125, 128] These include: *Lactobacillus rhamnosus, L. paracasei, L. gasseri, L. helveticus, L. plantarum, Bifidobacterium infantis, B. longum.* The plantarum strain has been shown to be especially helpful in repairing tight junction integrity, protecting against further rupture and promoting microbial diversity.

Researcher Zach Bush, M.D., has introduced a product called ION Gut Health, which helps to heal the tight junctions of the intestines and blood-brain barrier as well as increasing microbial diversity and bacterial communication by enhancing redox signaling.

Other supplements that have been shown to help heal the tight junctions and reduce intestinal permeability are: glutamine, quercetin, ginkgo biloba, curcumin, lipoic acid, vitamin D, and zinc. [125]

The next job is to increase the microbial diversity and repopulate the gut with healthy strains. What is healthy or unhealthy for the microbiome and gut? Eating and drinking foods that contain bacteria is helpful. Even though stomach acid kills most of these bacteria, some get past the stomach to colonize the intestinal tract. Examples are fermented foods like unsweetened yogurt and kefir, kimchi, sauerkraut, fermented pickles, miso, tempeh, and raw milk cheeses.

Probiotics are clearly helpful, especially when it comes to working with specific issues such as anxiety, stress, and depression, and the following chapters detail specific strains that have been shown to reduce anxiety and depression. For now, the larger issue is the diversity of the microbiome. How to increase the diversity of strains from the previously mentioned range of 1,000—10,000 up to 20,000—30,000?

If you rely solely on commercial probiotics, these only add 5 or 10 or 30 different strains. This method, when pursued to the exclusion of other things, results in a kind of monoculture. Monoculture is devastating for farming soils and habitats. In any ecosystem, greater diversity increases the resilience that ecosystem has to meet ongoing challenges.

One powerful way to increase the number of strains in your intestinal ecosystem is to eat fiber—lots of it. You need to feed these friendly bacteria well. To paraphrase what doctors tell pregnant women, "Remember, you're not just eating for yourself. You're eating for 40 trillion." Intestinal bacteria thrive on fiber.

One landmark study showed how the Western diet of low fiber, simple carbs causes a sharp reduction in microbiota diversity, and that increasing fiber in the diet had a formidable effect in increasing this diversity again. [129] Over several generations many strains of bacteria became extinct, and when this happened it required both probiotics and prebiotic fiber to re-establish diversity. But over a single generation, simply adding microbiota-friendly fiber was enough to powerfully increase diversity.

A second powerful way to dramatically increase your microbiome is to expose yourself to nature. Breathe in fresh air in a forest or beach or desert. Let water from the ocean into your mouth, let dirt from your garden stay on your skin for a while before washing it off so the bacteria can colonize your skin and work their way to your nose and mouth (and eventually your intestines).

Breathing air in nature allows hundreds of species of bacteria into your nose, mouth, and lungs, and from there they migrate to your intestines. If your intestinal environment is friendly, that is, not poisoned by glyphosate or other pesticides, not inflamed from inflammatory foods or anti-acid medication or stress, then they will make themselves at home and become part of your increasingly diverse health reserves. Remember, your best protection against disease—mental or emotional—is a healthy microbiome.

Providing a nourishing intestinal environment for your expanding and diversifying microbiome means eating plenty of the prebiotic food they need to thrive. As just mentioned, vegetables and some fruits are critical for this. You need a good amount of healthy fiber daily. Some types of fiber that are helpful include greens, sprouts, jicama, asparagus, onions, garlic, lentils, pistachios, cashews, avocadoes, kidney beans.

As I never get tired of reminding the reader, make sure food is organic whenever possible and especially free of glyphosate, otherwise you are taking antibiotics that kill your intestinal bacteria, effectively cancelling out your efforts to nourish them, as well as opening up your intestinal barrier and your blood-brain barrier to harmful toxins.

Some nutritional supplements with good prebiotic fiber which are helpful for increasing the number of strains of bacteria in your gut include: organic psyllium husks (4–5 capsules daily with a glass of water), FOS (fructooligosaccharides), GOS (gallactooligosaccharides), XOS (xylooligosacharides) which increases strains of Bifidobacterium, inulin, acacia gum extract, chicory root fiber, and resistant starch. Taking these helps nourish greater numbers of strains of bacteria.

The care and feeding of your microbiota is essential knowledge in holistic brain healing. Your microbiome will thank you with good brain health if you feed it properly.

Conclusion

Following these four dietary principles begins a process of healing and repair in the brain. This book uses these principles in two phases: healing and maintenance. Understanding the basic rationale behind these two phases allows you to have a better sense of what foods to eat or avoid and to navigate the second phase more skillfully.

Healing Phase. The first step is to support the healing and growth of the brain as quickly as possible. This is the most intense phase and usually requires some major dietary changes. Because it takes a month or two to adapt to the Healing Phase of the diet, try to hang in there while the body makes the necessary adjustments. Once you've made this transition, it becomes much easier to continue as your brain heals and strengthens.

Once your symptoms go away, it's advisable to stay on the Healing Phase for at least six months and preferably a year or, even better, two years. This allows the brain to grow strong enough to insure these changes remain firm.

Maintenance Phase. After you no longer have symptoms for 6–12 months of, for example, depression or cognitive decline, then you can experiment with switching into the maintenance stage of this program. This will take experimentation to see what your unique metabolism can tolerate, but most people can bring back in some foods that were restricted in the Healing Phase. Here again, everyone is different. Some may do best staying in the Healing Phase for much longer, while others can re-introduce foods and continue to feel good or operate at a high cognitive level. Some tests are recommended at the end of the Healing section to help better navigate this phase.

A Word of Encouragement

Incorporating the four dietary principles into daily life involves a significant dietary shift for most people. Your attachment to certain foods is the chief obstacle here. It's important to realize that your eating habits are only habits, and habits can change. It simply takes a conscious effort to try something new, persistence in the new eating pattern, and voilà! After a month or two you've instilled a new habit. It may seem impossible at first, but after several weeks it becomes automatic and you wonder what all the fuss was about.

Nevertheless, habits around eating are strong. To change, your desire to feel better and function at a higher level must outweigh your attachment to certain foods. When you really want to feel less depressed, anxious, stressed, or stop cognitive decline, then you will be successful even if it takes some false starts or you fall off the wagon at times. Sooner or later you'll overcome your attachment to one way of eating and establish a new, healthier pattern. Give yourself some time and don't expect perfection. It can be like turning an ocean liner—it just takes time. But if you earnestly persist, you'll soon be feeling so much better that your initial struggles will fade away.

The Healing Phase: Reach Your Neurogenic Potential

Both the Healing and Maintenance phases of the Healthy Brain Diet offer high degrees of neuroprotection. The Healing Phase is designed to trigger your brain's healing and growth, and the Maintenance Phase keeps it going.

The fundamental rationale of the Healing Phase is to heal and strengthen the brain as quickly as possible. The Healthy Brain Diet can be distilled into four principles:

- neurogenic
- ketogenic
- anti-inflammatory
- gut friendly (prebiotic, probiotic, and tight junction supporting)

In terms of what you actually eat, healing the brain involves getting the bulk of your food from vegetables and fiber but most of your calories from healthy, brain-enhancing fats. It also involves eating a colorful rainbow of anti-inflammatory and antioxidant foods as well as supplements that are neurogenic and anti-inflammatory.

Tests to Customize Your Diet to Fit Your Unique Needs

In order to determine how much to emphasize the anti-inflammatory portion of this diet, as well as to determine how to guide your diet in the Maintenance Phase, there are a few blood tests that everyone should have to better understand their current health status. These can be obtained either through an online service (such as Life Extension Foundation or Walk-In Lab) that gives you a physician's order for a local lab, or as part of your yearly checkup. While more detailed blood testing is often helpful, these are the minimal blood tests that establish a baseline for metabolic and brain health.

- **Fasting glucose**. After not eating for at least 12 hours, this test is a first indicator of elevated blood sugar and insulin resistance. Ideal levels are 70–85. Eighty-five to

100 is considered within a "normal" range by conventional medicine; however, most knowledgeable functional medicine and holistic practitioners view this as problematic as it indicates some insulin resistance (therefore accelerating cognitive decline). One hundred to 125 indicates a prediabetes trajectory that needs to be corrected as soon as possible. Over 125 indicates diabetes that needs immediate attention.

- **Hemoglobin A1c (HbA1c)**. This is the best overall picture of your glucose metabolism. It shows the average blood glucose level over the last three months or so. Ideal levels are below 5.2. Above this indicates a problem with insulin resistance that should be addressed immediately since it often leads to prediabetes. 5.7–6.4 indicates prediabetes; 6.5 or above indicates diabetes.
- **High-sensitivity C-reactive protein (hs-CRP).** This is an overall inflammatory marker. Ideal levels are below 0.55 for men and below 1.0 for women. Between 1.0 and 3.0 is considered average by conventional medicine but really indicates inflammatory levels that need to be corrected. Above 3.0 indicates either an infection or chronic inflammation that should be brought down immediately, as a host of diseases as well as brain and mental disorders can follow in its wake. Chronic inflammation is behind most chronic diseases, most neurological conditions, and the mental disorders this book focuses upon.
- **Vitamin D**. Also called the "sunshine vitamin" or the "happiness vitamin," vitamin D is proving to be a major player in brain health as well as overall health. There is much confusion and misinformation about this increasingly important vitamin (actually a prohormone). Older thinking was you needed to be careful you didn't overdose on it; current thinking is that it's very difficult to get too much. The existing guidelines have been shown to be based on an arithmetic error and are too low. Most people in the U.S. are deficient in vitamin D. Below 20 ng/mL is severe deficiency, 20–30 is considered deficient, and 30 is considered normal.

However, these figures are normative, not geared toward optimal health. Optimal vitamin D levels vary depending upon who is making the recommendation. Conventional ranges are 30–40, but most people who have studied this issue in the functional medicine and the holistic healthcare field recommend 60–100. It's hard to get enough from the sun unless you live in a warm place and spend time in the sun without sunscreen. Most people can benefit by supplementing with D3, 5,000–10,000 i.u. daily. Taking vitamin K-2 when supplementing with vitamin D is important to avoid calcium buildup in blood vessels and to make sure calcium goes to your bones. Keep supplementing until blood levels rise to the optimal range and keep testing every year to gauge your efforts.

- **Iron**. The accumulation of iron has a serious impact on brain health. Because the brain uses so much oxygen, it needs more iron to deliver this oxygen to neurons. But excess iron, especially in men and postmenopausal women, leads to neurodegenerative diseases including Alzheimer's, Parkinson's, and ALS. It increases inflammation and oxidative stress and lowers brain function. Ideal levels on the Serum Ferritin test are 40–80 ng/mL. To lower your iron, simply donate blood, avoid vitamins and foods that are "fortified" with iron, and don't cook in iron pots or pans. Too little iron (anemia) is remedied by taking supplemental iron, though it can take months to reach healthy levels.
- **Cardio IQ or NMR profile.** To get a better handle on your blood lipids, the standard cholesterol level is almost useless, as this alone is rarely a risk factor, despite the current fixation on it. Most relevant are triglyceride levels (preferably below 75) and particle size of LDL cholesterol. Ideally you want large, fluffy particles and few very small, dense particles. Triglyceride to HDL ratio is useful and ideally is below 2. Here again what we're learning is that lipid levels are determined mostly by carbohydrate intake in a complex dance with saturated fat intake. High lipid levels can usually be controlled through diet as well as medication.

- **Thyroid panel**. An overactive thyroid can bring anxiety, while an underactive thyroid can lead to depression. Descriptions of low thyroid are identical to descriptions of depression.
- **Omega-3 index**. About 90% of Americans are deficient in omega-3s. This test can be done at home. Healthy levels are between 8% and 12%.
- **Homocysteine.** This amino acid is formed as the body metabolizes methionine. High levels of homocysteine are associated with heart disease, blood-brain barrier permeability, cognitive decline, and dementia. A Dutch study showed that among normal people ages thirty to eighty, elevated homocysteine levels are associated with lower cognitive performance. [130] If your level is over 7.2 millimole/L, then you should work to bring it down as soon as possible. Folic acid, trimethyl glycine (TMG), vitamins B-6 and B-12 all work to lower homocysteine.

With the results of these blood tests you will have a baseline picture of your metabolic health and how to create a diet to optimize your brain. The first thing to understand is your hs-CRP level. Most people reading this book will have elevated inflammatory markers (again, above .55 for men, above 1.0 for women). If this is you, try to consume as many of the anti-inflammatory nutrients as possible daily. Test again in 6–12 months to see the effects.

The above list of anti-inflammatory nutrients contains some that were included on the neurogenic list because they are also such powerful anti-inflammatories (e.g., omega-3s, curcumin, green tea extract, blueberry extract). Additionally, experiment with the others to see how you feel. Some people may react to certain things and therefore should avoid them.

The Maintenance Phase: Maintaining Your Neurogenic Stride

The Maintenance Phase of this diet begins once you no longer have symptoms that cause distress. It's best to continue on the

Healing Phase of the diet for 6–24 months after your symptoms subside so you deepen the brain healing and strengthening that is occurring.

Once you've hit your neurogenic stride and your brain has healed to some degree, you can switch into the Maintenance Phase, which is less restrictive. You can gradually ease back into eating more carbohydrates, fewer anti-inflammatory foods, more protein, etc. However, this isn't permission to go wild with sugar again or resume the bad dietary habits that helped create the original problem. The idea is to bring your new eating consciousness into your ongoing life so that brain healthy eating becomes part of your lifestyle, not just a temporary emergency diet.

The best brain healthy diet for you is not the best brain healthy diet for someone else. There's no objective "right" answer here, just what's right for you. Finding the maintenance diet that's right for you means using the blood tests to see where you need to focus your efforts. For example, if blood glucose is high, indicated either by elevated HbA1c or fasting glucose, then in the Maintenance Phase fewer carbohydrates should be eaten, whereas if blood glucose and HbA1c are low and healthy as shown by these tests, then higher carbohydrate intake may be fine for now.

Some people can change their diet more easily than others. Some find it very difficult to give up the foods they love or feel a kind of addiction to carbs. It's important to remember that this addiction is simply a habit, reinforced over decades. With a willingness to stick with a new way of eating for six to eight weeks, you will install a new eating pattern. Taste preferences can and do change, they are not immutable.

What's most surprising is when a new way of eating becomes established, it seems easy and natural. Eating patterns are generally formed in childhood and young adulthood. However, they are malleable, far more malleable than you might think.

The one exception to this is sugar. A sweet tooth can be a lifelong addiction. That's why it's good to have healthy, sweet, no carb, non-caloric alternatives to sugar: stevia and monk fruit extract especially, as well as erythritol or allulose for some (although they cause too much gas in many people).

As you create your individualized diet, it is important to be experimental. Try different approaches, keep an open mind, and see what works. It may take a few months to see if something is working or not, so be patient and wait for a real result.

Food for Thought: Helpful Attitudes to Change Your Diet

In both the Healing and Maintenance phases of this diet, an important attitude is: *Be gentle with yourself.* Changing eating patterns takes time and persistence, especially after a lifetime of indulging in toxic but pleasurable delights. Move in this direction in your own time and way. Whether you jump fully into the Healing Phase or gradually adopt it makes little difference so long as you get there. Changing dietary habits is often slow.

A second attitude is: *Allow yourself to be human and to fail sometimes.* Don't expect or even aim for perfection, for this is a sure path to disappointment or giving up. Let yourself "fall off the wagon" on occasion without beating yourself up.

This said, it's also important to acknowledge the role of intention and willpower in changing your dietary habits. A third helpful attitude is: *Apply yourself.* Doing anything worthwhile takes a certain amount of discipline. It's necessary to rein in out-of-control indulgence in foods that degrade your brain. Stopping something that's hurting you, although it should be easy, can be difficult, especially when it's an addiction like sugar that feels really good in the moment.

What you eat is an existential choice. Like all existential choices, choosing one thing means not choosing other things. Do you want to feel better or worse? When you see it in these stark terms, a choice between weakening your brain or strengthening it, the choice is easier to make. In deliberately choosing what to eat, eating becomes conscious rather than what it usually is, an unconscious numbing by sugar and carbohydrates in the service of short-term pleasure.

It takes time to reach the place where you feel better than you've ever felt, but once you're there, things get much easier. The path to it takes a certain amount of willpower. When you really want something, you have the energy and discipline to accomplish it. What's important is moving in the right direction, not whether you go fast or slow.

Other Key Physical Factors: Exercise, Sleep, Eliminating Toxins

On the physical level of the body, there are other important aspects to healing the brain. The factors discussed below have profound effects on the quality and power of the brain.

Exercise. All types of exercise are good for your body and brain—aerobic (e.g., running), flexibility training (e.g., yoga), and strength training (e.g., weights). Exercise alters brain structures, increases brain volume, and reduces the number and size of age-related holes in the brain's white and gray matter.

Our brains evolved over hundreds of millions of years in an environment that, aside from sleep time, forced our ancestors to be continually on the move. There were no couches on the Serengeti plains to kick back on, no TV to watch for hours or computer games to play, no chairs to lounge in while you were foraging for food, no safety from predators in the wild. Continual movement and vigilance were required.

Our ancestors didn't need to exercise—their whole life was continuous exercise and motion. But most modern occupations involve long periods of sitting, which our bodies and brains were not designed for. To compensate for this, we are told, exercise will stimulate the muscles that would otherwise go flaccid.

It turns out, however, that research shows exercise does not compensate for long periods of sitting. It's suggested that everyone get up and walk around for a minute or two every half hour and certainly every hour. Sitting, as they say, is the new smoking.

That said, exercise is nevertheless the most potent single intervention to increase the health of your brain and body. Ideally a person gets all three types of exercise, although in practice very few of us actually do. Further, some people are physically limited in what their bodies are capable of. Sometimes exercise is not possible, in which case the idea is simply to do what you can, perhaps with the help of a physical therapist who can make modifications that will work.

But for the brain, some kinds are better than others. Recent research has looked at this question: What kind of exercise is best for the brain?

It turns out that the most neurogenic exercise is aerobic exercise. Aerobic exercise is anything that gets you breathing hard and your heart beating fast—running, fast walking, biking, fast dancing, hiking up a hill, swimming, etc. These kinds of exercise grow and strengthen your brain more than any other.

Leg strength is related to brain strength. The human species evolved with physical activity, especially standing, walking, running. Leg strength in particular is tied to emotional and cognitive benefits. Neurogenesis declined by 70% in a 2018 study that prevented animals from using their hind legs. [131]

According to the press release accompanying the discovery, "The research shows that using the legs, particularly in weight-bearing exercise, sends signals to the brain that are vital for the production of healthy neural cells, essential for the brain and nervous system. Cutting back on exercise makes it difficult for the body to produce new nerve cells—some of the very building blocks that allow us to handle stress and adapt to challenge in our lives." [132]

Aerobic exercise come in two forms: endurance workouts lasting a minimum of 20 minutes, but preferably 30–60 minutes or longer, and high intensity interval training (HIIT), where you go to 90% of capacity for 30 seconds and then slow way down for 2 minutes or so. Six to eight repetitions of this comprise a usual HIIT workout. While HIIT appears better than endurance training for certain metabolic functions, endurance training is superior to HIIT for neurogenesis. Both of these together seem to provide the best metabolic and neurogenic benefit (e.g., HIIT once or twice a week, endurance training three to four times weekly), but if you do just one type, do endurance workouts for 30–60 minutes. [133]

Sleep. One of the biggest brain health discoveries in the past two decades is the immense importance of sleep. Sleep increases neurogenesis, cleans the brain of toxins, and consolidates memory. But most of this only occurs in the last hours of sleep. Most everyone needs seven to eight hours every night. A very few people can do with six hours—almost no one does well on less than six. Reduced sleep is a major factor in emotional disorders, as it dramatically lowers emotional resilience, decreases neurogenesis and neuroplasticity, produces cognitive impairments and toxic residues in the brain. [134, 135]

Even a single night of four to six hours' sleep produces measurable declines in cognitive function the next day, including reduced ability to put facts together or attend to your environment.

With the introduction of electric lights about 100 years ago, the circadian rhythms of day and night established by millions of years of evolution got disrupted. With the possibility of light whenever we wanted it, people started going to bed later. Combined with a competitive work ethic, with each passing decade since, sleep time has gone down.

The National Sleep Foundation reports that most Americans get 6.5 hours sleep on weeknights. In the last decade, it's estimated that Americans get 38 minutes less sleep on weekends. Fifty to 70 million Americans have a diagnosable sleep disorder. One-third of Americans report getting less sleep than they need to function well, and only 40% report getting a good night's sleep most nights. In many circles, not getting enough sleep is like a merit badge or status symbol of how hard you work. But your brain and body suffer.

Because most people can function and get through the day with less sleep, it's easy to minimize just how critical sleep is for good health and good brain function. We hardly notice how much we've slipped in our cognitive capacity or emotional resilience, but it gradually adds up.

Many of the body's repair mechanisms work during sleep, and lack of sleep reduces immune function, is a recognized carcinogen, is linked to weight gain, elevated glucose levels and higher risk of diabetes, heart disease, high blood pressure, lowered melatonin production (which also lowers immunity), anxiety, and depression.

In 2013 scientists discovered how the brain cleans itself. Up until then it was a mystery, since the blood-brain barrier keeps the brain so protected and isolated. But just as an aquarium needs a filter to remove accumulated toxins, so the brain needs a way to clear the debris and toxic residue that build up with daily use.

The glymphatic system is the name given to how the glial cells and cerebrospinal fluid "wash" brain cells and clear synapses of toxic molecules that build up (especially beta amyloid, which accumulates in Alzheimer's disease, and stress hormones such as cortisol). The space between neurons increases by 60% during the later stages of sleep, which allows cerebrospinal fluid to wash through brain, providing a kind of internal shower or bath that clears out the day's metabolic waste.

A good night's sleep literally "clears your head." Without this, or with only a partial night's sleep, the brain slows down, neurogenesis diminishes, memory consolidation is impaired, and melatonin production and immunity are lowered; thus you become cranky, more emotionally vulnerable, and your quality of life suffers.

High on the list of best practices to heal the brain is getting a good night's sleep every night if possible. A single night of messed up sleep won't kill you, but it's important to organize your life so that you get seven to eight hours nearly every night. If you feel tired during the day, chances are you need more sleep.

Quality as well as quantity is important with sleep. We need to sleep in a dark room, as light in the room decreases neurogenesis and hurts cognitive performance. If you need a light or clock, make sure it's red or amber rather than the blue wavelengths of the spectrum, as these disrupt melatonin production and circadian rhythms. Keep cell phones, Wi-Fi, routers, electric alarm clocks, and other EMF exposure away from your head during sleep, preferably out of the bedroom altogether.

Practice good sleep hygiene to insure a full night's sleep:

- Go to bed about the same time every night.
- Don't watch stimulating movies or programs just before bed.
- Avoid caffeine later in the day.
- Limit naps to 20–30 minutes during the day.
- Don't eat at least three hours before bedtime.
- Limit alcohol, which interrupts sleep in the night as the body processes it.

- Turn on the blue light filter on your tablet, computer, or cell phone several hours before bed so the blue light wavelengths don't wake your brain up and prevent sleep.
- Keep cell phones and other EMF contamination out of the bedroom.
- Lower the temperature, ideally between 60–65 degrees.
- Try wearing red or amber tinted sunglasses an 30-60 minutes before bed to stimulate melatonin production.
- Make your room as quiet as possible, free from disturbing noise. Consider ear plugs or a white noise machine to prevent sounds from startling you.
- Make your room as dark as possible by blocking outside light with curtains.

If all else fails, try the natural sleep aids suggested in the next chapter, "Holistic Healing of Anxiety."

Physical Detoxification

We live in an increasingly neurotoxic world. Breathing smoggy air, inhaling mold, using common household cleaners and products, and ingesting lead, mercury, or aluminum are common ways we take in neurotoxins in today's world. They wreak havoc on the brain, producing all the disorders in this book and more. And they are just the tip of the iceberg.

This is an overview of the major toxins that grind down the brain and how to rid your system of these poisons.

Mercury. This potent neurotoxin enters the brain through eating fish, having dental amalgam fillings, and from pollution from smog and coal-burning factories and power plants. Aside from a host of physical ailments, neurological conditions such as anxiety, stress, depression, ADD/ADHD, and cognitive decline arise from mercury toxicity.

Even if you don't think you have high mercury levels, it's a good idea to check this out. The best test I'm aware of is through Quicksilver Scientific, which also identifies where the mercury is coming from.

There are numerous detoxification protocols to chelate, or pull the mercury out of the system, and each person needs to find what works best. Some poorly designed chelation protocols pick the mercury up in one part of the body but drop it off somewhere else rather than excreting it through sweat, urine, or feces. Common protocols use DMSA or calcium EDTA to bind mercury and excrete it.

Other approaches increase glutathione, which is the body's own defense against toxins like mercury. Increase your intake of glutathione-enhancing supplements such as the precursors NAC (n-acetyl cysteine) or cysteine. A Russian product called Modifilan was developed from seaweed after Chernobyl to rid the body of radiation and heavy metals. A mild chelator is chlorella, a type of algae that binds to mercury and other heavy metals and excretes them from the body.

Detoxing from mercury requires more space than can be given here, as well as the help of a health professional. Amalgam dental fillings (which are 50% mercury and release mercury gas into the system with every bite) require a qualified dentist to remove properly. High mercury level is a serious condition that needs sustained detoxification until levels fall.

Lead, copper, arsenic, and other heavy metals. The burden that lead and other heavy metals place on the brain can rapidly lead to cognitive decline, anxiety, stress, Alzheimer's, and other neurological conditions. They cause inflammation in the brain, free radical damage, demyelination of neurons, reduce mitochondrial function, and nerve disease. Testing for heavy metal toxicity can be done by many labs as well as the aforementioned Quicksilver. The detoxification protocols are very similar to mercury, and sometimes high lead levels hide high mercury levels, which then become evident when lead gets chelated.

Mycotoxins. Toxic mold affects the brain more than most people or physicians realize. Often it is growing in places where it can't be seen, so identifying it can be tricky. About one quarter of the population is sensitive to mold exposure, but everyone exposed is affected by an inflammatory immune response. Over time exposure inflames the brain, can create all the conditions in this book and make the person hypersensitive (allergic) to further exposure.

It's estimated that half of the buildings in America have some degree of water damage stemming from old drywall construction which absorbs moisture. Getting a mold inspection can reveal toxic mold contamination in your house. Finding a specialist to remove the mold will insure that it doesn't get worse while it's being fixed, which can happen with untrained contractors.

Detoxification consists of reducing your exposure to mold by getting the problem fixed, and then allowing the body's natural detoxification systems to clear out the mycotoxins. Here again glutathione is important, so taking supplemental NAC and/or cysteine is advised. The dietary guidelines in this book will help the body's natural detoxification systems and rapidly repair the damage.

Hormone imbalance. Having too much or too little of key hormones has a profound effect on mood. Anxiety, depression, and cognitive decline have been linked to birth control pills as well as too little estrogen (menopause) or too little testosterone (male "andropause"). An overactive thyroid is a quick road to anxiety, as is excess cortisol. Too little can lead to depression and cognitive decline.

Working with a physician who is experienced working with bioidentical hormones can be helpful. Getting tested for your hormone level allows you to see how much you have, though not how much you're able to use. Nevertheless, it's a good starting point to assess what's happening.

Smog. Air pollution lowers brain function. Smog contains heavy metals as well as tiny particles that cross the blood-brain barrier and are causally linked to Alzheimer's and cognitive decline. According to the World Health Organization (WHO), 92% of the world's population is breathing polluted air. [136]

If you live with heavy smog, try to move somewhere with less smog, whether it's another city or a part of the city with less pollution. If this isn't possible, get high-quality air purifiers for home and office that have HEPA filters, which can filter out 90% of the 2.5 micron particles (the most dangerous). On heavy smog days, a face mask for walking outside is useful, one that is at least N95 that can filter out 95% of 1.0–3.0 micron size particles.

Water. Much of the municipal water supply is contaminated with lead, other heavy metals, glyphosate and other poisons. A good water filter that filters out the toxins but keeps in the minerals is very helpful. Do your research, as there are many choices on types of filters.

Commercial meats, dairy, produce. By now every reader understands the importance of eating as organically as possible. Most of the foods sold in stores are contaminated with glyphosate and other pesticides. Commercial meats are loaded with glyphosate (from feed) as well as antibiotics and hormones that disrupt the body's natural systems. "Grass-fed," "organic," and "pastured" are words to look for when shopping. Paying a little more now saves both money and health in the long run.

Cell phones, computers, microwaves. The high EMFs (electromagnetic fields) emitted by cell phones and many computers open the voltage-gated calcium channels (VGCCs) in the body's cells, especially those in the brain and heart. A massive inrush of calcium ions produces inflammation, high levels of oxidation, depletes the body's magnesium in its effort to cope with the calcium ions and reduces mitochondrial function. The mitochondria in the brain's neurons, heart cells, and the testes are most vulnerable to EMF exposure. The result of this lowered brain function is both impaired cognitive function and emotional problems including anxiety, stress, depression, and other mental disorders.

In addition, some experts believe that the rise in autism, ADD/ADHD, schizophrenia, and male sterility result from EMF exposure. American males' fertility levels are down by 50%, with possible epigenetic effects being passed on to future generations. EMFs also damage the microbiome.

Use your cell phone's speaker whenever possible, and don't put the cell phone to your ear for longer than a few minutes if you absolutely must use it this way. Try not to carry it on you, or if you do, put it on Airplane Mode. There are sleeves available for cell phones which greatly reduce exposure. Keep cell phones away from your bed and reduce nighttime EMF exposure as much as possible by turning off Wi-Fi and keeping your bedroom clear from these forms of polluting electro-smog.

How Do I Begin? An Easy Way to Start

Everyone comes with their own beliefs and habits around food. Some people feel comfortable taking twenty or thirty supplements, while others can't imagine such a thing. If taking some number of supplements is a foreign idea to you, begin simply.

Start by experimenting with just a few supplements to see how you feel. It's impossible to know what the optimal combination for your particular brain is ahead of time. Start with what feels comfortable. Then add more as you feel ready. Below is a list of the ten most important supplements from my perspective. Start with as many or as few as you want, wait and see, then keep experimenting. This is not a cookbook or a one-size-fits-all approach. Each person must take responsibility for his or her own brain and learn what nourishes it best. Experimentation is the only way. It may seem overwhelming in starting out, but as you do it, it becomes a fascinating journey of discovery.

Top 10 Supplements (in order of importance)

1. omega-3s, 3-4 grams daily
2. curcumin, 200-1,200 mg daily depending on formulation
3. green tea extract, caffeine-free, 45% catechins, 300-725 mg daily
4. hesperidin (in the form of methyl chalcone), 500 mg, 1-2 times daily
5. quercetin, 500 mg, 1-2 times daily
6. ashwagandha, depending on concentration, 1-2 times daily
7. vitamin D, 5,000-10,000 i.u. daily as determined by blood test
8. magnesium (in the form of glycinate and l-threonate), 400-1,200 mg and 2,000 or more daily
9. carnosine or beta-alanine, 500 mg or 1,000 mg., 1-2 times daily
10. blueberries, one cup daily or, better, extract equivalent

Psychological Healing and Strengthening

The physical healing and strengthening of the brain involves many similar mechanisms in depression, anxiety, and cognitive decline. That's why this chapter is essential for all that follows. But the psychological aspects are very different in each of these disorders, so the following chapters address the psychological dimension.

In each of the following three chapters, the dietary information is adjusted to emphasize particular nutrients and supplements that research has shown to be helpful for that particular disorder. To avoid some repetition, the specific suggestions for each disorder is discussed in a separate appendix. Although appendices are often ignored by readers, in this case essential information will be missed. It's critical to read the corresponding appendix for each disorder in order to tailor the brain healing to meet your unique needs.

CHAPTER 3

HOLISTIC HEALING FOR ANXIETY

Anxiety has now replaced depression as the number one emotional disorder in the U.S. In any given year, about one-fifth of adults experience an anxiety disorder and many more come close. [1] A *New York* Times article entitled "Prozac Nation Is Now the United States of Xanax" (6-10-17) details how chronic stress, fear, panic, PTSD, and other forms of anxiety are so common they've come to seem more like a way of life than a disorder. The National Institute of Mental Health (NIMH) estimates that 80% of doctor visits are due to anxiety and stress-related disorders.

The growing brain and self of the young are the most vulnerable to the neurotoxic assaults of the modern world. The rates of anxiety in children are eight times what they were 50 years ago. [2, 3] Data from NIMH says 38% of girls and 26% of boys ages 13–17 have a diagnosable anxiety disorder. Treatment is ineffective, as most children with anxiety relapse. [4] A majority of college students experience overwhelming anxiety and 84% report feeling unable to cope. College counseling centers are overwhelmed with students seeking relief from anxiety.

If the same numbers were true of cancer or heart disease, a national emergency would be declared. In fact, anxiety is now 800% more prevalent than all forms of cancer. [5] But since anxiety is silent and often invisible, this disaster is only slowly coming to light.

What Is Anxiety?

Anxiety, stress, and fear are some of the most painful affect states we can feel. The DSM-V describes over a dozen different kinds of anxiety and anxiety-related disorders, including:

- generalized anxiety disorder (GAD)
- separation anxiety
- social anxiety
- post-traumatic stress disorder (PTSD)
- panic disorder
- agoraphobia

However, naming a disorder is not the same as understanding it.

Although anxiety, stress, and fear are technically different, it's often a difference without a distinction. Anxiety, stress, and fear share many common elements and operate along the same neural pathways. The sympathetic nervous system activates the ancient fight, flight, or freeze circuits of the reptilian brain stem and limbic system. As the amygdala is aroused, the hippocampus helps to regulate the intensity of feeling together with the prefrontal cortex.

While the higher brain centers try to modulate the feelings, their control can be overridden by the lower brain centers (sometimes referred to as an "amygdala hijack"), especially when hippocampal function is less than optimal. As we've learned earlier, problems with hippocampal regulation are widespread in the modern world, and weakened hippocampal function underlies anxiety, depression, and cognitive decline.

Stress or fear is when there is a known danger, and the intensity is usually proportional to the threat. Anxiety, however, can come out of nowhere and feels disproportionately strong. With anxiety it's hard to identify the threat. Anxiety is future-oriented.

Gestalt therapy was the first to point out that two things happen when someone feels anxiety. First, the person jumps into the future (mind). Second, the person holds their breath (body). In jumping into the future, the person leaves the present and starts to catastrophize about worst case scenarios. Sometimes these are conscious, while other times they are implicit, a vague foreboding of something bad happening.

In holding the breath and constricting breathing, the person reduces the flow of oxygen and disrupts the metabolic support needed for the situation. The word "anxiety" comes from the Latin *angere,* meaning "choke" or narrowing of the chest.

Any kind of arousal or heightened excitement needs the metabolic support of oxygen to fuel it. If you stay with the situation in the present and let yourself breathe, you have the energy to rise to the occasion and meet the challenge. However, in anxiety you choke and hold in your breathing. This cuts off the metabolic support of enough oxygen. Without oxygen to support your excitement, it becomes anxiety.

Gestalt defines anxiety as "blocked excitement." The life force of the person rises up to meet a particular challenge, for example doing a performance onstage. The actor begins with stage fright, but as the actor gets moving and breathes into the role, this stage fright turns into excitement, energizing the actor and producing a vivid performance. Without the excitement from his life force, it would be a dead, lifeless performance. When this life energy fuels the acting, it is compelling.

Because anxiety is connected to the life force, to the organism's basic excitement or energy, anxiety will never entirely disappear. You can learn to unblock it and allow it to flow more fully. You can get better and better at soothing it when it's too intense, or modulating, regulating, and transforming it into excitement. But there will always be times when anxiety comes. It can be reduced in daily life, but since it's so connected to our life energy, it won't disappear altogether.

In this way anxiety is very different than depression. Depression can go away and never return. While there will be times of sadness and feeling down, depression itself can be abolished. Anxiety, on the other hand, can be reduced so it's no longer a problem. Anxiety (and its underlying excitement) is a part of psychological life. It can be tamed but not eliminated.

Closely related to anxiety is stress. Stress and anxiety are often used interchangeably, as stress seems less shameful. The stress response is an adaptive mechanism in the face of challenge or threat.

Stress is activated by the sympathetic nervous system. When a car drifts into your lane while driving and you almost have an accident, the surge of cortisol and other stress hormones you feel when you jump into action to steer away from the oncoming car comes from the sympathetic nervous system. Afterward, when you're safe, you feel relief as your parasympathetic nervous system relaxes your body.

There are three types of stress, corresponding to which of our three "brains" are activated:

1. The reptilian brain stem that regulates the body and its fight/flight/freeze response
2. The mammalian limbic system that allows for emotion and bonding
3. The neocortex in humans responsible for the higher brain functions of abstract thought and executive function

When an antelope sees a lion, for example, the first type of stress causes the sympathetic nervous system to activate the brain stem's stress response and pour adrenaline into the antelope's system, energizing it to run away from the lion and survive. When out of danger later on, the parasympathetic nervous system kicks in. The antelope relaxes as its homeostatic balance is restored.

In primates, the second kind of stress appears corresponding to the limbic system: social stress. Monkey troops, for example, form a stable dominance hierarchy. Those at the top feel the lowest stress and those at the bottom of the ladder have the most stress. Frustrations of the higher-ranking monkeys get taken out on the lower members of the hierarchy, and over time this purely social stress is extremely damaging to the lowest-ranking, most-stressed monkeys.

In humans, in addition to the above two types, a third type of stress occurs, courtesy of our neocortex. People tend to rate giving a public speech or presentation as one of life's most stressful events. For someone about to give a speech before a large group, the neocortex allows the person to anticipate being in front of this large group. This anticipation creates stress over the upcoming event. Then afterward, if the presentation didn't go as well as hoped, courtesy of the neocortex's ability to remember, the person feels bad about it and experiences stress over past events. For humans, when your self-esteem or self-image is threatened, stress and anxiety are triggered.

In today's world, rather than confronting lions, we deal with the first form of stress in modern equivalents, such as commuting in heavy traffic, the physical stress of not enough sleep, poor nutrition, and overstimulation from cell phones and screens. Other stress is of the second and third kind—social stress and stress when our self-image is threatened.

Stress is usually talked about as if it's purely a negative thing. But stress is good as well. The brain and self need a certain amount of good stress. Good stress is when you are confronted with a challenging life event, and you are moderately stressed but rise to the challenge to meet it by bringing forth your inner resources to cope with it. Good stress is moderate and short-term.

Good stress makes you stronger. It brings forth new powers and abilities within. Just as stressing a muscle through exercise makes it grow stronger, so optimal stress strengthens your capacity to adapt and develop your inner abilities. Good stress challenges you to become more of who you are. Without challenges, you wouldn't grow. You'd remain a fluffy pile of stillborn potentials.

Bad stress, on the other hand, is stress that's either chronic or overwhelming. Chronic stress, whether low-level, moderate, or high, is unrelenting, lasting weeks, months, or years. This slowly erodes the brain and body, bringing anxiety, depression, cognitive decline, and a host of physical diseases. This is the type of stress that most people suffer from. Additionally, a single high-intensity stressful event, such as a sexual assault, can be devastating and result in PTSD, with profound effects over a lifetime unless treated and healed.

It's important to find the "sweet spot" of good stress and exciting challenge so your brain is optimally engaged. Too little stress results in boredom, disengagement, and lowering of brain function. Too much stress is overwhelming and also degrades brain function.

Like anxiety, stress will never disappear. The goal is to develop a brain and self that can meet the challenges of life so they are experienced as good stress or excitement. This brings peak engagement. When your brain and self are optimally engaged, your full potentials can come forth, which strengthens and enriches you and the world. You grow into your full self through meeting the stressful challenges of work, relationships, and life.

Why Are Chronic Anxiety and Stress so Damaging?

When you're anxious, the stress response is activated. The stress response produces a number of changes in the body and brain. You need energy fast (to escape from the charging lion), so adrenaline pours into the system. Glucose is released to raise your blood sugar and fuel your muscles. This energy needs to get to your body quickly, so there's vasoconstriction to raise your blood pressure as heart rate and breathing increase, getting this energy where it's needed.

The body prioritizes which systems need energy and which don't. Long-term jobs like reproduction, digestion, and immunity are downgraded. Sexual desire decreases in both sexes. Digestive problems like ulcers, colitis, and irritable bowel syndrome increase. Since getting away from the lion is more important than making antibodies against a cold or finding a tumor that can kill you in a few years, the body shuts down the immune system. This results in more colds, chronic diseases like cancer, and autoimmune disorders like lupus and asthma.

Adrenaline (epinephrine) and noradrenaline (norepinephrine) work within seconds to boost energy. Over the long term, however, these are backed up by glucocorticoids, a class of steroid hormone secreted by the adrenal glands. Glucocorticoids, such as cortisol, have powerful effects on the body.

Excessive levels of glucocorticoids produce heart disease in numerous ways, including the creation of both hard and soft plaque, and through increasing chronic inflammation.

Glucocorticoid excess turns on the "aging genes," as evidenced by telomere shortening in highly stressed mothers of kids with disabilities. Their telomeres genetically look five to ten years older than they are biologically.

The glucocorticoid excess from chronic stress or anxiety brings about:

- high blood pressure (hypertension)

- heart disease
- type 2 diabetes
- memory decline
- brain and hippocampal damage
- osteoporosis
- reproductive decline
- immune suppression
- thinning muscles
- fatigue
- heart disease
- anxiety and depression
- accelerated aging

Blood flow to the brain is altered during anxiety and stress. The blood flows into the primitive fight/flight/freeze brain regions and away from the higher cortical centers such as the prefrontal cortex. [6] This means a person literally cannot think as clearly when anxious or stressed. The person will often make poor choices that produce more stress and anxiety, which further erode quality thinking in a vicious downward cycle.

Chronic anxiety and stress damage the brain directly. Glucocorticoids are neurotoxic. They damage brain cells and can actually kill certain neurons in the hippocampus. Since the hippocampus is involved in regulating glucocorticoids, this produces another downward spiral; as more glucocorticoids damage the hippocampus, the hippocampus is less able to regulate glucocorticoid levels. As the hippocampus is attacked more and more, this glucocorticoid levels continue to increase, which is one reason they rise with age.

Excess glucocorticoid levels also produce inflammation. At first glucocorticoids reduce inflammation, but over time they increase inflammation, which then becomes chronic. As discussed earlier, the higher cytokine signaling involved in chronic inflammation is behind most major diseases and powerfully damages the brain. Cytokine signaling regulates many brain functions, including neurotransmitter metabolism and neuroendocrine function; it also reduces neurogenesis and synaptic plasticity, as well as affecting the neural circuitry of mood, producing anxiety, depression, cognitive decline, and brain fog. Purely social stress causes inflammation. [7]

Trauma is associated with a dramatic loss of hippocampal neurons. Brain-imaging studies of PTSD patients reveal a shrunken hippocampus, while the rest of the brain is intact. Some studies show a reduction of 25% of the hippocampus in cases of severe trauma. [8]

Since the hippocampus is centrally involved in emotion regulation—especially the regulation of anxiety, stress, and depression—the loss of hippocampal neurons dramatically interferes with a person's ability to self-soothe or self-calm. With one-quarter of the hippocampus gone, such a person would have immense challenges in regulating anxiety, stress, and depression. When trauma occurs early in life, the effects can be much greater.

Research into Adverse Childhood Experiences (ACES) reveals that the more stressful, adverse childhood experiences a person has, the greater the chances of later disease, drug and alcohol abuse, imprisonment, poor school performance, divorce, violence, depression, and anxiety. [9] The developing brain is extremely susceptible to emotional and physical stress.

Another neurotrophic signaling molecule, called fibroblast growth factor-2, produces powerful resilience when given to stressed animals, enabling them to bounce back quickly. When animals bred for high levels of anxiety received fibroblast growth factor-2 once at birth, they were hardier and more resilient for the rest of their lives. [10, 11] Higher levels of this molecule reduce stress, anxiety, and depression.

From Anxious Hypervigilance to Calm Alertness

Over time, chronic anxiety, stress, worry, and fear make the sympathetic nervous system dominant. This makes the person hypervigilant, anxious, always "on edge." Healing involves a shift from sympathetic dominance to a balance between sympathetic and parasympathetic parts of the nervous system. Restoring this homeostatic balance brings a sense of calm and peace, allowing you to relax, enjoy downtime without drugs or alcohol, and feel optimally engaged and challenged without feeling overwhelmed.

This requires healing the brain and self. It means bringing peace and calmness into the system, increasing the neurogenic capacity of the hippocampus and brain to grow new neurons and connections, reducing the circulating stress hormones and transforming a weakened brain into one that is strong and resilient. This produces a calm alertness that replaces anxious hypervigilance so you excitedly look forward to life's challenges as you engage life with your full capacity.

What If You're Anxious and Depressed (Or Experiencing Cognitive Decline)?

Read every chapter that applies to you. Many anxious people are also depressed, and most depressed persons are anxious. Someone experiencing cognitive decline often feels both depressed and anxious. Read all the chapters that apply to you.

The Psychological Side of Anxiety

This section examines various psychological approaches to anxiety, its emotional, mental, and spiritual dimensions.

The Emotional Level

Any discussion of anxiety must begin by acknowledging how scary it is just to be alive. The mere fact of living is anxiety producing. The existentialists refer to this as "existential anxiety," the knowledge we are fragile beings who live in a vast universe and could die at any moment. As the existential psychiatrist R. D. Laing once put it, "There is a lot more fear in life than anyone ever talks about." [12]

This is one reason why psychology doesn't talk about living an anxiety-free life. However, this anxiety can be powerfully transformed into vitality and excitement. Then it fuels your aliveness rather than constricting your life.

From the moment a baby is born, utterly helpless and unable to even lift its head, the newborn's fear and alarm need the mother or caregiver to hold and soothe the immature nervous system. As the mother strokes and holds the baby, she trains her baby's young brain, lets the baby participate in her calmness and steadiness. The baby calms down and feels safe and contented.

Over time, with many repetitions, as she picks up the crying baby and soothes the emotional storm, the mother's nervous system teaches the baby's nervous system to calm down. Slowly, this becomes internalized. When the child gets scared or upset when the mother isn't around, the child learns to do this on his or her own. The child develops the ability to soothe him- or herself when distressed. These internal self-soothing structures allow the growing child to modulate emotion and self-calm. This is how emotion regulation is learned in an ideal world.

Unfortunately, almost no one gets enough of this soothing and calming growing up, so strong, internal self-soothing structures are lacking in most people. Plus the growing diversions of cell phones, tablets, and computers to distract the mother's attention, and their use as an electronic babysitter, instead of a flesh-and-blood person, sets the stage for problems with emotion regulation—especially anxiety.

Experiments with monkeys showed that distracted mothers produced monkeys that grew up to be anxious, with lifelong high levels of stress hormones. If the mother didn't regulate the young monkey's nervous system, the growing monkey never learned how to do it. (However, people are not monkeys and *can* learn in adulthood.)

Additionally, no matter how internalized and well-developed a person's self-soothing self-structures are, everyone needs other people. We are relational beings. A person can do it alone for only so long before other people are required to regulate emotion and reduce anxiety. Having a friend put a reassuring hand on your shoulder in times of distress does wonders. Here again, the increasing online culture works against this. When cell phones and texting replace actual physical presence and touch, anxiety increases.

Traditional anxiety treatments have notoriously poor outcomes. Due to the number of psychological causes, treatment can be hit-or-miss. Many therapists are wedded to one or two theories. If the patient is experiencing several causes of anxiety, the others remain unaddressed. Add to this physical factors that are usually ignored such as poor diet, environmental assaults like glyphosate, smog, electro smog, and poor sleep, and it looks like the anxiety is "treatment-resistant," when it's really just untreated. To heal a fragile self and weakened brain, a holistic approach is necessary.

The Psychological Context

An integrated self that can regulate anxiety requires a healthy brain. But a well-nourished brain is not enough. You need nourishing psychological nutrients to grow such a coherent self. This is where the discoveries of psychology come in.

There are three major streams of psychology that chart the pathways to an integrated, coherent self.

- The first, psychoanalytic or psychodynamic schools, views the self as fundamentally relational. Early childhood wounding causes the self to fragment and become locked into repetitive patterns in relationship. It seeks to expand a person's relational freedom beyond the early attachment patterns that were ingrained during the formative years and heal the psyche's inner splits.
- The second stream includes humanistic-existential approaches, such as gestalt therapy, somatic schools of therapy and body work, existential therapy, and Rogerian therapy. Early wounding causes a person to leave the present moment by dissociating from the body and move into their head, which has become the norm in society. Coming back into your body and living a more embodied, present-centered existence is key in these schools.
- The third, a cognitive behavioral approach to therapy, looks at how changing your cognitions changes your feelings (e.g., going from depressive or anxiety-producing cognitions to more logical, undistorted ways of thinking).

This section focuses on the first two streams—the psychoanalytic and the humanistic-existential. These are considered depth psychologies, meaning that they work with the unconscious as the key to deeper change and healing. The third stream of cognitive behavioral psychology, which is not a depth approach, centers on changing thoughts or cognitions and will be considered in the next section on the mind.

Some people are wounded more, some less, but depth psychology has discovered that everyone gets wounded growing up. Early lack of empathic attunement to the baby's needs, separations, minor and major traumas, disappointments and losses—no one escapes childhood pain and wounding. This wounding causes the self to erect defenses against further pain by keeping large portions of itself repressed and out of awareness.

The child, in order to maintain parents' love, keeps down those feelings and parts of the self that threaten the parents (because of their parents' wounding and their parents' parents' wounding, going back for generations). The self is fragmented so its authentic nature is only partially realized, forcing the child to erect a false self or "as if" persona that is acceptable in the family but leaves out important parts of the self. The internal structures of the self necessary to self-soothe, self-calm, and successfully negotiate the outer world fail to fully develop.

Further, these early relationships—to mother, father, and other caregivers—become internalized as maps or attachment patterns that become the way to get the love and affirmation everyone needs. Due to the "primacy effect," where these early relationships become the template for what love looks like, other kinds of relationships barely register on the person's radar. The person becomes stuck in relationship patterns that are unsatisfying but keep the person forever hoping to finally get the love that they want, even when choosing partners who are clearly unavailable.

So, in this view two central things happen: The self fragments and constructs a false self that lacks solid self-structure. Second, the person relies on rigid relationship patterns that reinforce the false self and prevent true fulfillment in love and work. (Note that "structures" of the self refer not to "things" but processes that abide;

the ego, the self, and the unconscious are living processes rather than static things.)

In addition to this, according to the existential-humanistic schools, early childhood wounding causes the self to defend against early pain by leaving the body and dissociating into a mental plane. Since feelings emerge out of bodily experiences, to feel less pain the child constricts his or her muscles and tightens up. To further reduce painful feelings, the child constricts breathing, since high levels of feeling need high levels of metabolic support in the form of oxygen. Cutting down breathing cuts down feeling.

Through this double mechanism of holding the breath and tightening up, the person reduces painful feelings and moves into a mind space. This mind space is where most people live, with only minor excursions into the body during sex or exercise. Healing involves loosening up the tight musculature and freeing up the breath so the person can reclaim the sensory wonder of embodied living.

Although theoretical battles among the various schools of psychology are waged over which of these two approaches to the unconscious are better, an integral, holistic view doesn't see this as an either/or question but rather a both/and issue. Both streams of depth psychology describe essential parts of the elephant, and both are needed to fully heal the self.

Developing an integrated, coherent self means:

- Healing the early wounding.
- Working through the defensive structures that keep the authentic self submerged.
- Bringing forth the buried potentials and feelings and allowing them to develop and integrate into the structures of the self.
- Expanding the capacity for openness, intimacy, vulnerability, and connecting with a lover, friends, family on a deep level that nourishes the self.
- Re-inhabiting the body.
- Living more fully in the senses and the present moment.
- Expanding and deepening the ability to feel and resonate with others on all levels.

- Skillfully navigating and regulating emotion, using it as a guide in life.
- Maintaining good, clear boundaries that keep toxic relationships distant and bring good relationships close.
- Developing skillful emotion regulation, the capacity to self-soothe and self-calm when anxious or scared.

Healing life's inevitable wounding and allowing new aspects of the self to flourish is what psychotherapy is all about. Spending some time in therapy or counseling is a priceless gift for your own self and brain. Even if it seems you can't afford it, in most places low-fee counseling is available if you're willing to seek it out. Investing in bringing forth your full potentials is the best investment you can make.

What Causes Anxiety?

Depth psychology has uncovered several sources for problems with anxiety. A particular theory may fit one person perfectly, while someone else may find him- or herself reflected in several of these views. They overlap and influence each other, but each theory stresses one particular area of the psyche that leads to anxiety. It isn't either/or, rather it's a buffet, so work with any and all approaches that resonate for you.

Anxiety as a Result of Earlier Trauma (PTSD)

Early traumatic life events predispose the immature brain to anxiety. When such a frightened nervous system develops, fear and anxiety get almost hardwired into the nervous system. Someone with post-traumatic stress disorder (PTSD) grows up hypervigilant, on "high alert" for danger at every moment.

The amygdala is always scanning the environment for danger, and with a hyper aroused amygdala, danger lurks around every corner. As mentioned earlier, severe trauma is associated with up to a quarter less hippocampal volume, which means far less resources to cope with this ongoing alarm. At the barest hint of threat the person feels spreading anxiety that can quickly become overwhelming. The world feels unsafe. Life seems much scarier than it already is.

There are all kinds of trauma, ranging from "big T" Trauma to "little t" trauma. The more a person experiences either big T or little t trauma, the lower their set point for anxiety. The person walks around primed for fear.

Common causes of trauma include: enduring physical, emotional, or sexual abuse; a car crash or fall or other accident; bullying, harassment, living in a war zone or unsafe neighborhood; witnessing firsthand out-of-control behavior and abuse fueled by domestic violence, alcoholism, or drug addiction; economic stress; discrimination; traumatic birth; natural disasters; death or injury of a close family member or friend.

The damage of trauma is bad enough in adults. Multiply this many times over when it occurs in childhood or early adulthood. Ongoing, repeated trauma drills fear ever deeper into the brain. [13] Further, with a weakened brain due to early exposure to the many neurotoxins in our modern environment, what would otherwise simply be difficult or stressful situations can become traumatic.

Trauma treatment is its own specialization. Unbeknownst to most traditionally trained therapists, many of the basic practices of regular therapy can be retraumatizing with trauma patients. As most therapists are poorly trained in trauma, it's important to find someone who has special training in this area.

Trauma and its residue can be treated and resolved. When this occurs, anxiety goes down significantly. Some of the best studied approaches are:

- EMDR (eye movement desensitization and reprocessing)
- somatic approaches (including sensorimotor therapy, Hakomi, Peter Levine's Somatic Experiencing)
- cognitive therapy
- exposure therapy

Sometimes with specific traumatic incidents, trauma can be resolved relatively quickly. When trauma has been repeated and sustained over months or years, however, working through takes time.

The first requirement is to feel safe. Establishing safety within the therapeutic relationship is the first order of business. There is no telling how long this can take. The person shouldn't jump headlong into the trauma without first feeling safe. [13, 14]

Additionally, the person needs to be well resourced. The therapy needs to include ways for the person to self-regulate when becoming dysregulated. It's inevitable the person will have the trauma triggered, both in therapy and in life. When the person is triggered and becomes emotionally dysregulated and overstimulated, it's important to teach tools that allow the person to calm down once again and re-regulate.

Some of these ways of finding inner resources to re-regulate can be done internally, while others are more outward. These techniques involve such things as: focusing on breathing; focusing on the body or a particular sense to reorient; relaxation practices; leaving a situation and re-centering, either alone or by talking to a friend or therapist; mindfulness practices of witnessing and learning to tolerate emotional storms as they pass by; personal imagery such as visualizing a safe space, a protective figure or nourishing figure; taking a walk in nature; soaking in a hot bath; or listening to music.

The process of working through trauma, especially early, pervasive trauma, takes its own time. It can't be rushed, as this can trigger the person and be retraumatizing. Patience is necessary.

Anxiety as an Unconscious Signal

Ideally the mother, father, or caregivers encourage and normalize the child's entire range of feelings: fear, anxiety, distress, sadness, anger, joy, interest, shame, etc. When the parents are able to invite and hold the child's feelings, to play with and socialize them, the child is able to integrate and own the whole range of human emotion. However, in practice it doesn't work out this way.

Parents have their own wounding, blind spots, and neurotic avoidances. Some feelings are okay, while others are threatening to the parents. The parents convey to the child in many overt and covert ways that certain feelings can't be tolerated and disrupt the child-parent bond. These feelings quickly become threatening to the child.

Repression sets in along with other defense mechanisms such as disavowal, and the person walls off important feelings, impulses, desires, and areas of the self. The unconscious becomes filled with all the shadow elements of the self that are unacceptable. And the key to keeping these feelings walled off is anxiety.

One of Freud's most important discoveries is called "signal anxiety." When a forbidden feeling starts to emerge, the unconscious defenses go on high alert. Signal anxiety warns the person, "Be careful! Watch out! Here comes a forbidden feeling! Warning! Warning!" The defenses swing into action and push the feeling back down into the unconscious, without the person ever even realizing the feeling was there. The whole process is unconscious except for a vague feeling of anxiety, the source of which is mysterious to the person. [15]

This is what neurosis is. Neurosis and its defenses run on signal anxiety and fear. Neurosis is a state of chronic stress and anxiety. It's a state of being perpetually uptight, holding down the forbidden feelings. This is a major cause of generalized anxiety disorder.

At bottom, generalized anxiety disorder is the fear of being yourself. But learning to be yourself doesn't happen in isolation, rather it happens in relationship. Just as you learned certain feelings and parts of yourself were dangerous in relationship, so unlearning this occurs in relationship. In a deep, trusting, relationship (such as with a parent or therapist or mentor), when these forbidden feelings and parts of the self are seen and compassionately accepted and held, the person can begin to allow these feelings into awareness.

Depth psychotherapy is designed to deal with this. It's not something a person can do on their own, because no one can see their own unconscious—after all, it's unconscious. Therefore, it's helpful to work with someone trained in depth work who can point out what's unconsciously avoided and help bring it into awareness.

A depth therapist provides a warm, normalizing environment that was missing in childhood so that what seems unacceptable can now be owned and integrated into the self. Naturally, integrating what a lifetime of fear and avoidance has kept down doesn't occur overnight. It takes time and multiple experiences to accept "forbidden" impulses.

For example, if anger was forbidden growing up, even mild annoyance will set off the alarm bells of anxiety. No matter how successfully the person appears to be at not feeling angry, it's a losing battle since anger is a part of life. In counseling, the therapist is able to contain, or "hold," the patient's anger, which gives the patient permission to try letting the feeling in. Gradually the person can experiment with expressing it, initially tentatively, then with more and more assurance.

Old, unresolved anger can be worked through and detoxified as the person integrates unfinished angry feelings. Then outside relationships that elicit anger can be explored. Finally, anger toward the therapist can be examined, as this can be one of the hardest areas to examine. Over time, owning and feeling and expressing anger gets easier and easier. It may not feel pleasant, but it no longer feels scary or anxiety-provoking. The general level of anxiety goes down.

Slowly, as forbidden feelings are no longer forbidden but owned, the "holes" in the self are filled in and a new exuberance emerges. The need for signal anxiety disappears as the disowned feelings are integrated and become part of the whole self. The energy invested in anxiety becomes excitement to fuel the person's life energy. [16]

One particular type of signal anxiety is often referred to fragmentation anxiety. Here the signal of anxiety warns the person of impending fragmentation, so anything that sets this off is avoided like the plague. To understand this better, some brief context is helpful.

A strong, coherent self deals with life's challenges by responding to the event and growing stronger in the encounter. When confronted with obstacles, the person bends but doesn't break. When brought low by life's inevitable blows, such a self bounces back relatively quickly. This person has the inner resources to recover and learn from such blows.

In contrast, a fragmentation-prone self shatters relatively easily. Either a wounded, undernourished self or a weakened brain (and most often both) create a fragmentation-prone state where under stresses of various kinds the self fragments. The usual "slings and arrows" of everyday life throw the person back on their heels. When such a self fragments, it fragments into shame and anxiety. This person feels bad, not okay, but rather like something is fundamentally wrong inside them. The person with a fragmented self feels unlovable at their very core.

The word "fragmentation" is metaphorical and describes how the person feels like they are "falling apart." This isn't the sort of more literal or severe fragmentation seen in psychosis or schizophrenia, where the self is torn into different fragments. Rather fragmentation describes how the self feels shaky or wobbly when attacked or doesn't get the emotional sustenance it needs.

When self-structure is strong, the self coheres into an integrated whole. But when a weakened self fragments, it fragments along its "fault lines"—wounds, defensive structures, underdeveloped areas. The self then falls into shame, fear, anxiety, depression, guilt, and it loses capacity for emotion regulation. So further shame, fear, anxiety, depression overwhelm the self due to poor emotion regulation and reduced ability to recover from painful feeling states.

Stability and cohesion exist along a continuum. At one end is a high degree of coherence, integration, and cohesion. At the other end lies a fragmented, shame-filled self that feels bad and deficient. Minor interpersonal insults or fights may result in a small amount of fragmentation that leaves the person feeling bad and shaky but not demolished. Major blows to self-esteem result in a greater degree of fragmentation and shame.

The fragmentation-prone self that emerges from an "average" childhood is the neurotic personality of our time. Such a self has poorly developed self-structures that are brittle and shatter easily. Knowing at an unconscious level that the self can readily fragment into shame and feeling bad, the person tries to avoid situations that might produce this. Anxiety is the signal that warns the person of impending threat to the self. In this case, anxiety is the fear of feeling ashamed, of falling into a pit of badness or feeling not okay. Since almost any interpersonal encounter could lead to this, when the self is so fragile, fragmentation can happen anytime.

Marissa had been raised by a critical mother who always wanted Marissa to be better. She was never quite good enough. However she looked, however well she did in school, it could always be better. Marissa internalized this quest for perfection and sought approval from teachers and peers, adopting an outwardly "nice" persona that came from a strong need to be liked by everyone. Not surprisingly, she developed an eating disorder as a teenager. In college and early adulthood, Marissa was rather shy while quietly seeking approval from those she was close to. Her self-esteem was always on the line.

Marissa chose nursing as a career, hoping that her patients would give her the approval she so much wanted. But whenever she got feedback from other nurses that she needed to improve her performance, she crumbled. Critical evaluations from her supervisors upset her so much she entered therapy to cope with her upset.

Therapy showed how fragile her self-image was and how dependent she was on others' approval. It had led her to a very circumscribed set of behaviors where she never risked anything that might be disapproved of. Where others saw a "good girl" or girl scout, Marissa herself only saw her flaws and the ways she continually fell short.

Marissa was slow to trust that she and her feelings could be accepted in the therapeutic space. Her fears around her mother, her anger and hurt at her mother's rejection and father's absence, her avoidance of anything that risked disapproval, her secret attraction to "bad boys" as a way her shadow leaked out, all these and more became grist for the mill. Over time, she began to relax.

Marissa took small risks at first, then bigger and bigger ones, as she allowed herself to feel and express sides of herself she'd shoved aside to avoid her mother's disapproval. A big step came as she risked conflict with some friends and found she didn't fall apart. She began to see she was an adult now who no longer needed her mother's approval, which she'd probably never get anyway. As she welcomed back long-buried parts of herself, she started to feel more solid, more cohesive. Best of all, her anxiety receded.

When she ended therapy, Marissa still felt anxiety on occasion, but it no longer kept her captive in a very small cage of behaviors. She came into herself more and more, and as her self became more whole, her self-confidence expanded as her anxiety diminished.

Daily encounters with others who are angry or snide or insensitive shakes the self of such a person. Having a stranger be cold or unempathic sets off alarm bells. But such interpersonal insults are part of daily life. No one escapes this.

When every encounter is a risk for fragmenting into shame and feeling bad, the person goes on guard against looking bad or feeling ashamed. Life requires anxious vigilance to protect against assaults to the self and the resulting fragmentation into shame.

Most of the clients I see in my clinical practice don't have low self-esteem, they have fragile self-esteem. This is another consequence of a fragmentation-prone self. Life becomes a continual effort to manage the self-image, to present the most perfect, ideal picture for others to admire. Since such a self-image is delicate and shatters easily, curating the self-image to the world is a never-ending task. Sensing this fragility, such a person is continually hypervigilant, wary of the next interpersonal assault. A pervasive feeling of anxiety that appears to have no particular cause is the result.

Enter depth therapy. Therapy is a kind of retrofitting for the self, like retrofitting a house to be earthquake-proof. Therapy shores up faulty, failing self-structures and allows new structures to grow so the person becomes stronger and more resilient.

In the safety of the inner exploration of psychotherapy, over time the early wounding can be surfaced, felt, expressed, and healed. The widespread defensive structures of the self that protect against unacceptable feelings get eroded, paving the way for more solid, enduring self-structures.

The growth of the self into greater resiliency and flexibility allows the person to tolerate emotions that had previously been warded off. Since the person feels more solid within, the outside is no longer so anxiety provoking, so doesn't need to be controlled as much. Other people can be unkind or jerks, but it doesn't throw the person off kilter. Contact with other people is no longer fraught with danger but becomes a source of pleasure and emotional nourishment.

Anxiety as a learned response

The behaviorists have discovered that fear and anxiety are learned, conditioned responses. Thus they are best transformed through exposure. For example, if a woman has a bridge phobia, the best way to cure the bridge phobia is by approaching a bridge. However, if she approaches the bridge too quickly, her fear gets triggered, and then her phobia is reinforced. Conversely, whenever the woman avoids a bridge due to her fear, this also reinforces the fear.

The solution is neither to avoid bridges (which reinforces the fear) nor to rush onto them (which has the same result), but to approach the bridge slowly, carefully, and with full control. The behaviorists importantly note that it's not just exposure to the feared stimulus that extinguishes fear but *safe and controlled exposure.*

Behaviorism realized early on that relaxation and fear were mutually exclusive bodily states. When a person is relaxed and calm, fear and anxiety are not present. What this means for a bridge phobia is that this woman slowly approaches the bridge. When she starts to feel fear, she stops walking, maybe even takes a few steps back, while she calms down and re-regulates. Then she takes a few more steps toward the bridge. When she feels her fear rising again, she stops, calms down, and backs up a little, and proceeds only when she again feels calm. After doing this multiple times, the woman will find herself standing calmly in the middle of the bridge. Safe and controlled exposure cures the phobia.

When anxiety is the result of a clear situation, unlearning the fear response through exposure is a ready solution. For example, addressing a phobia with a clear stimulus, this is the treatment of choice. However, with signal anxiety or anger or fragmentation anxiety, the stimuli are so varied, so multi-leveled, so changeable and complex, involving past people and associations amalgamated with present day, that it's not possible to do a simple behavioral desensitization protocol.

This requires depth therapy, where these many images, levels, and changing targets of fear can be worked with in the safety of a controlled therapeutic environment. Depth therapy works to calm fears along the same principles of safe, controlled exposure but does so over time and with the different parts and planes of the psyche. [17]

Anxiety as a Result of Inadequate Self-Soothing Structures

Anxiety can also stem from not having experienced adequate soothing and calming as an infant and child. As previously discussed, a child learns emotion regulation from the mother or caregiver. Only when the mother is highly attuned, empathic, and available to soothe and calm the immature nervous system of the infant can the growing brain and self develop internal structures to self-soothe and self-calm.

All too often this doesn't happen. Actually, it rarely happens optimally.

Some experiments with monkeys illustrate this. The first experiment, memorable to anyone who's had an introductory psychology class, involved giving a baby monkey the choice between a wire mother and a cloth mother. Both "mothers" had a photo of a monkey's face on its head, but the body was made of either wire or cloth. Not surprisingly, the baby monkey clung to the cloth mother over the wire mother. But this baby grew up profoundly disturbed, highly anxious, and never able to mix successfully with other monkeys.

The second experiment involved eroding the monkey's mother's attention. The researchers gave the mother less food than she was used to, keeping her slightly hungry. This left her always scanning the environment for more food, unable to pay full attention to her new baby monkey like she otherwise would. She was distracted. Without this adequate mothering, her offspring grew up highly anxious, with lifetime elevated levels of stress hormones, even into old age.

Now think of what the human equivalents of this might be. A mother, father, or caregiver who is perpetually distracted by a cell phone, texting, playing online games, talking, checking email, etc., is hardly the well-attuned, available presence the baby and child need. In paying attention to her screen rather than her child, the mother deprives the child's brain and nervous system of the touch, the warm gaze, the caring attention necessary to grow a calm nervous system. Is there any doubt such a child would become anxious?

To make matters worse, when the child of such a parent starts to cry in distress, or otherwise seek the parent's attention, the parent hands the child an iPad or smartphone. Enter the wire mother. Only this is a wire mother that comes with colors, lights, sounds, and moving pictures, not just a still photo of a face. But it is not a human being, with the warmth, smells, touch, and responsiveness of a human face. A cell phone or tablet is but a fancy wire mother. In a culture like this, how could anxiety disorders not skyrocket?

Aside from our culture of exploding screen time, the causes of mothers' or fathers' lack of attention are many. The mother or caregiver may have been depressed. The mother may have been traumatized or anxious herself or never received sufficient soothing from her mother. She may have had to work and simply not been around. She may have been poorly attuned to the emotional needs of the child or unresponsive to the child's anxiety. There may have been insufficient holding and physical touch to soothe life's fears. If the mother is anxious, she passes this on to the child. If her body isn't calm, she can't fully calm the child's body. When her nervous system is anxious, she teaches the child's nervous system to be anxious. The list goes on.

As a consequence, the child never learns to calm down. When self-soothing structures of the self are underdeveloped, lifelong anxiety often results without psychotherapeutic work. [18, 19]

Ann had a thin body and nervous demeanor that reflected her struggle with anxiety. She entered therapy when her drinking started getting out of control, which was the only way she'd found to cope with her anxiety. She also took Klonopin, and at times appeared drugged and like her mind was working more slowly.

Ann's mother was an anxious woman with a traumatic childhood who'd lost her own mother at age 13. Lacking anyone who could soothe her, Ann's mother was unable to give Ann what she'd never received herself—a calm nervous system. When Ann would turn to her mother for comfort, her mother wouldn't know what to do. She'd stiffen, feel inadequate, and hurry Ann on her way, telling her to be a big girl.

Over three years in therapy, Ann learned to sit with her anxiety rather than try to immediately escape from it. She learned different relaxation strategies, ways to breathe into her anxiety and to observe it arise and pass away. With time, she was also able to trust me and feel reassured that her feelings were normal, not scary monsters that she needed to run away from.

Aside from dietary changes, she made use of massage to calm her body down, and she was able to ask her partner, Mary, to hold her for hours on end. She was finally able to get the holding and comforting she'd missed as child, and her body soon responded to Mary's soothing touch. Rather than watch TV at night, they spent long hours holding, touching, playing, and being physical with each other. Ann was able to receive this and soaked it in like she'd never before been able to.

Gradually, Ann's body and nervous system came out of the "high alert" she'd grown up with. Her anxiety didn't entirely disappear, but it shifted into excitement at work and for her relationship. She began to form other relationships and enlarged her circle of friends. Drinking decreased on its own. When her partner wasn't around or she wasn't in therapy, Ann knew she could calm herself down and re-regulate when she got overstimulated. She internalized new ways to manage her affect. New life challenges arose, but anxiety was no longer crippling.

Being with a therapist who is a calming presence and can settle down the patient's fears is a new opportunity to internalize something that was missing in childhood. Over time in therapy, as the person feels soothed during sessions, this ability gets internalized. The person becomes better and better able to calm themselves when scared or anxious. This usually facilitates new relationships in the person's life that also help regulate anxiety and provide needed physical touch.

Finding a romantic partner to touch and be touched by, hug, spend hours cuddling with on the couch, etc. is also a powerful way of filling the touch gap in the person's life. For those who are single, massage and bodywork can be a big help.

Anxiety as Insecure Attachment or Attachment Disorder, Leading to Insufficient Social Support or Isolation

Closely related to inadequate self-soothing structures is a poor attachment to the mother or caregivers. All baby mammals need their parents to feel safe and to care for them. A baby antelope will run toward its mother when faced with a lion, even if it means running near the lion to get to the mother. It will run *toward* danger in order to feel safe.

Human infants are similar. The child becomes attached to the mother, father, or caregiver to provide safety in a dangerous world. This attachment bond forms early, in the first 6–18 months. The child attaches to the mother or caregiver and wants to spend time around her to feel safe. As the child grows up, this basic sense of safety then allows the child to explore the world and become adventurous.

For example, when at a playground, the child starts off close to the mother. As the child feels secure, he or she will begin to wander off and explore the playground. Sometimes the child will look back toward the mother. If the mother meets the child's eye with a reassuring, approving nod, this builds his or her confidence. The child is emboldened to explore further. The mother's confidence instills the child with confidence.

But if the mother is anxious or looks worried as the child moves away, this scares the child, who then comes back closer to the mother. The mother's anxiety instills the child with anxiety.

The attachment bond brings the child as close to the mother as is safe. If the mother turns away from the child at times of distress or is rejecting or ambivalent about closeness with the child, the child pulls away. He or she needs to stay at a safe distance, not too close to the mother or caregiver.

An insecure attachment develops that only lets the child get so close to the mother. Fear and anxiety are never fully soothed, as there is an emotional distance between mother and child, and closeness itself becomes dangerous.

This sets the child up for later intimacy issues, so the person keeps other people at a safe distance. This in turn limits how much soothing and calming a person can get from friends and intimate relationships due to interpersonal anxiety. Most anxiety has an interpersonal component, but some is focused on fear of closeness or contact with other people. Attachment problems set a person up for interpersonal anxiety.

It's probably clear how this is related to poor self-soothing structures. Without a secure attachment figure to bond with and feel safe with, there's less opportunity to internalize strong self-soothing structures (internal). With intimacy and connection fraught with danger, there's little chance for deep, authentic, close relationships to develop, so the person remains relatively isolated and anxious (external), even if surrounded by lots of people and apparent friends. [20] The isolation and excessive distance in relationships is the outer manifestation of insecure attachment. The ensuing lack of social support creates anxiety. Being either too close or too distant from people creates anxiety.

According to the newest models of the psyche, the basic nature of the self is relational. We grow up and exist in a web of relationships. When these relationships are toxic or absent, the self feels anxious and shaky.

From birth to death everyone (repeat EVERYONE!) needs loving, empathic, supportive relationships to feel good. Creating authentic, positive relationships in your life is job #1. It's essential to be able to be emotionally vulnerable and open with other people you can trust, to find people in your life who love you for who you are rather than a curated image. Receiving genuine emotional support from other people is the oxygen the self needs throughout life.

Look no further than our monkey relatives to illustrate this. When a monkey is alone and given a mild electric shock, it shows the classic stress response. But when this same monkey has monkey friends that it knows are nearby and watching, there is a much lower stress response. On the other hand, if there are monkeys who are strangers nearby, the stress response is higher. This points to the double-edged nature of relationships: Positive relationships help emotion regulation, whereas negative relationships cause emotional dysregulation.

The research with people is similar. Living in a loving support system creates strong resilience in a person. Living without such a support system creates emotional fragility and anxiety.

People with spouses or close friends have longer life expectancies. When a spouse dies, the risk of the surviving spouse dying within a year or two skyrockets. Death rates from those with heart disease is three times higher for those who are single and isolated as opposed to those who are married or have close friends. [21] Loneliness is linked to higher anxiety and even high blood pressure in people over 50, as big a risk factor as being overweight or sedentary. Loneliness is linked to higher levels of the stress hormone cortisol. [22]

Social support supplies an outlet for life's frustrations. It's not just the reassurance and warmth you get from a good friend but the chance to express your frustrations after a hard day. When mice are given a wooden peg to chew on after a frustrating, stressful event, this lowers stress levels. When the mice are given another mouse's leg to chew on instead of a wood post, this also reduces stress.

Taking your frustrations out on others is not the goal here, although this happens far too much in society. The goal is to vent your frustration in non-harming ways with a sympathetic ear. Not having such a spouse or friend increases anxiety.

However, it's not just any kind of spouse or friend that helps. Those in a bad marriage show no such protection and die at the same rates as singles or isolated people. Toxic relationships of all kinds—angry, bullying, stress-producing, hostile, predatory, mocking—produce anxiety. To confer emotional resilience and an immune system boost, relationships need to be genuinely positive and supportive.

Obviously, the role of early family experience is huge. In a study begun in the 1950s at Harvard University Medical School, the incoming class was sorted into two groups: Those who had a positive childhood and those who had a negative childhood characterized by some degree of psychological abandonment, neglect, lack of love and support. Forty years later researchers looked at their patterns of relationship and health.

In pairing each participant with a warm, emotionally positive interviewer and tracking the brain waves of both, those with a positive childhood showed remarkable matching, coherent synchronization with the brain waves of their interviewer. Those with negative childhoods had weaker, slower-forming signs of synchronization, indicating unresponsiveness to close personal relations and reflecting the lifelong sense of isolation and emotional poverty with which they had begun. This group also had major health problems, with 89% suffering from the chronic diseases of age versus 25% in the other group. [23] The great impact of stress and anxiety on the immune system has been discussed earlier.

Isolation and loneliness create a fragile self that is not being shored up or strengthened by contact with others. Lack of this essential emotional nutrient leads to fragmentation and anxiety. Anxiety leads to avoiding contact with others and further isolation. The two reinforce each other in another vicious cycle of increasing isolation, loneliness, and anxiety.

> *Bob felt right at home in the tech world. He'd grown up with computers and had a high-paying job at a major tech company. Having always considered himself a computer nerd, he'd been a bit of a loner all his life. His father was an engineer who stressed the importance of hard science, while his mother had been mostly involved in her career. She'd kept Bob at a distance due to her own mother's avoidant attachment style.*
>
> *As a result, Bob never had a chance to learn about closeness in relationships. He'd had friends in school and college, but none that close. His use of pot brought him into therapy, for although marijuana calmed him down at night, it interfered with his memory and lowered his job performance.*
>
> *It took a good couple of years for Bob to let down his guard and start to trust me, and more time to really let me in to his world. We worked over and over again, at deeper and deeper levels, on his fear and anxiety at being vulnerable and sharing his feelings. Simply learning to identify his feelings took time, and then sharing and expressing them were further steps.*

As he opened up and let me in, his original feelings of rejection around his mom surfaced, together with his lifelong longing for deeper connection and intimacy. As his bond with me strengthened and he allowed himself to be seen and warmly accepted in therapy, he began to reach out to co-workers and create new friendships. He risked getting closer, sharing more deeply with his new friends than he'd ever done before. As his capacity for emotional intimacy with friends expanded, his pot use decreased and eventually stopped altogether. As he let in the nourishment he received from his friends, anxiety stopped being an issue. Becoming bolder, he started dating seriously.

To feel less anxious and more excitement, it's necessary to have a good deal of positive, warm relationships in your life, at least your personal life even if it isn't possible in your professional life. Too little contact (isolation and loneliness) or too much contact of the wrong kind (stressful, angry, toxic relationships) brings anxiety. Even being surrounded by lots of superficial relationships creates a sense of isolation.

Early life experiences mold us to create certain kinds of relationships. Since these attachment patterns are usually unconscious, depth therapy is helpful in bringing them to light and allowing new relational possibilities to develop. Remember, you learn about relationships in a relationship. You can't learn new patterns on your own. This is why therapy can help, by providing a new relationship to explore relational patterns and try on new ones.

Here again, there is no instant transformation. Unlearning old patterns that keep you populating your social life with toxic relationships or isolating and steering clear of close friendships takes time. It takes time to take risks and reach out to form new, nourishing relationships.

Depth psychotherapy is an environment where all this can shift. It's a chance to explore the deeper fears around intimacy and what keeps the person at a safe distance from others. The therapeutic relationship safely permits a secure attachment with the therapist to develop. [24] This can be a corrective emotional experience and a chance to create what's called "earned secure attachment."

When the person can then form safe, deeply intimate relationships with others in outside life, these relationships then become an ongoing source of calming that soothe anxiety and free the person's life energies. In this new view of the psyche, life is a team sport.

Anxiety as Chronic Stress

The earlier part of this chapter examined some of the effects of chronic stress. Aside from the immense toll it takes on so many systems of the body, it can also result in anxiety. Chronic stress has gone beyond epidemic proportions to practically a lifestyle these days.

As noted before, stress is a problem when it becomes chronic or severe, with no break or chance to recover and reset. When stress becomes a lifestyle, you need a lifestyle makeover. It's essential to find ways to step away from the stresses, to relax, refresh, and allow your body to come into homeostatic balance once again. Your body and emotional being need to slow down, to calm down and renew.

> *Dave loved the first few years of his job at a promising start-up. As he rose to higher positions, however, and even after they'd gone public, the stress grew more intense. After five years, working long hours and often on weekends, Dave had become a nervous wreck. The demands of the job had escalated to an unsustainable level.*
>
> *He had trouble sleeping, he'd stopped working out, he had little time for recreation, he was always checking his phone at home. Work had become his life. Although it was financially rewarding, the stress was killing him. He entered therapy complaining of anxiety attacks and stress.*
>
> *While everyone has emotional "stuff" from childhood, sometimes it's the present situation that needs to change. The first order of business was for Dave to learn to incorporate stress reduction strategies into his life. Making time for yoga classes, reducing caffeine, taking time away from screens, making boundaries around work and sticking to them, giving himself downtime and time with friends so his body*

could re-establish homeostasis, all these provided needed relief.

The game-changer, though, came as Dave realized he needed to make big changes in his work life. Though outwardly successful, he was miserable. He knew he didn't want his entire life to be work. With his experience with this start-up under his belt, he made a move into another tech company that was more established and had better boundaries around work.

This job change brought about a big shift in his life. He found he enjoyed many of the things he'd been doing to reduce stress and incorporated them into his life. As his stress went down to a manageable level, he found himself enjoying life once again.

The first step is to identify the sources of stress in your life. Change what you can and learn how to get relief from what you can't. If your job can be modified to be less stressful, do whatever you can to make it so. If you are in a stressful job that won't change, then finding ways to de-stress outside of work is key when changing jobs isn't an option.

No matter how much stress you're able to reduce, it's important to find ways to recover from the stress that's still there, to shift out of sympathetic nervous system dominance (fight-flight-freeze) into parasympathetic nervous system dominance (relaxation). What activities work for you to de-stress?

Stress reduction practices:

- exercise
- take a yoga or tai chi class.
- walk, preferably in nature
- meditate (see Appendix B)
- dance
- breathe deeply (see later section)
- listen to music
- eliminate or reduce caffeine and stimulants
- visualize … a relaxing scene or nature or a soothing, safe place

- journal, write down your thoughts and feelings
- watch good movie
- spend time with a close friend or family member
- cuddle with your lover
- get a massage
- read a book
- watch a sporting event
- spend time with a pet
- play cards with friends
- go offline, take a digital vacation
- knit, fish, or enjoy your favorite types of recreation
- learn to relax, such as progressive relaxation (see later section)

Relaxation and enjoyment are key, as is the ability to lose yourself in a state of flow.

It may be necessary to focus on positive, nourishing relationships and de-emphasize toxic, stressful relationships (say with an abusive boss) in order to keep your sanity. Being a support person for a family member, a Sunday school teacher or yoga instructor, a valued member of a community apart from your work can provide the affirmation and soothing that a toxic work situation doesn't.

Do a technology assessment. While technology can provide stress relief ("Netflix and chill"), the always-online culture contributes to chronic stress. The screen wire monkey entrains the nervous system to a faster and faster pace, revving up your body with ever more hits of adrenaline and dopamine to keep eyes on the screen.

Research shows a direct link between screen time and anxiety. Higher amounts of time people on social media correlate with higher rates of anxiety and depression. The more time a person relates to digital images of people instead of real, flesh-and-blood human beings, the greater their emotional poverty and anxiety.

Most people today don't understand just how strong their own interpersonal needs are. Technology is a wonderful tool but it is not a substitute for other people. The brains of average people have been hijacked by algorithms that reward screen time with hits of neurotransmitters. Cell phones, tablets, and computers are the wire monkeys of our age. When you spend too much time with these simulacrums of human beings, your anxiety levels will inexorably rise.

Take a digital holiday and see how dramatically different your nervous system feels. It's liberating! But digital detox is only half the answer. Replacing screen time with your own being and real people completes the healing. Finding the optimal balance between screen time and non–screen time, where your brain and self thrive, is perhaps the major challenge of our times.

The importance of switching off stress can't be overstated. Without relief from chronic stress, the body, brain, and heart wear out. Finding optimal stress or optimal engagement is ideal. But short of this is at least getting downtime so your brain and self can repair and rejuvenate. Good diet, enough sleep, and exercise are of course invaluable. But emotionally recharging through whatever activities work for you is also necessary.

Existential Anxiety

As mentioned at the beginning of this chapter, the existentialists emphasize that just being alive is scary. Human beings know they are mortal and will die, and this produces "angst," anxiety or existential dread. Additionally, human existence entails facing certain things that come with the human condition, which creates further anxiety. These include:

- **Being alone.** We are born alone and die alone. No matter how connected we are to other people, the fundamental nature of being human is that we live our life alone. The simple fact of existing in this vast universe all alone creates fear.
- **Existential freedom.** A human being is free to choose whatever he or she wants to do in life. The possibilities are endless. Facing these infinite possibilities is overwhelming and scary, often to the point of paralysis and escaping into diversions.
- **Existential choice.** In the face of freedom's endless possibilities, a person must choose what to do, what

direction to go. But this means choosing not to do other things, choosing not to go in other directions. The necessity of choice means that choosing one thing entails choosing not doing everything else. But saying no to everything else is hard, since we want many things and fear missing out in choosing one. FOMO (fear of missing out) is really a form of existential anxiety. But as the saying goes, "You can't have your cake and eat it, too." You need to choose, and choosing means not choosing all the other possibilities. Even not choosing is a choice. There is no escaping the necessity of choosing, and this produces anxiety.

- **Responsibility.** We need to take responsibility for our actions and choices. But taking responsibility is anxiety-provoking. If we are responsible, it means accepting the consequences of our actions and choices. This is frightening, for there might be negative consequences that follow. Often responsibility is confused with blame, but blame is entirely separate, a judgment or critical evaluation. Rather, responsibility means owning our current state of existence, whatever we're feeling, thinking, sensing. We are then able to act and respond. We become response-able. Yet this state of responsibility involves anxiety.
- **Meaning.** In the existential view, life has no intrinsic meaning, each person is adrift in a meaningless universe. This existential meaninglessness makes for alienation, uncertainty, and anxiety. The individual must forge a meaning to make life livable. Only by finding and creating meaning out of life's vastness can this alienation and existential confusion be remedied.
- **Death.** The founder of existentialism, Soren Kierkegaard, saw human existence as a conversation between life and death. Only humans know we'll die, and death anxiety is part of the human condition.
- **Intimacy.** The existential dilemma here is that we desperately need intimacy with another, AND we are terrified of it. The need for deep connection together with the fear of intimacy and being seen creates yet another form of existential anxiety.

All of these are part of the human condition and create existential anxiety. Most people cope with this anxiety by avoiding it and fleeing into an inauthentic existence. [25, 26] Examples of an inauthentic existence are: a lifestyle of consumerism; escape into compulsive entertainment; addiction to alcohol, drugs, work, shopping, video games; compulsive socializing; nonstop activity and busy-ness.

Such activities make up much of modern society. Contemporary culture is profoundly shaped by escapes into mindless activity and mass media entertainment. From this perspective, existential anxiety drives much of civilization.

The solution to existential anxiety is to face these central human issues head-on. Rather than avoiding key existential concerns, it's necessary to confront the basic human conditions like aloneness, freedom, responsibility, and choice. In directly facing, for example, the angst that comes with freedom and the need to choose and take responsibility, each person must look inside to fashion his or her unique response.

> *Anxiety drove Ben into therapy, after his brief use of benzodiazepines dulled him to the point where his work suffered. In his early thirties and single, he was addicted to distraction: video games, movies, surfing the Web, anything online. His anxiety became overwhelming when he was alone or took a break from his computer. He only half-jokingly said he wanted to have a port installed in his skull so he could download information directly into his brain.*
>
> *In therapy he realized he'd been avoiding the central questions of his life: What was he running away from by being continuously occupied with online activity? Who was he? What did he want to do? What was truly important to him when he put aside his online distractions? Could he find true love and relieve his haunting loneliness?*
>
> *As Ben started learning about himself, he became fascinated by the depths he discovered within. He saw how fear was driving him in directions he didn't really want to go, and how his distraction-filled life only covered his fears but didn't really solve anything. Realizing how much of his life was a gigantic escape was sobering.*

As the months rolled by, Ben started experimenting with different ways of relating to his existential emptiness. He became curious about meditation and learned to mindfully observe this emptiness and sit with it. He learned to tolerate it rather than immediately try to fill it. He even had glimpses of the emptiness transforming into fullness. He also reached out to others at work and joined a running club.

Over time, he risked opening up with his newfound friends. He started online dating and didn't let his anxiety cut his dates short as he had in the past. He found his work was part of his distracting lifestyle and decided to go back to school to become a teacher, as he'd always enjoyed working with kids. In short, he began to fashion a life from the inside out, one that reflected his authentic desires and values.

Two years later, Ben's life had transformed. Fear of missing out no longer drove him to distraction. Instead, he was in charge of his life, a life that increasingly expressed his real self, in relationships, work, and play. "It feels so good to be living my own life, not looking outside all the time." Life became fulfilling as he engaged his deeper self with the world.

Inward searching results in the person discovering authentic inner values. He or she can then use these values to forge an authentic life, one that reflects inner truth rather than an inauthentic, surface persona. In facing these existential issues directly, the person becomes real, making choices that genuinely reflect who the person is.

This process takes time, and dialogue with others helps, particularly an existentially oriented therapist. The result is that existential anxiety diminishes considerably. By no longer avoiding key existential concerns and developing an authentic life that reflects inner values and meaning, by finding authentic intimacy, anxiety fades more into the background. However, it never goes away. Anxiety is part of existence in this view, and while it can be reduced and tolerated, it never vanishes forever.

Putting These All Together

By now it's probably clear that all these psychological approaches are related but different, emphasizing distinct aspects of a person's psyche that lead to anxiety. All of these approaches require time and sustained therapy to detoxify, repair, and transform the self. Issues that are years or decades in the making take a few years to heal. Putting in the time and effort to work on yourself enriches your life and relationships in unexpected but deeply satisfying ways. You reap the dividends for the rest of your life.

The Mental Level

The mental level sees how your cognitions lead to anxiety. If you think you'll be rejected by someone, you'll feel anxious approaching them. If you think this person is secretly in love with you, your anxiety level will probably go way down. How you feel is strongly influenced by how you think. Changing how you think changes how you feel.

This is the basic rationale behind cognitive therapy. However, what the depth psychology schools point out is that what we think is often determined by deep unconscious feelings not accessible to immediate introspection. These require time and a more gradual opening up to these buried hurts and emotions to change. Then the thinking can shift. But all three schools acknowledge that some degree of change is possible simply through changing cognitions at the conscious level.

An integrated, coherent self is able to think clearly, logically, and creatively. But as we get socialized in growing up, we come to think that life just "is" a certain way. That is, we internalize beliefs, ideas, and "shoulds" about how we're supposed to relate to other people and be in the world. These unexamined assumptions restrict our actions, limit our possibilities and can lead to anxiety.

All systems of therapy address how the self organizes or frames the world, but cognitive therapy specializes in this area. Cognitive therapy points out numerous thought distortions, often called errors in self-talk, that set you up for anxiety. Cognitive therapy works on first identifying anxiety-producing thoughts, then replacing these cognitions with more realistic, rational cognitions.

Here are some major cognitive distortions that can be identified, challenged, and corrected.

- **Overgeneralizing** takes one bit of information and decides this represents the whole picture. For example, after getting turned down for a date, you conclude no one will want to be with you. This conclusion naturally leads to anxiety when approaching someone else. Reducing this anxiety involves recognizing this cognitive distortion and replacing it with a more balanced, rational view, such as that although some people aren't interested in you, there are other people who are. Knowing you need to make an effort to find them doesn't eliminate anxiety but rather reduces it so you can reach out to find them.
- **Critical self-talk** involves putting yourself down and always falling short. This is a plague in today's world and a recipe for anxiety, a mental auto-immune disorder. It needs to be recognized and rooted out whenever you see it, for this is poisonous to well-being. Critical self-talk can be replaced with compassionate seeing that empathizes and understands you were doing the best you could at the time. Giving yourself permission to make mistakes and fail is essential to growth and learning. It doesn't mean you're a bad person, just that you've had the courage to take a risk. In the process you've learned something.
- **Minimizing the positive and maximizing the negative** involves, for example, thinking, *I'm the worst person in the world with no redeeming qualities,* which leads to feeling anxious. The remedy is to first identify this mistaken way of thinking, and then substitute a more rational thought, such as, *I'm average in my bad qualities, no worse than most, and I also have good qualities as well, just like everyone else in the world.* This new cognition provides perspective and reduces anxiety.

- **Catastrophizing** is always expecting the worst. This blows out of proportion minor events that you believe signal doom. For example, doing poorly on a project at work and fearing this means your team and supervisor will hate you and you'll be fired. If this is what you think, of course you'll feel anxious. The remedy is to see this as a worst-case scenario and to replace it with more reasonable thinking that recognizes everyone makes mistakes, it's part of any job, and it can be corrected as well as counterbalanced by all your positive contributions. Less anxiety follows these more realistic cognitions.
- **Shouldism,** or mental "must-urbation," is unexamined rules that you take in from society that make it harder to follow your own inner guidance. It substitutes an outer standard for your own sense of the situation. Living from shoulds means always falling short of some imaginary ideal. Shoulds clog up your sense of what you want to do or are willing to do, which are the true basis for action. Identifying, questioning, and deconstructing shoulds then leads to replacing shoulds with your own values and sense of what needs to happen. Getting yourself out from under the pressure of shoulds minimizes anxiety and allows your self's full energies to meet the world head-on.
- **Disqualifying the positive.** Disregarding the positive or saying, "It doesn't count," is a sure path to anxiety. It's important to note this tendency and to actively replace it with appreciation for the positive and allowing yourself to feel nourished and strengthened by positive feedback, to consciously enjoy feeling good and stay with this feeling rather than rushing past it. Focusing on the negative creates anxiety, whereas letting in the positive reduces it.

These are the most common cognitive distortions. There are others, and to identify, challenge, and correct faulty thinking takes some effort and focus. This is a form of mental detoxification. Cognitive therapy works to eliminate these mental neurotoxins, to challenge them and replace them with undistorted thinking.

Other cognitive factors are control, predictability, and optimism. When a person feels loss of control, this is stressful and anxiety-provoking. Finding ways to achieve some degree of control in a stressful situation helps significantly. Similarly, predicting when stress happens and when it doesn't lowers anxiety. Find ways to increase predictive information about your stressful circumstances.

Optimists live 19% longer than pessimists—and no wonder. Pessimists are always bracing for the worst. This floods their bodies with stress hormones and anxiety, significantly shortening their lives. If you can foresee things getting better, this helps lower anxiety and stress. This is closely related to catastrophizing, a mark of all pessimists.

There are many free, online resources to assist in examining and reframing your cognitive biases. It may be helpful to see a cognitive therapist to assist in this process.

The Spiritual Level

No school of psychology speaks of eliminating anxiety. Only the spiritual traditions—whether traditions of the Personal Divine (Christianity, Islam, Judaism, bhakti schools of Hinduism) or traditions of the Impersonal Divine (Buddhism, advaita Vedanta in Hinduism, Taoism)— speak of a state entirely anxiety-free. The ultimate solution to anxiety is spiritual, for from spirit comes "the peace that passeth all understanding," as the biblical phrase expresses it.

The spiritual traditions point to a state of vast peace, silence, and quietude beyond all fear and anxious worry. This, they say, is the nature of our true being, soul or spirit beyond ego, that partakes of the Divine and the Divine qualities of inner peace, silence, light, love, joy.

Divine peace and joy and love are intrinsic to the soul or spirit, not dependent upon any outer circumstances. The spiritual literature is full of testimonies that proclaim this inner state of peace, bliss, and love far surpasses any pleasures of the surface ego.

Spiritual Practices to Help with Anxiety

There are two major forms of spiritual practice that work toward peace and reduce anxiety: Mindfulness practices that are emphasized in traditions of the Impersonal Divine, and heart-opening practices that are emphasized in traditions of the Personal Divine. Actually, both traditions utilize both kinds of practices, but each tends to focus more on one or the other.

Mindfulness practices. Anxiety is about the future. Mindfulness practices work to bring you into the here and now, into this present moment right NOW. The traditions of the Impersonal Divine teach that the only reality that exists is this present moment.

The past exists here and now as memory, history, regret, nostalgia—but only as thoughts and images about the past in the present. The future exists here and now as anticipation, rehearsing, hoping, or dreading—but as thoughts and images about the future in this present moment. To pursue the future is to run after a continually retreating phantom. Only living in the present moment is fulfilling, because this is all that actually exists. However, this doesn't mean a disregard for the future or the need to plan. It means living *in* the present, rather than *for* the present.

There are two main types of mindfulness practices that bring a person into the here and now:

- concentration practices
- open awareness practices

Concentration practices focus awareness on one particular aspect of experience. For example, in focusing upon the breath, the person lets go of all other objects of attention and continually comes back to the sensations of the breath. In doing so, the subtler and subtler sensations of the breath in the body appear. The person realizes that there is a vast amount of sensory information that is ordinarily disregarded. In tuning in to these subtler realms of experience, the person's mind settles down, the present moment opens up, and as a result, anxiety reduces.

Open awareness practices, on the other hand, do not restrict attention to one thing but pay attention to everything that arises in consciousness: thoughts, feelings, images, sensations. By paying exquisite attention to everything that arises, the person first realizes just how noisy and continually active the mind usually is (monkey mind). But with continued observation of what is, this noise begins to diminish. The dust of the mind starts to settle, and the present moment opens up. There is an alert but quiet awareness and aliveness as thoughts and anxiety recede.

Heart-opening practices. The traditions of the Personal Divine maintain that the soul, our ultimate individuality, exists in a relationship of love with the Divine. Opening the heart is necessary to awaken the soul so it can come forward into the outer consciousness and suffuse this surface living with its peace, silence, love, light, and ineffable joy. All trace of anxiety and fear disappear in this effulgence.

The obstacles to this are evident: the vital ego, desires, identification with the body and outer nature, attachment to the mind's prejudices and limited ideas. All spiritual traditions begin with purification practices to bring some initial calm to the surface ego. Ethical principles exist in all religions, for it is not possible to have a calm, quiet mind if the person is stealing, killing, and otherwise behaving badly.

Once there is a basis in ethical living, heart-opening practices start to work on raising the vibration of the person by bringing in higher energies of love, devotion, compassion, gratitude, and joy. The soul's aspiration, not the ego's desire, increasingly becomes the central motivating force in the person's life.

The soul calls on the Divine for union, for the light, power, love, peace, and silence of the Divine to transform the ego and purify it so it becomes a transparent, luminous instrument of the soul within. This soul-infused spirituality raises the heart to its highest peak, releasing fear, anxiety, and worry in a surrender and opening to the Divine.

The nature of the soul is light, love, bliss, peace, and silence. Whatever the outward circumstances, this light within is not dimmed. It may be eclipsed by the ego's storms, anxieties, and upheavals, but it remains steady, calm, and loving throughout, even when the surface self feels defeated by life's turmoil. To bring the soul's unerring guidance and light, peace and love and joy to the surface self is what heart-opening practices attempt to do.

Full relief from anxiety comes only in discovering your deeper being. Since soul or spirit is the hidden source of peace, tuning in to this source brings solace from anxiety's troubling fear. When this inner peace overflows into your outer self, you approach life with a newfound vitality and assurance. Life becomes an adventure that you meet with enthusiasm and joy rather than fear and dread.

The directions for these meditation practices are in Appendix B: "Meditation Practices."

Finding Your Soul's Mission

When you don't know your mission, life is an anxious, confused whirl. What direction should I go? What should I do? What people should I hang out with? The person is driven by the environment, however inspiring or mediocre or degrading it happens to be.

Not knowing your mission or direction in life creates a spiritual void that is hard to tolerate. The person attempts to meet the family's or peer group's expectations, to do what they think they "should" do, and to fill this spiritual void through distraction, entertainment, consumerism, or addictions. The person becomes lost in the outer world of sensation and pleasure seeking, tossed about by random forces like a cork in the ocean. Such a life leads directly to anxiety, stress, and depression.

When you find your soul's mission, so many things in life become clear. Your path in life appears in retrospect as a meaningful obstacle course that helped you bring forth your hidden strengths. What needs to happen so you can move forward and realize your destiny becomes apparent, even though it may take years of preparation and training to get where you need to go. But when the goal is clear, putting in the time and effort to get there may be inconvenient but presents no insuperable problem. The type of people you need to attract into your life (and the type of people you need to keep out of your life) comes into focus. The discipline needed to get where you want to go suddenly is there, in fact can be almost effortless when the vision ahead is clear.

Peter had been lucky to be on the ground floor of two tech start-ups that made it big when they went public. As a result, by his mid-thirties he didn't have to worry about money. He took a few years off, bouncing around for close to a decade from project to project before his funds finally began to run low. A pervasive sense of anxiety had been creeping over him for much of this time.

Peter was open to trying different types of meditation as a way to deal with his chronic anxiety. Breathing through waves of intense fear and anxiety was a new experience, and he found it liberating. Focusing on the breath allowed him to feel the anxiety but not get thrown by it, and at times it receded entirely. What resonated most for him, however, was focusing in his heart area and tuning in to his deeper aspiration for God's love. Heart meditation brought him to spaces of inner peace and joy that seemed like a miracle.

Initially, Peter had no idea what he wanted to do with his life. As the first part of therapy focused on his difficult childhood and rocky romantic life, his interests and passions only slowly emerged. He was very health conscious, loved the outdoors, and had frequently gone on river-rafting expeditions. At some point he realized that he could use the rest of his savings to set up a river-rafting company in Oregon.

As he played with this fantasy over the next few months, he realized how it brought together many of his interests, his desire to turn others on to nature and respect for the earth. His excitement exploded as he decided to take a risk and pursue his vision.

Two years later he returned to check in. His anxiety was no longer a problem. He had hired people who shared his values and love of the outdoors. He was being a steward of the earth and helping adults and children learn to love nature. He almost leapt out of bed each morning in anticipation of a new day's quests.

In therapy I've seen many clients' problems simply fall away when they find their soul's mission. Problems of excessive drinking or drugs, of wrong choice of jobs, school, friends, mentors, leisure activity, or whatever else can all evaporate when your vision is clear.

Granted, this usually takes time and focus. It takes most people a few years of moving slowly, finding the right next step, then the next one, and so on until the larger path forward comes into focus. Sometimes a vision quest can produce this opening. If someone doesn't believe in Spirit or the word "soul" is problematic, substitute "authentic self" instead. Finding your authentic self's mission is essential to feeling good and optimal functioning.

Here again therapy can help, both in detoxing from internalized messages from parents or culture that throw the person off-track as well as in learning what your true interests and abilities are. When the soul's mission is discovered, however, a person often takes off and anxieties take a backseat. Finding your soul's mission strengthens both the self and the brain.

The Physical Side of Anxiety

For anxiety, there are some critical tweaks to the Healthy Brain Diet laid out in Chapter 2, The Solution, that it's important to highlight. There are specific supplements to heal long-term anxiety as well as supplements for short-term, immediate anxiety relief that are extremely helpful, even crucial. To avoid repetition, these are in Appendix C, The Physical Side of Anxiety. After finishing this chapter, read this appendix.

It's clearly a two-way street between the health of your brain and how you feel: The state of your brain has a great impact on your emotional state, and your emotional state has a great impact on your brain. Chronic anxiety, stress, and depression all shrink the brain. [8, 21] And brain atrophy makes emotion regulation much more difficult, resulting in anxiety, stress, and depression.

Many years ago I noticed in my clinical practice that a disproportionate number of my most anxious, fragile patients were vegans. I didn't understand the significance of this at the time. Only later did I come to understand how a vegan diet, unless pursued with great care, lacks some of the most important fats, vitamin B-12, and other nutrients necessary to build a healthy brain. For example, a 2012 Australian study showed that not eating red meat doubled a person's risk for anxiety. [27] (The all-important distinction between grass-fed and conventional meat needs to be noted, although it's usually overlooked in studies. Australian cattle are almost entirely grass-fed.)

As mentioned earlier, this division into physical and psychological factors is artificial and only for the purposes of discussion. The first principle of holism is the unchangeable wholeness of the human being. Physical and psychological factors work together as an integrated whole. In order to understand different aspects of this whole, it is convenient to focus on how different parts relate together. However, it is always to the unified whole of brain and self to which these distinctions point.

Why Medication Is Rarely the Answer

In the middle of an anxiety attack, anti-anxiety medication can be a godsend. But rarely is medication the solution to anxiety. As noted earlier, the overmedication of the west has numbed the brain of millions, creating a nation of dulled zombies.

The first line of medication for anxiety are SSRI's, the same medication used for depression. However, serotonin's role in anxiety is questionable. As the next chapter details more fully, the "serotonin deficiency theory" is a myth.

SSRI's work with depression not by providing more serotonin but by boosting neurogenic capacity through increasing the rate of neurogenesis and neuroplasticity, as the chapter on depression explains in detail. It's similar with anxiety. Anxiety (and stress) is a state of reduced neurogenic activity.

Research from the University of Colorado further confounds the simplistic view of serotonin. Researcher that showed chronically stressed rats actually had higher serotonin levels, while rats with less stress had lower serotonin levels. [28]

One big drawback to SSRI use is that over time, the brain, through its myriad protective mechanisms, downregulates serotonin production and serotonin receptors. This makes it very difficult for many people to withdraw from the medication. It takes time for the brain to upregulate once again to achieve healthy levels of neurotransmitters and receptors.

The second line of medication for anxiety are benzodiazepines (Xanax, Klonopin, Ativan, Valium, Halcion, and others.) These medication work on the GABA system of the brain. GABA (gamma-aminobutyric acid) is the main inhibitory neurotransmitter, and it produces calmness and relaxation. However, benzodiazepines also dull the consciousness, and have numerous side-effects, including memory problems, drowsiness, slurred speech, REM sleep impairment, confusion, physical addiction and depression. Benzodiazepine addiction is extremely difficult to recover from, and I've worked with patients who struggled for years to break free. Research published in JAMA Internal Medicine concluded that one in four seniors is taking this form of anti-anxiety medication. [29]

Just as SSRIs downregulate serotonin, serotonin receptors and can produce dependence, so benzodiazepines downregulate GABA and GABA receptors, as well as downregulating gene expression of GABA. [30, 31] This makes feeling relaxed without medication very challenging, and some experts believe the brain never recovers completely from this downregulation.

Pharmaceutical interventions can help in a crisis, but the long-term costs of continued use are still barely recognized. This book advocates natural ways of increasing calm and peace that work to heal the brain instead of hammering it with powerful, brain-altering chemicals. It begins with correcting the underlying causes of anxiety and Appendix C presents safe, natural remedies for immediate anxiety relief.

Please turn to Appendix C, The Physical Side of Anxiety, to read the complete dietary, exercise and other information for healing anxiety.

Conclusion

Moving beyond anxiety requires developing a strong brain and an integrated self. Without the foundation of a strong, resilient brain, even the most coherent self will falter and suffer from anxiety. Similarly, with even the healthiest brain, a wounded, fragile self is anxious. The diagnosis: a weakened brain and self. The prescription: heal and strengthen the brain and self.

The psychological work to strengthen a weakened self is really psycho-spiritual work, for the self is not only psycho-physical but psycho-spiritual as well: body-mind-spirit. The physical work to heal the brain means a nutritional plan that stops poisoning the brain and builds it up for peak performance. Most people need both physical dietary support as well as psychological healing, but once again it's important to note, many do just fine with simply one or the other.

CHAPTER 4

HOLISTIC HEALING FOR DEPRESSION

Depression causes immense pain around the world. The number of people diagnosed with depression has increased by five to eight times in the last fifty years. According to the World Health Organization (WHO), depression is now the leading cause of disability and ill health worldwide, with over 300 million people suffering. [1]

According to Blue Cross Blue Shield (BCBS), it has spiked by 33% in just the past five years (2013–2018), across all age and gender groups. Since most of those who are depressed also battle other conditions such as anxiety, chronic illness, or substance abuse, BCSC ranks depression behind high blood pressure as "the second most impactful condition on the overall health of … Americans." [2] A 2017 Harris survey found two out of three Americans are not happy.

America is following the worldwide trend, as people who are depressed live an average of 9.6 years less, and the chief medical officer for BCBS predicts that "by 2030 depression will be the No. 1 cause for loss of longevity of life." [2] The young are especially vulnerable. Between 2013 and 2018 depression has gone up 65% for adolescent girls, 47% for adolescent boys, and 47% among millennials.

What Is Depression?

Many people confuse occasional sadness or unhappiness with depression. Contrary to the images projected by modern media that there's something wrong if you don't feel happy all the time, feeling sad sometimes is a normal part of life. But depression is well beyond this, an almost unbearably painful, extended dark mood that continues for months or years.

On the inside, feeling depressed is a continuum. On the mild end depression is a prolonged, severe mood of feeling despondent, down, and despairing. As depression intensifies it moves into feeling worthless, hopeless, with difficulty concentrating and loss of pleasure in activities (anhedonia). It affects sleep and eating (vegetative functions), so the person sleeps either more or less and eats either more or less. There may be thoughts of suicide or death. As depression worsens it gets progressively bleaker, darker, more isolating and painful. Toward the more severe end it descends into complete darkness, utter futility, and loss of motivation. It becomes hard to move or get out of bed. At the far end it becomes deadness and complete numbness.

From the outside, while "depression" is often used as a catch-all to include any type of not feeling well, the *Diagnostic and Statistical Manual,* 5th Edition (DSM-V) identifies numerous types of depression. A depressed mood or loss of interest or pleasure must be present for at least two weeks.

Diagnosis is based on how a person feels and behaves. There is no blood test or brain scan to diagnose depression. For this reason, it's always advisable to get a complete medical checkup to rule out any illness that may be presenting as depression. For example, low thyroid or chronic fatigue syndrome can look identical to depression.

Types of depression include:

- major depressive disorder
- persistent depressive disorder (dysthymia)
- adjustment disorder with depressed mood
- seasonal affective disorder (SAD), now a subset of major depressive disorder (with seasonal pattern)
- premenstrual dysphoric disorder
- postpartum depression, now a subset of major depressive disorder (with peripartum onset)

There are a number of subtypes within these classifications, but even these provide only limited information over a very broad category. It needs to be acknowledged that depression is not simply one thing or even fifteen things.

There are as many types of depression as there are people. Each person's depression is unique, a distinctive pattern of physical, emotional, mental, and spiritual elements. This makes the healing journey an individual path for each person.

What Is the Meaning of Depression?

Depression is often talked about as if it's a random event, something you "catch" like a cold. I believe this is fundamentally wrong.

Depression is a kind of feedback, a signal that something is wrong. The person is not getting what they need on physical, emotional, mental, or spiritual levels—usually some of each. All depressed people have an individualized physical and psychological signature to their depression.

But, it is commonly objected, isn't there a genetic predisposition for depression in certain people? Yes, of course, everyone's genetic dice are loaded in certain directions. Which genes get expressed, however, depends upon the epigenetic switches that turn on or turn off certain genes. Lifestyle, diet, and environment control the epigenetic expression far more powerfully than anything else, and this has overthrown the old paradigm of a deterministic, genetic narrative. The new epigenetic research shows just how malleable the genome is for any individual, depending upon a person's lifestyle.

The big questions are: What is the significance of this depression? Why is this person depressed?

The holistic healing of depression means addressing every level of a person's being—body, heart, mind, spirit—to discover what is needed to feel good again.

What If You're Depressed AND Anxious?

It used to be believed that depression and anxiety were polar opposites, that you either had one or the other but couldn't have both. This was proved wrong. In fact, most depressed people also struggle with anxiety.

Neurologically, anxiety and depression are related. They are regulated through similar neural pathways along the hippocampus. Stress and anxiety are almost always precursors to depression, and anxiety continues after depression sets in, often becoming worse.

Because depression and anxiety are related, their treatments overlap, especially in the area of diet. If you struggle with both depression and anxiety, focus both on this chapter and Chapter 3, "Holistic Healing for Anxiety."

Further, cognitive decline often accompanies depression (as well as anxiety), with brain atrophy directly tied to length of time depressed. [3] While cognitive decline involves a different region of the hippocampus, the holistic functioning of the brain ties all three together—depression, anxiety, and cognitive decline. The basic plan to heal and strengthen the brain is similar for all three. This chapter applies the basic plan with some specific tweaking, followed by different psychological interventions for each.

The Psychological Side of Depression

First we look at the psychological dimension of depression: What it means on emotional, somatic, mental, and spiritual levels. The psychological side of depression brings out the deepest longings of the human heart and soul: for genuine intimacy and connection, for meaning and purpose, for engaging work, for mourning earlier losses, for self-expression and becoming our fullest self. When these deep needs are not met, depression is a natural response.

The meaning of depression is often physical in our neurotoxic world. As we've seen, the world is drowning in physical neurotoxins. Yet emotional neurotoxins are no less damaging to the self and brain.

Not getting your emotional needs met, being subject to toxic spirituality ("God is punishing me") or lack of spiritual fulfillment, noxious mental standards of perfectionism or shoulds—all these lead to profound states of despair, emptiness, and depression. The psychological roots of depression are many.

The Emotional Level

Healing depression involves seeing what needs aren't being met, working through the unfinished inner (often unconscious) blocks to meeting these needs, and then changing to meet these needs. For example, it's probably no surprise that chronic loneliness often leads to depression. But it's not enough simply to suggest that someone find friends. The ways a person may hold back from reaching out, deflect genuine contact, or cut short interactions with others must be addressed, and this means exploring the unfinished past as well as what relational skills need to develop.

There are a number of key themes or emotional meanings in depression. Try to discover which of these emotional meanings apply to you. They aren't mutually exclusive, and there is some overlap between them. As you read these, see what resonates internally with your own experience. Even if nothing does, remember it usually takes some time to discover the deeper meaning of depression since the causes are often unconscious.

That's why it's very difficult to explore these on your own. It's far easier to do this with a guide—a depth psychotherapist who is well trained in working with the unconscious and can point out areas where your awareness is blocked.

Let's discuss each in turn.

Depression as a result of an inauthentic existence

From the perspective of humanistic-existential psychology, depression results from an inauthentic life: not following your true calling, not actualizing your potential.

The existentialists emphasize how difficult it is to confront the basic issues of life: the existential anxiety of being alive, the freedom to choose and the fear of choosing the wrong things in life, the fact of our existential aloneness and how to create real intimacy with others, the inevitability of death. Rather than face these issues directly and fashion an authentic life that expresses the deeper self, most people escape into an inauthentic, off-the-shelf life of consumerism, mass entertainment, drugs and other addictions, workaholism, compulsive internet distraction, superficial relationships—in short, much of regular life for many people. [4, 5]

Sooner or later this inauthentic escape stops working. The person feels an existential void and inner emptiness. The deeper levels of the self are not engaged with the world, and the result is anomie, listlessness, and depression.

The solution is to deal with life head-on, for example, to accept and feel the anxiety that comes with needing to make choices and the fear of making wrong choices. To choose one thing means not choosing other things, which creates fear. (FOMO, or fear of missing out, is one form existential anxiety takes.)

In facing life's challenges directly, a person takes risks by making life choices that could fail and result in disappointment. But such failures do not collapse the self, they strengthen the self when dealt with and then let go of. Finding your true calling and true vocation is a key existential task necessary for a fulfilling life. Finding authentic relationships with others is another. Discovering your genuine interests and values and developing these is another. By pursuing your passions, life becomes intrinsically interesting, exciting, joyous, and meaningful. Sadness at times is inevitable but depression is not.

The psychologist Abraham Maslow once said, "If you deliberately plan to be less than you are capable of being, then I warn you that you'll be deeply unhappy for the rest of your life." [6] This is exactly what happens in existential depression.

I have worked with many, many clients in this boat. An early coping strategy led them to choose what was safe rather than what they truly wanted. Often their fear is, "If I really go for what I want and I don't get it, I'll be devastated. I can't handle that, so I'll play it safe and settle for what I can get." This strategy of "settling" for second or third best leads to diminished energy, whether it's in the choice of friends, a lover, a school, or a profession. This leads either to a "life of quiet desperation" or depression.

Jan's working-class parents told her, "The world's a rough place. Be thankful for what you get." They dissuaded her from trying out for sports, telling her she wasn't athletic enough. They told her she "wasn't smart enough for college" and barely let her attend the local community college to learn basic accounting skills. The message she got growing up was that she didn't have what it takes to succeed and should just be happy finding a job, any job, with benefits.

When it came to dating, the message was the same. She wasn't pretty enough to snag the cute boys, so she should just find a good husband and settle down. Reaching for the stars was out of the question. She'd be lucky if she found anyone to marry.

So Jan was understandably depressed when she entered therapy. It took some time and much encouragement to begin exploring her interests and to try things she'd always wanted to do but hadn't out of fear she'd fail and look stupid. She always wanted to try ballroom dancing but was afraid she'd look clumsy. When she finally tried it, she found she loved it.

It even turned out she had a talent for it, which she developed over several years of lessons and then competitive dancing. She ended up meeting an entirely new social group, people who saw and admired her dancing ability. And it was in this community she met Bill, the sort of guy she always avoided for fear of rejection. But as she came alive in other parts of her life, she opened to Bill and ended up marrying the "man of her dreams."

"I never realized how safe I'd played it until I began to take chances and try new things," she said as therapy came to a close. "All my life I felt insecure and like I'd never make it. I was depressed because I didn't have anything I really loved in my life. I never knew I could enjoy life so much."

When you go for what you want, this has energy behind it. If you don't get it, you mourn this loss and move on, making this energy available for the next thing you want. When you do get whatever is next, it feels great. Life is energized. But when you "settle" for what's available rather than what's most energized, the thrill is gone. You live with diminished vitality, a shrunken world, and lowered hopes for what's possible.

Humanistic-existential therapy focuses on peeling away the layers of inauthentic living to discover the deep, inner values and potentials that need to come out and be expressed. It means designing your life from the inside out, so that the inner self can come forth and create a life of meaning and authenticity. As this occurs, depression fades away.

The psychoanalytic equivalent to this is not realizing the self's nuclear ambitions, failing to develop one's skills and talents, or not following one's ideal. The language is different, but the process is similar—a failure to actualize one's deeper, authentic nature.

Depression from failing to get what was needed emotionally much earlier in life

In the psychoanalytic world, Heinz Kohut described a depleted, depressed self that emerges after the surface, defensive grandiosity is either worked through in therapy or else crumples from life's blows. This occurs when the young self didn't receive enough attuned emotional support in its early years, usually insufficient confirming, affirming, loving mirroring from mother, father, or caregivers. As a result, the self, rather than expanding and growing with self-confidence, deflates. [7, 8]

The healthy vitality that should energize the self never comes online, and the people around the child never recognize what's missing or needed. To cope with this the child disavows these feelings of deflation and develops a coping strategy to compensate for this inner lack through an outer show of grandiosity and superiority. But this is a very brittle, fragile persona that the world sees and is easily punctured by life's arrows.

Sooner or later some event or series of events pierces the brittle shell of the false self and the early depressed, depleted self emerges. The person has no idea what's going on. To them, it is a complete mystery why they are depressed. Because this is so unconscious and from such an early period in life, it takes time and deep exploration to uncover the roots of the depression and heal the early deficits.

However, when this dismantling of the defensive shell occurs in therapy, the person can feel and heal the depleted core, releasing the psyche's innate vitality underneath. As these healthy energies emerge, they become structured into the self and infuse it with joy and excitement. The psychic environment shifts to a more fulfilled and fulfilling life as the person's inner resources become accessible, providing greater resilience in daily life.

Another psychoanalytic writer, James Masterson, writes of the original "abandonment depression" in not only borderline personalities but to some degree in most people. [9, 10] The mother or caregiver is not sufficiently available, sometimes physically but usually emotionally, to nurture the child. The self collapses without this nurturing. This collapsed, sad, abandoned self looks in vain for support, and not finding it soldiers on as best as possible. Later life circumstances, such as the ending of a relationship, trigger this early wounding, creating a depression that is far more than simply mourning the end of a relationship.

Here again, because the childhood roots are so early and deep, it takes time, usually years, to uncover and heal the early wounding. As the self re-experiences the original feelings and integrates this loss, a psychic renewal occurs and the person is able to move on with fresh energy.

Depression as chronic inhibition

From the somatic side of humanistic-existential psychotherapy comes this contribution by Alexander Lowen, founder of Bioenergetics, an offshoot of Reichian body therapy. Depression results from a personality and body structure that chronically inhibits the free expression of feeling. [11]

Emotions are the main guides in life. Although some feelings should not be expressed in daily life (murderous rage, for example), most other feelings do seek for outward expression. Feeling sadness and crying, feeling love and expressing it, sensing anger when boundaries have been crossed, feeling touched by a friend's hardship and providing comfort, feeling interest in something and pursuing it—what we do in life is guided by feelings. Feelings are the primary basis for action.

When parents don't adequately see, support, and encourage the child's feelings but instead suppress and discourage self-expression, this makes expressing feelings dangerous. Out of fear of disapproval, the child dampens his or her feelings by inhibiting breathing and tightening up muscles.

Gradually this creates a structure of chronically contracted muscles known as "character armor." This armoring systematically squeezes down feelings and stifles aliveness. The person clamps down on the energy that should be going outward into the world for expression. The person's fundamental aliveness isn't expressed but suppressed and held in. The life force is choked. Over time this chronic inhibition and held-in vitality leads to depression.

The solution is to reverse this flow and bring out what is held in, to express rather than suppress. But this is easier said than done. The early messages and prohibitions around the free expression of feeling need to be brought to light and deconstructed on cognitive, emotional, and somatic levels. The person needs to feel—not just rationally know—that it's okay, natural, and good to express themselves. Since these early prohibitions were learned in relationship, they need to be unlearned in relationship, such as the safe container of therapy.

Over time, through repeated experimentation and initial awkwardness, the course of the person's life current can be reversed and these life energies can flow into acting in the world rather than being constricted and jammed up internally. The result is an explosion into life rather than a suffocating depression that kills the person's life energies.

Mary's parents believed that "children should be seen but not heard." Her parents had their own busy lives with little time for kids. Mary felt she was an annoyance more than anything to her mother, who was quick to anger whenever Mary spoke out of turn or "bothered" her by wanting her attention.

As an adult, Mary's voice was constricted. It was as if she didn't want to be heard. Her world was limited to work, Netflix, and the internet, and a few friends she occasionally saw. She avoided the limelight at her job and had given up on online dating.

It took time for Mary to feel safe enough to explore how she held herself in. She knew how much she wanted to be otherwise, but her fears of offending others took time to subside. By taking small steps and gradually exposing her feelings and desires, she began to come out more in conversations with friends.

At some point she tried to become an extrovert, which led to a few embarrassing moments. But she then realized that expressing herself meant expressing her real *self, not someone else's self or even her own idea of who her self should be. As she came forth, gradually at first, then more and more, her circle of friends widened. She went back to school to pursue an old interest in computers and programming, something few women were into. This brought her into contact with more men than she'd ever known in her life and opened new social avenues.*

Over the years, she found that her way of expressing herself was unique to her. Reversing her inhibition didn't mean getting a new personality. Rather it meant adding more life and self-expression to who she already was. She was still soft spoken and rather shy, but she became capable of asserting herself, reaching out to others, and achieving what she wanted the world—without getting criticized or judged. This was a revelation to her. As her depression melted away, she enjoyed becoming herself more, sharing herself with friends and taking chances with the men she began to meet.

Depression as anger turned in

One of Freud's great insights is that in some kinds of depression, anger originally felt toward an outside person is deflected back onto the self. The self attacks itself, and the result is depression. There may also be a loss or partial loss of the person who the self is angry at, and this contributes to the depression.

The clinical literature as well as research literature has supported this as one aspect of depression. [12, 13, 14] The goal in therapy is to bring these feelings into the light of awareness so they can be consciously felt, expressed, and worked through.

Cognitive therapy deals with the mental level of this negative self-talk, but depth therapy deals with the underlying emotional dynamics. Good results have been reported in the literature in working therapeutically by getting the person to express outwardly the anger that is currently turned back against the self. It takes an emotionally attuned and accepting therapist to bring forth and encourage expression of these forbidden feelings.

Since these feelings tend to be unconscious, it may take some time to work through the defenses against these forbidden impulses. In the accepting, exploratory atmosphere of psychotherapy, these inner barriers give way in the light of awareness. When the anger finds its appropriate target and can be expressed (not necessarily to the person but in the therapist's office) and released, and any deeper feelings of loss felt, the depression dissipates.

> *Jack didn't feel anything when his father died. Instead he felt kind of numb and just continued on with his life. But after several months he realized he was depressed. At the beginning of therapy he was mystified as to why he could be depressed since there was so much good about his life.*
>
> *In raising the issue of his father's death and his apparent lack of feelings, it soon came out that Jack had a great deal of suppressed anger toward his father. Over several months he was encouraged to feel and express his anger toward his dad, in fantasy, in words, and sometimes through hitting pillows. At some point as his anger surged forth, the classic grief reaction came, and he wept with abandon at his father's passing.*
>
> *When he allowed his mourning its due and let himself feel his sadness and loss, his depression soon lifted. He missed his father, acknowledged feeling angry toward him, but in spite of this he realized how much he'd gotten from his dad and found a new level of love and appreciation for him. This freed up his blocked energies so they flow into life once again.*

Depression as an ungrieved loss or losses from earlier in life

The classic example of this is when a six-year-old child's mother dies but the family barely acknowledges the loss. After a quick funeral, the father keeps on working, relatives may help out and the family returns to "normal," leaving no space for grieving or dealing with the child's immense loss. Later on, when this person reaches their twenties or thirties, depression sets in.

The therapeutic task is clear: Deal with the original loss. Here again, due to the decades of denial and family repression, the person often doesn't realize the strong effect this early death had. In the emotionally warm and accepting environment of therapy, the frozen affects surrounding this profound, early loss can begin to thaw.

Although the inner child part of the person may have been shut away for decades, it is really not so far away, often just beneath the surface. Sometimes simply having permission to feel what was not allowed earlier is enough to elicit the buried feelings of sadness and grief, loss, devastation, fear, and even shame around feeling such things.

This illustrates the difference between grief and depression, which has gotten obscured in the recent DSM. The wisdom of sadness shows us we've lost something vital to the self—a relationship, an unfulfilled need, a cherished goal. Feeling the sadness and mourning this loss is essential to move on. When this grieving doesn't happen consciously and in the open, it operates behind the scenes and pulls the person down from inside.

As the original loss or losses are felt, the person moves on and can lay down the heavy burden carried for years. There is no longer any reason for the depression after this early wounding heals.

Depression as a result of chronic stress and anxiety

One of the surprising discoveries about depression is how closely linked it is to anxiety and stress. As stated throughout this book, anxiety, stress, and depression are regulated by many of the same neural systems in the brain, particularly through the hippocampus, BDNF levels, and rates of neurogenesis and neuroplasticity. A large body of stress research now shows a direct line from chronic stress and anxiety to depression. [15]

Researchers use mammals in their experiments since all mammals share the same brain structures—a reptilian brain stem that runs the body, the mammalian limbic system that processes emotion, and a neocortex capable of higher cognition (highly developed in humans, not as well developed in other mammals). When researchers want to understand depression, they induce this condition in mice or monkeys or other mammals. They do it by putting the animal under chronic stress.

The first response to stress is heightened anxiety, fear, agitation. But the system can't keep this going. Chronic stress undermines so many of the body's systems that things break down from within. The animal slumps, becomes apathetic, shows little interest in food, sex, or other animals, becomes lethargic and looks very depressed.

A period of anxiety or chronic stress precipitates most episodes of depression. In humans, adrenal fatigue is one common diagnosis, but there are more body systems involved. Stress hormones prepare the person to fight, freeze, or flee. But the body can only maintain a state of constant threat or stress for so long before breaking down. The ongoing surge of stress hormones damages numerous systems—hormonal and neuroendocrine, immune, cardiovascular, insulin regulation, digestion, and metabolism.

Depending upon a person's specific vulnerabilities (based on genetics, lifestyle, microbiome, past history), different systems within the body crash, creating heart disease, diabetes, cancer, ulcers, backaches, etc. In many people, the ensuing breakdown turns into depression.

The remedy is to reduce the stress or at least take breaks from it if it can't be eliminated. Some chronic stressors may remain part of life, so it's essential to learn how to reduce stress and have periods of no stress—hours or days or weeks away from the stress so the body and brain can reset. Regaining the body's and brain's natural homeostatic balance is critical to healing.

For more information, see the previous chapter, "Holistic Healing from Anxiety." It details different stress reduction strategies so you can tailor your lifestyle to the optimal levels of stress and build in rest, recuperation, and serious breaks from stress.

Depression as a result of learned helplessness

Psychologist Martin Seligman introduced the concept of learned helplessness, which came out of his initial research into dogs. [16, 17] In one set of experiments, dogs were placed in a box over an electrical grid. When the dogs were given a mild electric shock, they had no choice but to endure it. Later, when placed in a box with a barrier they could jump over to escape the shock, they continued to stay there and helplessly endure the shock. In contrast, dogs who were initially placed in the second box with the barrier quickly jumped over the barrier and escaped the shock.

The first set of dogs had learned that nothing they did could stop them from being shocked. Even when the conditions changed so they could escape the shock, they continued to suffer. They had learned they were "helpless." Soon, they appeared very depressed.

The theory of learned helplessness expanded to human depression and describes the situation many people find themselves in. Such people believe nothing they do can change how they feel. What therapy seeks to instill in such patients is a sense of agency and self-efficacy. This empowers them to take risks and act to make their circumstances better rather than stay resigned to a depressing situation.

All forms of therapy try to bring about a more empowered self. Cognitive behavior therapy works to restructure cognitions to be more empowering and utilizes behavioral programs to reinforce a sense of self-efficacy. Depth therapy works through the early experiences of defeat and attempts to unleash the natural assertiveness buried underneath these early defeats. Whatever approach is used, the result is a self that no longer feels helpless and passive but instead an active, effective self that can act even in adverse circumstances.

Depression as a result of poor emotion regulation

When you are in touch with feelings and use them as the main source of inner guidance, you are led to people, work, and life situations that provide joy, love, and fulfillment. When you are out of touch with feelings, you stumble into unrewarding, toxic situations and relationships. Anxiety, depression, anger, and suffering of all kinds ensue. [13, 14]

Most people are out of touch with their feelings to some degree. But some people are more out of touch than others and thus are led further astray. These blind spots shape everything—perception, life choices, relationships. When people have impaired inner guidance, they veer far off track. Poor, faulty emotion recognition and regulation is rampant in today's world.

Our feelings guide us. Some feelings we need to follow; some we simply need to feel, consider their input, and then put aside. Knowing which feelings to follow and how to follow them is life's most important skill, an essential part of skillful emotion regulation.

If your feelings guide you due north, but you were raised in a family that blocks out important emotions, you grow up moving northwest or even west rather than due north. After a few years of this—far from heading straight toward due north—you'll be heading west more and more, and soon you'll be traveling due south. Do this for a few decades and you'll be traveling in circles. You won't know where the hell you are. Of course you'll feel depressed and lost.

> *"I have the perfect life," Debbie announced when she entered therapy. "I don't understand why I'm depressed. I have the perfect family, the perfect husband, and the perfect job. I should be happy. My depression must be biological."*
>
> *Debbie insisted she wanted antidepressants, so she started a course of Prozac for the first part of therapy. This helped a little, but after two years it stopped having much effect, so she stopped. By then it was clear that her perfect life was far from perfect.*
>
> *She discovered she had many more feelings about her life than she'd known. As the safety of the therapy process allowed her to sense into her experience more fully, to name and explore hidden feelings, she saw how her relationship with her husband was actually quite emotionally abusive. It replicated her relationship with her emotionally abusive dad, a demanding figure who minimized her needs and feelings, put her down continually, and led her to minimize her own emotional needs. Her husband was a new version of her familiar father. She'd internalized the attachment pattern she grew up with.*
>
> *Debbie entered couples therapy for a period, long enough to understand her husband wasn't interested in changing but just wanted her to go back to being the compliant doormat*

he'd married. So she left the marriage and filed for divorce. She wasn't thrilled about becoming a single mom, but she couldn't continue to be mistreated so badly.

She also discovered she didn't really like her job. As she examined how she got there, she saw how she'd acceded to her parents' wishes to get a job that paid well. But the more she worked, the more difficult her job became.

Eventually she started to connect to her earlier interests. She had been an art major in college and wondered if she could do something with her degree. She found a position as curator of a small, local museum. It didn't pay well, but she soon realized that she loved it.

On a field trip with her son's class, Debbie met Meg, another mom she was drawn to. As they got to know each other, she found herself falling in love. Amazed she could have feelings like this for another woman, she eventually accepted her attraction, and the two moved in together, madly in love and together raising their two kids of the same age.

It took a few years for these changes to occur. As Debbie's self-awareness increased, as she followed her feelings rather than her "shoulds," or what her parents had told her to do, her life blossomed. Her depression evaporated like a morning mist as her new job and new life with Meg unfolded. "I didn't know just how far away from myself I was," she said toward the end of therapy. "It seems like magic to see how I can trust myself rather than need advice from other people."

Most people who are depressed don't know why they're depressed. When people are out of touch with their feelings, it takes time, focus, and the desire to come into contact with the full range of their emotional lives. It takes real inner work to get in touch with their emotional nature and the guidance it provides. Psychotherapy is designed for precisely this sort of inner exploration and learning.

As this happens, people make new life choices, choices that serve them better and gratify their needs more fully. Depression disperses as vital and rewarding relationships, work and recreation displace the old, unrewarding, depressing choices from before.

Depression as a lack of social support

Interpersonal therapy sees depression coming from interpersonal difficulties such as personal conflicts, loss of a relationship (grief), loneliness (lack of relationships), as well as role disputes and transitions. Interpersonal therapy involves resolving these interpersonal problems. [18]

When the problem is the loss of a relationship or the loss of several relationships, the task is to grieve, to honor the meaning and importance of the person(s) while also letting go and moving on. When the problem is a role dispute or transition, the person feels worthless in the dispute, humiliated or unable to survive the loss of face. The therapeutic task is to support the patient in acknowledging the humiliation and recovering a sense of self-worth in other relationships.

The research literature is clear in showing that loneliness directly contributes to depression. Isolated and lonely people experience depression at a much higher rate than those who are married or have close friends and social relationships. [19] Loneliness is becoming an epidemic in the West. One in three adults over fifty lives alone. An English study showed one adult in eight had no close friends, a rise from one in ten in 2015. Those without close friends were 2.5 times more likely to feel depressed or hopeless "all the time" or "often" compared to those with friends. [20]

When the problem is loneliness and lack of relationships, the goal is to find new relationships that can provide sustenance and emotional support. This is no easy task. Loneliness tends to reinforce itself through the avoidance of opportunities to meet others. As avoiding relationships gets further ingrained, it becomes the default mode for relating (or not relating) to others. Reaching out gets riskier and scarier the longer the person is alone.

Here again therapy is helpful. In the safety of a human relationship with the therapist, the relational barriers can be explored and worked through. The person can explore the early messages and conditioning around being with others, to feel rather than disown the deep needs for relationship, to reach out, to actively initiate contact with others, to risk rejection and not be immobilized by the fear of being devasted by it, to tolerate greater intimacy and not be so threatened by it that it gets cut short.

Interpersonal therapy contends that dealing with present relationship issues is the key element to recovering from depression. The aim is to find nourishing relationships and to assist people in creating healthy boundaries, so they can function on their own when appropriate and merge with others at times of deep intimacy. Learning to more skillfully navigate the interpersonal world steers the person out of depression.

Depression as a result of a deficient self

The core wounding of most people involves a wound to the very sense of self. This creates a sense of a deficient self and the feeling of shame—the feeling that underneath it all you are bad, not okay, unworthy, or wrong. Shame is so painful because it's the deep feeling you are unlovable.

Various approaches to depth psychology describe this deficient self in different ways. Kohut's psychoanalytic self psychology first articulated this as a narcissistic wound in which shame is the predominant feeling to defend against. Defensive structures shore up the deficient sense of self but create an as-if or false self that must be worked through for genuine vitality and self-esteem to develop. Only then will the self become more coherent, integrated, cohesive, and stable.

Other psychoanalytic writers depict similar features. Existential and gestalt theorists explain how the existential void inside the self must be confronted and gone through in order for the authentic self to emerge. Somatic therapists point to the dissociation from the body and resulting overly mental self that is responsible for this feeling of being unreal, vague, or insufficient. Reconnecting with the body and somatic reality brings the needed sense of being real.

Whatever vocabulary or school of psychology one chooses, there are similar features to the modern self that come into view. The sense of a deficient self is a common understanding across many different depth approaches.

Greenberg's emotion-focused therapy highlights this in depression. [21] Greenberg asserts, with much research validation to back him up, that the root of depression is a core insecure self. This insecure, deficient self is under constant threat of fragmentation. Given the near universality of the core wounding to the self first described by Kohut, it makes sense that this inner deficiency is central in depression. What's not clear is how much poor diet and other physical factors contribute to exposing this vulnerability.

Treatment entails first tuning in to this core sense of deficiency at the center of depression. To transform it, it must first be experienced. After entering into a relationship with this state of insufficiency and with the help of an attuned therapist, the person experiences more fully the early experiences that led to this state. The supportive therapeutic presence allows the patient to tolerate what were previously intolerable emotions and be able to symbolize them in words.

In deepening the person's inner experience, primary emotions are accessed. Love and self-compassion replace shame and fear allowing healthy vitality to emerge. The person and the therapist provide what was missing in childhood, the affirmation and love everyone needs. Therapy's second chance for internalization of new, stronger psychic structures fortifies the faltering self as shame and the collapse into depression recede.

The process of depth therapy takes time. It doesn't happen in a single session or two. But as the healthy, vital self comes out and develops, the person feels better, the sense of self grows stronger and firmer, and depression fades away.

Discussion

Depth psychology takes into account the unconscious ways you create suffering in life. One of the most humbling experiences in life is to comprehend that you have an unconscious, that you are not fully in conscious control of your life, your life choices, or how you feel. Once this is grasped, there is a natural desire to understand your deeper, unconscious self and to integrate your life with your greater self's potentials.

The different schools of depth psychology each bring a unique lens to understand depression. No single school explains it all since there are so many different forms of depression. Like the blind men describing the elephant, these therapeutic approaches each contribute something important to understanding the emotional currents that culminate in depression.

There is considerable commonality among these various schools, yet also wide variation and difference. How any one person resonates with these themes is entirely individual. These are themes to be explored, preferably with a skilled therapist, to see what, if any, of each approach corresponds to your unique depression. When you find something that corresponds to your situation, these can be road maps to help guide you out of the dark woods of depression and into the sunlight of fulfillment.

The Mental Level

An integrated, coherent self is able to think clearly, logically, and creatively. But as we get socialized in growing up, we come to think that life just "is" a certain way. We internalize beliefs, ideas, and "shoulds" about how we're supposed to be and to relate to other people. These unexamined cognitions and beliefs restrict our actions, limit our possibilities, and can lead to depression and anxiety.

Cognitive therapy deals with depression at the level of mind. In cognitive therapies such as cognitive behavioral therapy (CBT), depression is viewed as a result of distorted cognitions. Negative cognitions (negative beliefs and thoughts) make a person depressed. Recovering from depression involves changing cognitions. Other cognitive approaches to therapy hold similar views. [22, 23]

All cognitive therapies first identify the faulty cognitions. Negative views about the cognitive triad of self, world, and future are first identified, then subjected to critical review and reevaluation.

Here are some major distortions about this cognitive triad of self, world, and future that can be identified, challenged, and corrected.

The self:

- **Overgeneralization,** which takes one bit of information and thinks this represents the whole picture. For example, after getting turned down for a date, you conclude no one will want to be with you, which is pretty depressing. The remedy is to see this as a cognitive distortion and recognize that although some people aren't interested in you, there are other people who are.
- **Critical self-talk,** putting yourself down and always falling short. This is a plague in today's world, a mental auto-immune disorder. It needs to be recognized and rooted out whenever you see it, for this is poisonous to well-being. Critical self-talk can be replaced with compassionate seeing that empathizes and understands you were doing the best you could at the time. Giving yourself permission to make mistakes and fail is essential to growth and learning. It doesn't mean you're a bad person, just that you've had the courage to take a risk.
- **Minimizing the positive and maximizing the negative,** for example, thinking, "I'm a horrible person with no redeeming qualities." The remedy is first, to identify this mistaken way of thinking, and then second, to substitute a more rational thought, such as, "I'm average in my bad qualities, no worse than most, and I also have good qualities as well, just like others."

The future:

- **Catastrophizing,** or always expecting the worst. This blows out of proportion minor events that you believe signal doom. For example, doing poorly on a project at work and fearing this means your team and supervisor will hate you and you'll be fired. The remedy is to see this as a worst-case scenario and to replace it with more reasonable thinking that recognizes everyone makes mistakes, it's part of any job, they can be corrected, and they are counterbalanced by all your positive contributions.

- **There's no hope,** which involves killing any possible positive future in order to avoid possible disappointment. Asking, "Do I really know absolutely for sure what will happen?" brings the honest answer, "No." Seeing that killing hope negates any positive future allows the person to unhook from this bad mental habit.

The world:

- **Fairness myths,** involve understanding that life isn't perfect, that sometimes bad people succeed and good people fail, that the universe doesn't owe you a living, that people have a right to be obnoxious and irrational, and that expecting life to be fair is utterly irrational.
- **All-or-nothing thinking or mental filtering** has you see the world or yourself as all bad if something is less than perfect—all the good aspects are filtered out and only the bad mistakes seem real. This black-and-white thinking reduces the complexity of life to simple either/or categories. The remedy is to identify this overly simplistic thinking and recognize the gray nuance in life's complexity, and to learn to hold different, even opposite views of a single situation. It substitutes both/and thinking for either/or.

To identify, challenge, and replace faulty thinking is a kind of mental detoxification, for these cognitive neurotoxins are eliminated when you see them, challenge them, and replace them with undistorted thinking. Depressogenic cognitions lead directly to feeling bad and depression. Seeing the world and oneself more clearly and realistically, with positive as well as negative aspects, leads the person to feel better.

There is a good deal of research support for the utility of cognitive therapy for depression. The big advantage of cognitive therapy is that it is relatively short-term. The downsides are that many people find it doesn't go deep enough for significant change and there are many people it doesn't work for.

Also, for unknown reasons cognitive therapy works about half as effectively as it did during the 1980s. One proposed reason is that as its techniques became more widely known, more people already have changed their cognitions in the direction cognitive therapy prescribes. For some people it works wonders, for others not so much.

From the perspective of depth therapy, distorted cognitions are the result of feeling depressed, not the cause of it. Nevertheless, distorted cognitions clearly make depression worse, so adopting logical, undistorted cognitions can only help, even if it doesn't entirely resolve the depression.

Since the protocols for cognitive therapy have been standardized, you can find many free resources online, through articles, podcasts, YouTube videos, DVDs, and free webinars. However, finding a good cognitive therapist to work with in person is ideal.

The Spiritual Level

There are a number of spiritual causes of depression.

Lack of meaning. One of the primary spiritual and existential tasks in life is to discover meaning. Not finding meaning in life causes a person to live in an existential vacuum that creates a kind of "sickness of the soul." A life without meaning is empty and sad.

In such a meaningless life, the person drifts into anomie, depression, and despair, and the only respite is to grab whatever passing pleasures can be found. But such desperate grabbing only numbs the pain. It doesn't touch the root of it, so the pain increases. It becomes an existential, or spiritual, depression.

The only solution is to engage in a spiritual quest to find or create a meaningful life. The simple intention to find this sets in motion forces that, with persistence, bring this about. However, this takes time, inner searching, questioning others, and reflecting on what life is about.

Some people find meaning within a religious tradition ("religious and spiritual"), while more and more people find it outside a tradition ("spiritual but not religious"). The quest to find meaning usually takes time, but sometimes it happens in a flash. Finding what makes life meaningful for you changes everything. When you align your life with this greater meaning, you enter into a greater harmony with the universe.

Not knowing your soul's mission. Related to this is not finding your soul's mission. The world's spiritual traditions declare that this universe is fundamentally a spiritual creation, and only in aligning with this greater Reality does anyone find peace, joy, love, and fulfillment. To the degree that a person's life is out of alignment with this spiritual reality, there is suffering.

Part of aligning with this Reality is finding your soul's mission. Each person is born into this world to learn, to grow, to work out certain things, and to contribute something to the world. What is your soul's mission?

Some of this is psychological, that is, discovering your innate talents, interests, and abilities. But finding your soul's mission is more than this, for it situates your talents and abilities into a larger context—"why" as well as "what" you do. This also takes time and much inner reflection. But the aspiration to discover this brings teachers, books, and guides of all forms into your life so that, in time, your deeper purpose can be found.

Once you find your soul's mission, everything else begins to fall into place. Setbacks will happen, but when your vision is clear, even great obstacles can be overcome.

Not following your spiritual vision. This is another cause of depression. Having a glimpse of the spiritual life but not following it, seeing a higher or better way of living and turning your back on it, or having a sense of your spiritual destiny or possibilities and not pursuing them leads to deflation, a sinking sensation where you lose your way in life.

Here again the solution is simple, though not always easy. It involves bringing your life into alignment with this higher purpose. Otherwise this other kind of "soul sickness depression" will continue.

The Dark Night of the Soul

The most common form of depression stemming from spiritual causes is "the dark night of the soul." This phrase was coined by the fifteenth century mystic St. John of the Cross in his spiritual masterpiece *The Dark Night*. It describes the spiritual journey of the soul's gradual awakening by first being purified and cleansed in a fire that is dark.

Although the phrase "dark night of the soul" is bandied about rather casually these days, St. John of the Cross was describing an intense, years long process of inner purification, in which a person's life is turned inside out as a preparation for a life of infused spirituality. It is a painful, difficult journey that involves confronting many uncomfortable truths about yourself, which can be very depressing. But the promise of spiritual awakening it holds keeps the soul moving forward, first into greater darkness but then into the light.

A psychological parallel is what Carl Jung first described as a crisis in midlife or later (ages thirty-five to sixty-five). Jungian psychology holds that in the first part of life (birth to about thirty), the ego emerges from the collective unconscious and encounters the world. Pulled outward by the senses and outward flow of life energy (libido), the young ego generally isn't so conscious of its deeper subjectivity and fashions a life based on family, cultural, and peer pressures. A certain degree of outward success is the reward for this outer movement, but since it has ignored the inner depths, it must eventually collapse.

In midlife, the outward flow of libido ebbs and begins to flow back into the collective unconscious. The person follows this flow of life energy and turns inward, perhaps for the first time or, if not, with renewed interest in the psyche's interior. The person's subjectivity and inner life come alive.

This midlife reversal of psychic energy is an about-face that brings the ego into deeper relationship with its source. It's the start of an individuation process in which it's reunited with its original wholeness, the archetypal Self. This means the self must integrate its split-off aspects and confront its disowned, unconscious parts.

The parts of the self that were cast aside and repressed growing up in the person's family system need to be recovered and integrated. A new order or synchronization between inner self and outer life calls forth as the old order falls apart.

This culminates in a life of higher meaning, creativity, renewal of vitality, and deeper, more authentic relationships. In bringing a psychological and Jungian interpretation to the journey of the dark night, several Jungian writers show just how psychologically sophisticated St. John was in this classic work. [24, 25, 26, 27]

There are some common features to this journey.

People usually begin this journey when they feel like they've "made it" in the world. There may be the two-car garage, family, kids, job, and some degree of financial stability. At midlife they may feel at the height of their powers. But just at this moment, the rug gets pulled out from under them.

In psychological language, the focus is on narcissism. That is, a prideful, narcissistic person has a vague sense of emptiness and lack, but these are consciously denied and covered over with assertions of self-worth or superiority. The irony of narcissistic pride is that outward appearances mask their opposite. The greater the person's outer show, the greater the inner emptiness. The more the person asserts superiority, the more the person feels less than.

This confusion of outer appearances and inner reality is present throughout the journey. Things are the opposite of what they appear to be. Pride goes before the fall but this leads to redemption. The seeming outer strength at midlife betrays an inner weakness. Although this is a journey into joy, deeper connection, and light, the person feels greater shame, isolation, and darkness than ever.

So just when the person believes they've finally made it at midlife, they are really the most lost and out of touch with their inner self. When the person feels most lost and in the dark, it's actually the beginning of finding themselves. This is exactly how many people enter therapy, lost and at the end of their rope.

First stage. A common image across the world's spiritual traditions likens the spiritual journey to crossing a desert. The first stage of the desert represents a phase of purification in which the pleasures of the world fade but the fruits of the spirit haven't yet appeared. St. John of the Cross details how one of the first signs of the dark night of the soul is this drying up of worldly satisfactions, creating a sense of aridity.

The usual life pleasures the person had been getting satisfaction from begin to dry up. In psychological terms, the cathexis (libidinal charge or life energy) withdraws from the world as it starts to flow back into the unconscious. When the world is no longer energetically charged (cathected), it seems flat, neutral, or dead.

St. John is quick to point out how this aridity creates a thirst for Spirit, although the person may not recognize this. The person wants something but often doesn't know what. It may take time to realize this searching is the soul's searching for the Divine.

In the words of St. John, "Because the enkindlings of love in the spirit increase exceedingly, the longing for God becomes so intense that it will seem to such persons that their bones are drying up, their nature withering away, and their ardor and strength diminishing." [27]

Second stage. This leads to the next stage in the dark night of the soul. Along with aridity comes lassitude and a loss of motivation. The usual motivations and desires of the person begin to flag. There is a loss of willpower. The dark night depletes a person's energy.

Naturally this loss of willpower alarms the person, who fears losing everything that up until then has provided pleasure—career, family, intimate relationship, friends, community involvement. It all begins to seem meaningless. The person tries harder and harder to force themselves to carry out their duties, but these efforts soon fail. Resistance is futile.

Instead, St. John counsels surrender. The person needs to do whatever possible to fulfill life's responsibilities and at the same time let go and allow this process to carry them inward. The person needs to hang in there, accept that a higher power is at work, and trust that a greater strength and delight lie ahead.

Third stage. As the person is drawn inward, there is greater self-awareness. The person sees himself or herself more clearly, which St. John calls "the bitter pill of self-knowledge." In Jungian terms this signals the confrontation with "the shadow." The ego is drawn down into the underworld of the psyche.

As anyone who is familiar with this aspect of the psyche knows, the underworld of the psyche is not a pretty picture. It can be very disconcerting, for it's the repository of the person's unacceptable impulses. Yet this is an essential aspect of knowing yourself more fully.

St. John describes this beautifully. "The aridities and voids of the faculties in relation to the abundance previously experienced and the difficulty encountered in the practice of virtue make the soul recognize its own lowliness and misery, which was not apparent in the time of its prosperity.

Now that the soul is clothed in these other garments of labor, dryness, and desolation, and its former lights have been darkened, it possesses more authentic lights in this most excellent and necessary self-knowledge." [27]

In Jungian psychology, the shadow has no particular content, rather it consists of everything that is not in the light of consciousness. For St. John and the fifteenth century monks and nuns he was writing for, the personal and cultural shadow at that time and what tortured him most deeply, were sexual impulses and blasphemy. In today's world, these things hardly raise an eyebrow.

In our very different cultural and historical context, the modern shadow consists of shame around a defective or deficient self, not feeling worthy, conflicts around anger, dependency, or other forbidden feelings, and early trauma.

Journeying into the underworld alone is treacherous, but in St. John's time it was the only way. Today, psychotherapy is a journey into the underworld of the psyche, and having a guide (therapist) can be of great assistance.

Fourth stage. As the person gets more and more lost crossing the desert, losing willpower and the pleasures of life, in encountering the shadow and getting drawn down into the underworld, suddenly there is a joyous breakthrough. An oasis appears in the desert.

What was troubling recedes, and the person enjoys a respite from the pain and engulfing depression. Serenity and light replace the darkness. The person feels huge relief and believes the worst is over and the goal is reached.

What this actually signifies, however, is the beginning of the much darker night of spirit, which St. John views as a separate, second phase.

Phase 2: The night of spirit. In this second half of the journey there is a more direct spiritual action to purify the soul. The temporary reprieve of joyful exhilaration at the oasis soon gives way to a feeling of sinking into a black hole. Everything seems dark and unknown. St. John compares this to the biblical story of Jonah being swallowed up in the dark belly of the whale.

There is a descent into utter darkness, where the soul feels lost, alone, abandoned by God and by friends. People seem far away. There is a terrible sense of having been forgotten by everyone, even the Divine. The soul is stripped bare.

As this is happening there is a de-repression that occurs in the psyche. The defenses in place for a lifetime loosen and seem to crumble. As a result, there is a return of the early, unhealed wounds from the past. This takes several forms as the early wounding gets activated.

- Bad or deficient self. The core wounding to the sense of self comes up, a feeling of inner "badness" or deficiency, together with an ocean of shame that is part of this core wounding. When this early wounding is activated, everything is seen through the eyes of this bad, deficient self—both past memories as well as present day life.
- Vulnerability. Without the usual defenses in place, the person feels exposed to everyone's gaze. It seems like everyone in the world is able to see their badness or deficiency. In one sense the person is right, because without the usual defenses operating, the person is indeed more exposed, lacking protection and open to everyone's gaze. But in another sense the person is mistaken, for since everybody's else's defenses are still in place, no one notices. Nevertheless, a feeling of vulnerability and a sense of "nowhere to hide" plagues the person.
- Angry, judging, negative father. The early family relationships get activated, and wounds the person may have experienced

with the condemning, raging oedipal father take hold. Old memories resurface to be felt, experienced, and worked through. Present-day relationships with teachers, mentors, bosses, and other authority figures are lit up in the person's life, as the negative-father filter colors these relationships and may create conflict and serious difficulties.

- Abandoning and engulfing bad mother. Wounds emerge around the pre-oedipal mother who was either abandoning or engulfing or both. Here again early memories arise that need to be felt and emotions that need to be experienced as the person was unable to acknowledge them back then. The psyche is cleansing itself, and it must experience now what it was unable to bear back then to be free of it. As with the bad-father wounds, the bad-mother wounds also color present-day relationships that are nurturing or sustaining, such as with a wife or partner, women friends and colleagues or others.
- Working through. As the bad self and the wounding around the bad mother and bad father re-emerge, the early feelings that were too much for the young psyche to feel are now re-experienced. The lowering of defenses makes this process easier in some ways but more painful and uncomfortable in others. But the adult psyche is able to tolerate feelings that were intolerable as a child; so however painful it is, if the person can persevere, gradually an inner shift occurs.
- Resolution. In working through and healing the early wounds around self and parents/caregivers, the person gets in touch with parts of themselves that were previously inaccessible. Not only are painful parts recovered but lost potentials and buried talents are unearthed. These buried capacities can now be integrated into the self. New talents and interests emerge. New possibilities appear in life.

The light emerges. As more and more oases appear, the past is no longer colored by negative memories and wounding. Positive early experiences emerge along with positive, joyful, and creative sides of the self. The person realizes that when growing up there were both positive and negative experiences of mother, father, and self, and all have been important to becoming a whole person. The desert starts to bloom.

Then the desert progressively gives way to a moist, lush landscape. As new aspects of the inner being come forth, the person's relationship with the outer world changes. The task is to align this new, enlarged inner self with one's outer life. This may take time and cause some disruption. But to create a new balance between inner self and outer life is the whole meaning and purpose of the midlife transition.

As this occurs there is very often a profound spiritual awakening. Spiritual joy and exaltation, states of inner peace and tranquility, heart openings of love and compassion and gratitude for being alive, replace the darkness of the previous period. A more soul-infused self transforms relationships, work, and daily life. Greater creativity, mature meditation and prayer, and gratitude for life's abundance become the keynote of daily living.

Relationships take on a new hue, more authentic, affirming, and loving. The person sees how important relationships are. He or she is more present in relationships, better able to give and more open to receiving love and nurturing.

Work and play are transformed. Work is renewed by changing the outer form so it's in closer alignment with the person's inner values and self. Alternately, the person's inner attitude toward work changes, and when its inner meaning shifts, the previous alienation subsides.

Life's difficulties and setbacks still occur, but banished are the depression and spiritual darkness that accompanied it. A new stage of more sustained joy, light, love, and peace are the spiritual foundation on which the person can build their life anew.

> *Andrew's mother had been traumatized by the Cultural Revolution in China, where her husband had been killed. Andrew had only been a baby when she'd immigrated to the U.S. and been overwhelmed from the start.*
>
> *When Andrew was six, his mother left Andrew and his younger sister with an aunt for three years, telling them she couldn't handle them anymore. When his mother brought*

them back to live with her, she let them know that if they acted up, they'd be sent back to their aunt immediately. Naturally, Andrew became utterly compliant to avoid any possibility of another traumatic separation from his mother.

Deeply scarred from his own mother's abandonment, he wanted to be sure nothing like this ever happened again. So Andrew married a woman who he knew was never going to leave him. However, after twenty years of marriage and two kids, Andrew was bored and depressed. He and his wife had stopped having sex a decade earlier, and Andrew found himself attracted to several women at work. After a failed affair, in his mid-fifties, he entered therapy more depressed than ever.

I suggested he start couples therapy with his wife, which he did. However, after six months of trying to revive their dead relationship, he left his wife and filed for divorce. In our individual work, Andrew focused on his early years with his mother and the horrific time after she left. His uncle had been a kind of surrogate father figure for Andrew, but an unreliable one, and that played itself out in our relationship of the transference, where he felt betrayed when I was vacation a few times.

At one point Andrew joyfully strode into the office and declared he was in love with a co-worker he'd been obsessed with and had started to date. Little did he know, this was but an oasis in the desert, not a solution. When she dumped him a few months later, he fell even further into despair.

Over the next couple of years as Andrew worked on his feelings about his mother and uncle, early feelings of shame and worthlessness emerged. Over time, as he detoxed from shame, he was able to lovingly hold this young part of himself and discover a source of vitality and intrinsic value inside. New interests grabbed his attention, which he explored. Most didn't pan out but some did.

He began to risk going out with a number of different kinds of women, not just women who would never reject him as had been his pattern. This led to a new excitement in his relationships.

He also recognized that he was burned out with his work. It didn't make sense economically for Andrew to start over in another profession, although he was tempted to. Instead he retooled his current position so that instead of dealing with screens and written documents, he had more contact with people. This, he found, gave him more satisfaction at work than he'd had before.

As Andrew brought his outer life into harmony with his inner self, his depression lifted, not at once but in waves. The dark nights became less frequent and the bright days in the oases outnumbered the nights. He also began a yoga practice, which brought him deep states of relaxation and peace and stirred an interest in attending church once again.

"Living in the sunshine is so much better than living in darkness," he said toward the end of our work together. "Just surviving my childhood was a major feat, but now I feel like I can live and enjoy my new love and other people in a way I never could."

This process can be slow or fast, depending upon how the person relates to it. For most people, who have a primarily externalized orientation, the midlife transition is halted partway through. The caricature of this is the middle-aged man who buys a new sports car, divorces his wife to marry a younger woman, and starts a new company. But dealing with the dark night merely in outward terms means recycling old wine in new bottles—a replay of the old forms with new characters, while the underlying structure remains the same. The renewal of the dark night remains stillborn or only partially realized. Only in embracing the dark night of the soul as an inner process will the psyche be able to re-create a life of genuine fulfillment.

The dark night of the soul does not only occur at midlife. There are quarter-life crises as well as other-life crises. The dark night of the soul is a pattern of renewal that most people experience at some point. Having your life crash and burn, then to rise from the ashes, Phoenix-like, to re-fashion your life is an archetypal cycle in which the psyche can re-align with its spiritual source.

This is hard to do without a guide or talented therapist. But when the journey of the dark night is fully embraced and gone through, the psycho-spiritual transformation builds the capacity for bearing life's inevitable suffering without falling into depression.

Spiritual Practices to help with depression

The idea behind spiritual practice is to discover the spiritual foundation of consciousness—the Divine or God or Emptiness or Love, whatever word or symbol for Spirit you prefer. The soul and/or spirit within each person is a source of intrinsic peace, joy, love, light, guidance. To find your loving center of peace within is to have a safe harbor amidst all life's storms.

One of the worst parts of depression is that it often keeps the person focused on the outer, external world and out of touch with the inner being, soul, or spirit. That's why spiritual practice can be lifesaving. In connecting internally to an intrinsic source of value, peace, love, and joy, depression is easier to bear and may recede.

All spiritual practices are helpful in this journey, and some are being used in therapy as important aids in coping with depression. Two forms of meditation now have a good deal of research evidence behind them to show they are helpful in depression as well as support brain health.

Heart-opening spiritual practices and mindfulness practices open consciousness inwardly to the Divine source. Both appear to increase neurogenesis and neuroplasticity along the entire length of the hippocampus, an unusually strong effect compared to most other things that only affect one side or the other. These neurogenic effects support the healing and growth of the brain and self, as well as being strongly antidepressant.

Appendix B: "Meditation Practices" at the back of the book details instructions for these two practices. There are a number of variations of each. Experiment with the different forms to see which resonates with you. Then stick to that practice as it deepens and opens the riches of your inner being.

Psychological Detoxification

Psychological toxins come in many forms: toxic people or circumstances, toxic cognitions, and poisonous spiritual beliefs. Detoxification involves eliminating these from your life as much as possible. Although this is implicit in many of the previous sections, it's worth discussing it on its own.

Situational depression. This is the clearest case of toxic circumstances pulling a person down. While many of the situations described earlier may be mysterious at first or unconscious, in situational depression it's usually clear why you're depressed. Most often it's due to some kind of toxic environment—emotionally abusive or unfulfilling, relationship deficiency, financially or emotionally stressful, toxic work environment, etc.

Toxic relationships are a fact of life, but some people invite such relationships or fail to erect firm boundaries around themselves to protect against such intrusions. When you come away from spending time with someone and feel drained, foggy, bad about yourself, or deflated, chances are you've been emotionally poisoned.

Some people suck the energy out of others like a psychic vampire. Other people demand all the attention and create a one-way relationship that requires others' constant attention. There are those whose caustic, constant put-downs of others create around them a cloud of negativity. The list could go on … innumerable are the ways toxic people drain others emotionally.

In contrast, with other people you come away feeling nourished, with more energy, more love, feeling better about yourself and the world. The goal is to get more nourishing people in your life and reduce your toxic exposure.

Of course, it's too simplistic to say someone is toxic or nourishing. Everyone has both nourishing and toxic sides. While personal growth lies in developing the nourishing sides and letting go of the toxic sides, some people live primarily on one side or the other.

When someone is primarily toxic for you, the relationship either needs to change or be minimized. If you can confront the person on what isn't working, the other person can hear you nondefensively, and the relationship can transform, great. If not, developing clear boundaries is essential. Sometimes this means limiting contact, sometimes it may mean ending the relationship.

Chronic stress is one toxic circumstance, as discussed in the previous chapter on anxiety.

Another toxic circumstance is loneliness. Chronic loneliness afflicts a growing number of people, especially older adults, and it leads to depression, anxiety, and other health issues. It's a greater risk factor for heart disease than smoking. Finding ways to reach out and establish meaningful relationships is essential, but as mentioned before, this is easier said than done. The help of a therapist is often needed.

As noted earlier, another great help is meditation, which can transform the emptiness of loneliness into fullness of aloneness. Meditation can be seen as training in how to be alone, going deeply into oneself to discover the bounty of the inner life. Most people don't know how to be with themselves and try to continually distract themselves in an attempt to fill their inner void. Spiritual traditions teach that this is an impossible task, as the emptiness of the ego can never be filled. Rather, spiritual traditions suggest this emptiness is a gateway into deeper being if can learn how to make this inner journey. Meditation and prayer are the way.

Toxic cognitions are the focus of much of cognitive therapy, but one form appears under the guise of spirituality. Toxic spiritual beliefs can be oppressive, stressful and depressing. For example, believing, "God is punishing me," or "This proves I'm a bad person," while depressed or when bad things happen reinforces the depression. The ensuing blame, guilt, shame, and self-judgment lead to depression.

Healing lies in the opposite direction: taking responsibility but not self-blame or judgment, compassion for your struggles and mistakes, appreciation for what can be learned and gratitude for the learning, even when it's hard on the ego.

Another psychological toxin is too much technology. Although the electro smog produced by the EMFs of cell phones, computers, and Wi-Fi has powerfully damaging physical effects on mitochondria and neural cells, the other form of poisoning is the emotional deprivation they create.

Technology assessment. Do an appraisal of how much time you spend with screens: cell phone, tablets, computers, TVs, watch—any form of screen. Now estimate how much time you spend with actual people, making in-person contact and genuine connection. What do you find?

Remember, the recent discoveries of depth and developmental psychology show we are relational beings. Your nervous system was developed in relationship with other people. Your brain and self require a steady stream of emotional nutrients. Without real relationships, the self becomes fragile and fragments into shame, anxiety, and when the deficit grows large enough, depression.

The cure is clear: more people, less screen. Simple. Easy physically, but maybe not so easy emotionally. Here is another place a good therapist can help sort out priorities and work with subtle ways you may be avoiding relationships as a way to avoid the anxiety of contact.

Conclusion. The profundities of the psyche revealed by the different schools of psychology, the dark night of the soul, and spiritual practices point to a different way of relating to depression's pain. These encourage the person to open to it rather than avoid it, to discover its deeper meaning. The quest is to find out, "What is the significance of this depression?" By entering into deeper relationship with it, depression can then reveal itself.

The depressed patient is likely to reply to this by saying, "What? I'm already drowning in the depression. I need to keep it as far away as I can, and even then I'm already overwhelmed by it. Opening to it sounds like disaster."

It turns out that nearly all the depressed patients I've worked with were indeed drowning in it, but they had turned away from it. They were resisting it with everything they had, but it was pulling them under, and the more they struggled to break free of it, the more it dragged them down.

A shift happened when they stopped resisting it. In turning and facing it, letting themselves float downstream and surrender to the darkness, they entered into a new relationship with their depression. This critical shift allowed them to sense into and inquire into their depression.

Paradoxically, when they stopped resisting it, stopped judging themselves for being depressed and accepted the painful feelings, they usually felt better. They weren't immediately cured, of course, but they realized that resisting their depression only added to the pain. As the saying goes, "Pain times resistance equals suffering." Letting go into depression's pain and exploring it allows the person to investigate the self's depths.

Establishing a relationship with the pain, learning to better tolerate it, is an individual process of experimentation, best done with a therapist. Some people prefer to sense their pain from a distance and lean into it. Others prefer to identify with the pain completely and "become it" as their way of exploring it. However close or far, engaging with the darkness begins to illuminate it.

The faith that helps support this is understanding that depression is meaningful. No matter how meaningless it appears at first, there is a deeper or higher self, a more authentic or truer self that is emerging through this pain. As terrible as the dark night of depression is, there is a greater dawn awaiting. The psyche moves naturally in the direction of healing and wholeness when we stop resisting it and harmonize with its greater movement.

The Physical Side of Depression

For depression there are important tweaks to the basic plan outlined in the Healthy Brain Diet in Chapter 2. There are specific nutrients, supplements, strains of bacteria, and forms of exercise that must be emphasized for their specific role in helping depression. These are detailed in Appendix D. This contains important information that anyone who is depressed should read.

Why Medication Is Rarely the Answer

The "serotonin deficiency" theory of depression has been pretty well discarded by the research community. But doctors and patients are so well indoctrinated in the serotonin deficiency theory, and since old paradigms in science die slowly, it will probably be at least another twenty years before this one fades away.

Remember, most studies show depressed patients have normal levels of serotonin, while some studies show higher than normal levels and only a few show lower. New understandings of the brain reveal that low levels of neurogenesis and neuroplasticity are involved in depression. Low rates of neurogenesis and neuroplasticity are associated with depression, while high rates reverse and protect against depression. [28] SSRIs and other antidepressants work by stimulating neurogenesis and neuroplasticity, though only to a limited degree. I believe the neurogenic-enhancing program offered here is more natural and robust.

An experiment that proved to be one of the final nails in the coffin of the serotonin deficiency theory was done by Luca Santarelli, Ph.D., at the Columbia University lab of Rene Hen, Ph.D. Santarelli increased serotonin levels in depressed mice but prevented neurogenesis from occurring. There was no change in depression, even with elevated serotonin levels. Only when neurogenesis and neuroplasticity rates were increased did the depression lift. The level of serotonin was not relevant, rather it was the rate of neurogenesis that was determinative. [29]

This study has been replicated, as have similar studies in which the progenitor cells involved with neurogenesis are ablated (which prevents increased neurogenesis and neuroplasticity), showing that increasing serotonin levels via SSRIs has no effect on depression. [30] According to the authors, such studies show that "the behavioural effects of chronic antidepressants require hippocampal neurogenesis and are mediated by an increased synaptic plasticity ..."

From a neurogenic perspective, a depressed brain is a sluggish brain. The brain's movement can be increased by enhancing neurogenesis and the rate at which it creates new neural connections, restores health and emotional resilience. When this is done by aligning with the brain's natural mechanisms, it avoids medication's side effects.

As mentioned earlier, antidepressants also come with a host of side effects, including loss of sex drive, weight gain, brain fog, memory problems, insomnia, suicide, and violence. They are effective less than half the time (about 44% or less in most studies), only slightly more effective than placebo. The NIMH-sponsored trials of the mid-2000s revealed only a 30% response rate after one year, half as effective as previously thought.

Psychiatrist Dr. Peter Breggin, author of *Talking Back to Prozac* and *Medication Madness,* believes that medication simply masks the symptoms of depression and that antidepressants are "about as good as a placebo ... there is no promising medical treatment [for depression]." [31]

Although most of the research shows that depressed patients do not have lower serotonin levels, depressed patients do have lower levels of BDNF, the brain growth factor most involved in neurogenesis and neuroplasticity. BDNF levels rise as depression lifts. BDNF levels are so tied to depression that they have been proposed as a marker for severity of depression. [32] Gene expression is also altered in depression, and the main genes that are disrupted in depression code for brain growth factors such as BDNF and fibroblast growth factor-2. [33]

This lowered neural movement and neurogenic capacity in depression led researcher Dr. Huda Akil to remark, "We came to realize that depressed people have lost their power to remodel their brains. And that is in fact devastating because brain remodeling is something we need to do all the time." [34]

Lower BDNF levels are also associated with cognitive decline. And there is an association between depression and cognitive decline. [35, 36]

As explained in Chapter 2, chronic inflammation lowers neurogenesis. One study showed that even chronic intestinal inflammation lowered neurogenesis. As the authors describe in their abstract, "Adult neurogenesis ... is involved in learning, memory, and mood control. Decreased hippocampal neurogenesis elicits significant behavioral changes, including cognitive impairment and depression." [37]

As the first chapter explains, fiddling with levels of one or two neurotransmitters out of over fifty mood-regulating brain chemicals (in continuous feedback loops that upregulate and downregulate in response to changes in one, and with multiple redundancies) is woefully simplistic. Serotonin receptors are downregulated in response to SSRI use, and this is one reason getting off antidepressants can be so difficult. Prescribing a solution (increased serotonin) for an imaginary problem (serotonin deficiency) throws a wrench into the brain's enormously complex gears.

It's possible that in a few decades we will look back on these early days of pounding the brain with powerful, blunt-force psychiatric drugs with the same astonishment as we now view lobotomy or bloodletting.

This book proposes a radically different approach: Restore the brain by harnessing its own intrinsic healing power; stimulate neurogenic capacity by increasing BDNF levels, neurogenesis, and neuroplasticity naturally; and in the process strengthen the general health of the brain.

The general strategy is to heal and strengthen a brain weakened by poor diet and toxic environmental poisons. Diet is the first step to build up the brain. It is important to discover if there are neurotoxins that need to be detoxed, together with avoiding further exposure. Other physical factors also play important roles.

For antidepressant supplements and tweaks to the Healthy Brain Diet, exercise and other physical factors that are specific to depression, be sure to read Appendix D, The Physical Side of Depression,

Conclusion

As with anxiety, for some people depression is mainly physical—a weakened brain suffering from inadequate nutrition or a toxic load—and physical healing and strengthening is needed. For others psychological work to heal and strengthen the self is what's most needed. For most, both are optimal for healing.

CHAPTER 5

HOLISTIC HEALING FOR COGNITIVE DECLINE

A tidal wave is coming. The rise of cognitive decline, mild cognitive impairment, Alzheimer's, and other dementias is just beginning. While Alzheimer's was relatively rare a hundred years ago, currently one in three seniors currently dies with some form of dementia. Soon, half of all eighty-five-year-olds will have Alzheimer's. Since most people can now expect to live to eighty-five, that gives you a fifty-fifty chance of developing Alzheimer's.

Women get Alzheimer's at twice the rate of men (two-thirds of Alzheimer's patients are women). African-Americans have double the rate of whites and Latinos have about one and half times this rate.

If there was a cure or a drug to prevent this, it wouldn't be so scary. Unfortunately, Alzheimer's is the only major disease for which there is currently no cure, no treatment and medically approved way to slow its progression..

As an article in the journal *Neurology* put it,

> "Despite great scientific efforts to find treatments for Alzheimer's disease, only 5 medications are marketed, with limited beneficial effects on symptoms, on a limited number of patients, without modification of the disease course. The prevalence of Alzheimer's disease doubles every 5 years, reaching an alarming rate of 50% in those aged 85 or older." [1]

Wait, it gets worse. A recent meta-analysis of ten studies involving over 2,700 patients showed that the two main classes of drugs currently being used to treat Alzheimer's actually hasten cognitive decline. The study's authors report that those receiving the cholinesterase inhibitors and memantine had a "significantly greater annual rate of decline" than those not taking any medication. [2] This study shows that the very medications currently being used to treat symptoms of Alzheimer's actually make things worse, hastening the very thing they are supposed to stop.

As pointed out before, pharmaceutical companies have spent billions of dollars trying to find the "magic bullet" for cognitive decline and Alzheimer's. Hundreds of clinical trials have been run in this effort to discover the next patentable, blockbuster drug. The failure rate has been total. Nothing has been successful.

Science follows the money as surely as flowers follow the sun. When the economic model rests on creating drugs that can be patented, this shapes the entire field. Without research dollars to support it, science doesn't grow in the direction of natural, non-patentable nutrients, even when these show great promise.

What if Mother Nature has already provided what we need to heal the brain? What if nature's bounty of plants and nutrients could stimulate the innate intelligence of the body to do what these drugs are supposed to do? After all, the body has far, far greater wisdom to heal itself than any drug company.

Luckily, there are a few nonprofit centers doing research along more holistic lines, both in the U.S. and Europe. One of these is the Buck Institute for Aging in California. Researchers there have been able to reverse the cognitive decline associated with Alzheimer's. This research shows that success has come from natural remedies and a lifestyle approach. That protocol primarily consists of many of the things in this chapter, though it fails to include much of this chapter's nutritional information and gives much less attention to the psychological side than this book does.

Other research centers doing cutting-edge nutritional, psychological, and neuroscience research fill out the picture much more fully. A diet and lifestyle along the lines of this book activates the anti-aging genes, clears toxic brain buildup, and stimulates the brain's repair and renewal capacities. The idea is to work with the brain, not against it.

The brain, as previously stated, is incalculably complex. With its multiple feedback loops and redundant protective mechanisms, its vast number of interacting and mutually regulating neurotransmitters, hormones, and neuropeptides, the belief that a single drug will inhibit one particular neurotransmitter and solve the problem is hopelessly naïve.

In contrast, the holistic approach of this book enlists the body's own immense potential to heal. By working with the brain and body, by supplying nutrients and natural herbs that help stimulate the brain's intrinsic detoxification and neurogenic abilities, we unleash the organism's intelligence to heal the brain.

Will you hear about this from most physicians? No, because medical education is focused on drugs, not nutrition, and most medical education material and advertising is developed by drug companies, not blueberry farmers.

A holistic approach, because it is based on natural, non-patentable nutrients, will take time to develop into the fullness of what's possible. If a natural remedy "moon shot" were funded along these lines, even greater success would come much sooner. If only …

What is cognitive decline, or Alzheimer's?

There is a difference between cognitive decline, mild cognitive impairment, and Alzheimer's and other dementias.

Cognitive decline begins when certain types of memory become harder to retrieve. Names are often the first thing to go due to their arbitrary nature. Certain things like fluid intelligence decline slightly, while others, such as crystallized intelligence, empathy, impulse control, don't reach peak performance levels until well into the fifties and sixties. This is why we want fighter pilots to be in their twenties or thirties but politicians and wise elders to be in late middle age and beyond.

Mild cognitive impairment (MCI) is the term used to describe the intermediate stage between cognitive decline and the dramatic decline of dementia. Over 90% of people diagnosed with MCI progress to Alzheimer's or other dementias within ten years if they live that long. The conversion rate is 10–15% per year, depending upon the study. [3] Sometimes other conditions are diagnosed so that, when these clear up, the MCI is resolved, but MCI is generally the first step in a progression to Alzheimer's.

MCI shows itself as problems with language, memory, thinking, and judgment. The most common form of MCI is memory loss, called amnestic MCI. This form is usually degenerative and leads to Alzheimer's.

Dementia comes from the Latin "de" ("without") and "mens" ("mind"), and it literally means "without mind," or the overall loss of cognitive functions and mental abilities.

Dementia comes in different forms. The most common is Alzheimer's, which comprises 60–80% of dementias. Other common types are: Lewy body dementia, vascular dementia, Parkinson's disease dementia, Huntington's disease, and mixed dementia.

Memory loss is most common and usually the first symptom. Memory plays a central role in cognitive abilities and your sense of self. Memory is necessary for most all higher cognitive functions, such as executive function, working memory, fluid and crystallized intelligence, even emotion regulation.

Memory holds together your sense of "self" so you have the experience of being a person who is continuous in time and space. In Alzheimer's disease, as memory fades, the whole sense of self crumbles. In interacting with an Alzheimer's patient, there is often a sense that he or she isn't "all there." Without memory, the personality shrinks to a ghost of its former self, and the patient can seem childlike and undeveloped.

There are seven stages of cognitive decline in the progression to Alzheimer's.

Stage 1 is normal cognitive function (no impairment or memory loss).

Stage 2 is very mild cognitive decline, also called "normal aged forgetfulness." There are "senior moments" but no impairments in daily life.

Stage 3 is mild decline or early confusion, the first stage of MCI.

Stage 4 is moderate decline or late confusion. Early symptoms of Alzheimer's disease begin to show. Routine things like banking or shopping become overwhelming.

Stage 5 is moderately severe decline or mid-stage Alzheimer's. The person needs help with everyday tasks such as dressing properly for the season or occasion.

Stage 6 is severe cognitive decline or mid-stage Alzheimer's. Here people tend to wander and get lost, forget much of their own personal histories and may have a hard time remembering the names of their spouses or children.

Stage 7 is very severe cognitive decline or late-stage Alzheimer's. At this final stage of deterioration patients lose awareness of their environment and are unable to have a conversation.

The development of MCI and Alzheimer's is tragic. Conventional views are that once this begins, nothing can be done to stop or slow it. Like a person falling off a cliff, once cognitive decline progresses to MCI, the downward momentum is inevitable if the person lives long enough. However, recent research shows this conventional view is incorrect. Many people can recover fully or much of their cognitive capacity if they make the right lifestyle choices.

The sooner you take responsibility for your brain's health and change your diet and lifestyle to support rather than damage it, the better. Remember, the brain changes in MCI and Alzheimer's begin decades before symptoms emerge. The adage "an ounce of prevention is worth a pound of cure" is nowhere so true as here.

What brings cognitive decline and dementia?

This is the million-dollar question. Closely related is: What is healthy aging, and what produces unhealthy aging? Increasingly, it's clear that lifestyle is the key.

In healthy aging, the body and brain maintain a balance between damage and repair to keep most diseases at bay. There is a certain amount of atrophy, but it's not yet clear how much can be prevented. Inevitably there is decline as damage slowly outruns the body's ability to repair, but this decline is gradual.

When people remain engaged, active, optimally nourished, and exercise their abilities, their muscles, organs, brain, and cognition stay at relatively high levels well into advanced age. However, when people eat poorly, become sedentary, or hardly use their bodies or brains, decline sets in rapidly.

The brain has a remarkable ability to withstand decline for a long time compared to other bodily systems when it's well cared for. Nevertheless, given the neurotoxic world in which we live, the brain is under continual assault and often degrades faster than it should. Additionally, certain types of assaults appear to bring about brain diseases such as Alzheimer's, Parkinson's, and other kinds of dementias.

Aging is a result of many factors, such as: glycation and accumulating cross-links (AGES), rising inflammation and a declining immune system, buildup of amyloid between cells (in the brain and other organs), rising genetic damage and mutations, lower levels of neurotrophic factors such as BDNF, declining autophagy and lysosomal activity (which removes toxic waste), the buildup of senescent cells (which produce toxic material and inflammation), and other things not yet understood. As this damage accrues, sooner or later it results in things like cancer, heart disease, diabetes, or other diseases that finally result in death.

One approach of this book is to reduce the speed at which these factors affect the body and brain and increase the cleanup and recycling of damaged cells.

This book's second approach is to increase the body's and brain's capacity for healing and regeneration. This means raising and maintaining a high level of neurogenic activity. Reduced neurogenesis is a hallmark of aging across species. Only recently has it been discovered how to increase the brain's neurogenic rate, which this book details. Further, in Alzheimer's, neurogenesis rates fall even more. In a July 2019 paper, the rate of neurogenesis was proposed as an early biomarker of the disease. [4]

Another 2019 study showed that in brains of people with an average age of 90.6 years, neurogenesis was occurring, although at a significantly lower rate in those with cognitive decline and Alzheimer's. In contrast, those who scored higher on cognitive tests had higher rates of neurogenesis. The researchers commented, "***if we can find a way to enhance neurogenesis, through a small molecule, for example,*** **we may be able to slow or prevent cognitive decline in older adults,** especially when it starts, which is when interventions can be most effective." [5, 6] (Emphasis added.)

Well, guess what? As every reader knows by now, there already are already *numerous* molecules that enhance neurogenesis, detailed in Chapter 2. However, since they are naturally occurring, they can't be patented and marketed by pharmaceutical companies, so they aren't widely known. Hence this book.

The goal is to keep cognition and the brain sharp, operating at a high level into advanced old age with only negligible declines. This means preventing or reversing significant cognitive decline and the mild cognitive impairment that leads to Alzheimer's or other dementia.

Current theories about Alzheimer's

Two of the most prominent brain changes in Alzheimer's are the accumulation of amyloid plaques *outside* neurons and the accumulation of abnormal tau protein tangles *inside* neurons. Amyloid plaques kill neurons by interfering with brain cell communication at the synapses, while tau tangles destroy neurons by blocking nutrients and other essential molecules inside neurons. As beta-amyloid accumulates, a critical level is reached where abnormal tau spreads throughout the brain. The tau neurofibrillary tangles cause most of the damage in Alzheimer's, after accumulating amyloid plaques have started damaging the brain.

The amyloid theory. The most well-known is the amyloid theory, as the buildup of amyloid plaques is a hallmark of Alzheimer's. This has been the focus of the most intensive research, but until recently it has been a universal failure. Dozens of trials have ended in disappointment after removing amyloid plaques failed to reverse or slow degeneration in Alzheimer's patients. More recently, however, there has been some success with amyloid-clearing drug trials at earlier stages of the disease, so the amyloid theory has gained new life.

Amyloid beta has important health functions for the brain and body, including antioxidant activity, modulation of synaptic plasticity, neurogenesis, and other neurotrophic activity. The healthy brain regulates amyloid production so it doesn't accumulate, but this fails in Alzheimer's, and the brain overproduces it. The overproduction of amyloid in the brain is thought by many to be part of the brain's attempt at healing itself gone awry.

Current thinking is that as the brain tries to repair itself through increased amyloid production, this failed effort results in amyloid accumulation. The accumulated amyloid sets the stage for later production of tau neurofibrillary tangles, which do most of the damage. The failure of amyloid-clearing drugs in the later stages of Alzheimer's is probably too little too late, so tactics have shifted to trying to clear amyloid earlier in the process.

Two major strategies to deal with excess amyloid are *preventing* amyloid beta fragments from aggregating and *clearing* aggregates after they've formed. Prevention involves keeping certain brain signals either high or low. Increasing a substance called alpha secretase keeps amyloid levels low, but so does decreasing levels of beta and gamma secretase. A number of natural substances that either increase alpha secretase or decrease beta or gamma secretase are detailed later in the Diet section.

Clearing away amyloids that have already accumulated (taking out the garbage) means ingesting nutrients that can rid the body of this excess. There are a number of natural substances and nutrients that are listed in the Diet section.

The tau theory. Neurofibrillary tangles are twisted fibers inside brain cells, formed primarily of tau, which is part of a structure called a microtubule. Microtubules transport nutrients and other substances from one part of a neuron to another. In Alzheimer's, the tau becomes highly phosphorylated, causing the microtubule to collapse, which then becomes highly toxic to brain cells. Tau is responsible for most of the destruction in Alzheimer's. It is the synergistic interaction between amyloid and tau which predicts progression to dementia. [7]

The number of neurofibrillary tangles is tightly linked to the degree of dementia. [8] Recent research has shown that while tau tangles cause great damage, the mere presence of tau proteins suppresses neural activity. The synergistic effects of tau and amyloid work to multiply the destructive effects beyond either one alone. [9] Strategies to prevent the hyperphosphorylation of tau or removing highly phosphorylated tau are the two main strategies being pursued. A number of natural plants have this effect, and several do double duty as neurogenic substances. These are described later in the Diet section.

Low levels of acetylcholine. The neurotransmitter acetylcholine is centrally involved in memory. Low levels of acetylcholine have been noted in Alzheimer's patients. The main drugs used in medicine today are those that target a brain chemical that inhibits acetylcholine. These drugs, called "cholinesterase inhibitors," have FDA approval and are being taken by millions of patients. Yet recent research shows that these drugs (such as Aricept) not only don't work, they actively make the problem worse by increasing the rate of cognitive decline. [2]

By working with the brain, however, the body can naturally and safely produce more acetylcholine though its own mechanisms. There are a number of natural substances that do this described in the Diet section.

Excess glutamate. Glutamate is the major excitatory neurotransmitter in the brain. Too much or prolonged excitation is toxic to neurons. Problems with glutamate reuptake and recycling in Alzheimer's result in early cell death. Memantine is a medical drug that blocks overstimulation of receptors by glutamate that could lead to excitotoxicity in Alzheimer's. Unfortunately, here again, research shows that the drugs that do this exacerbate the problem and speed up cognitive decline. [2]

There are, however, natural ways to calm neural overstimulation that do not block glutamate receptors. See Chapter 3, "Holistic Healing of Anxiety."

Toxicity. Brain performance declines swiftly in the presence of neurotoxins. Heavy metals such as mercury, lead, arsenic as well as mycotoxins in the form of mold can produce symptoms that look like Alzheimer's. Since cognitive impairment is due to toxins rather than brain damage, this is more properly referred to as an

"Alzheimer's mimic" condition, though it often is diagnosed as Alzheimer's. If treated there can be complete recovery.

Inflammation. By now every reader understands that chronic inflammation is behind most major diseases and is highly damaging to the brain. Studies show that cognitive decline is directly linked to levels of inflammation. [10] One study showed that mid-life (average age fifty-three) inflammation levels indicated twenty-four years later the degree of cognitive decline and brain shrinkage, especially in the hippocampus (memory and emotion regulation) and other key brain centers. Even inflammation in the gut decreases neurogenesis and "elicits significant behavioral changes, including cognitive impairment and depression." [11] Reducing levels of inflammation is key to both preventing and reversing cognitive decline.

Infections. The body's and brain's attempts to fight off infections can cause an overproduction of amyloid. Common infections that can cause this are: herpes virus 1 and 2, cytomegalovirus (CMV), chlamydia, helicobacter pylori, Lyme disease, and chronic gum disease. Amyloid accumulates and tau becomes hyperphosphorylated as the brain struggles to deal with these infections. By treating these infections directly, symptoms of cognitive decline can improve.

Insulin resistance. Alzheimer's is often called "type 3 diabetes." A failure of glucose metabolism in the brain produces glycation, higher levels of blood sugar and insulin, as well as inflammation. This cascade of higher glucose, insulin, and inflammation wreaks havoc in the brain. In response, the brain overproduces amyloid and tau, and this doomed attempt at repair brings further brain cell destruction in its wake.

One of the best predictors of cognitive decline is a person's blood sugar levels. The higher the glucose level, the faster the rate of cognitive decline. [12, 13] Not only is cognitive decline directly tied to blood sugar levels, so is the size of brain's memory center (the hippocampus). Higher glucose levels are directly related to both brain shrinkage, or atrophy, as well as cognitive decline.

Even mildly elevated glucose levels, those that most physicians believe are "normal" and well below prediabetic levels, were shown to be correlated directly with failing memory and smaller brain size. [13]

As the researchers put it, even in the absence of "diabetes or impaired glucose tolerance, chronically higher glucose levels exert a negative influence on cognition."

This is yet another reason why knowing your HbA1c level is critical. This blood test shows your blood sugar level over the past three months. Anything above 5.2 should be corrected with the dietary changes recommended in this book.

So Many Theories, What to Do?

Since all of these theories have evidence to support them, it may well be there is truth in each. Increasingly, Alzheimer's is viewed not as a single disease but, like cancer, a collection of several different disease processes at work. There are different types of Alzheimer's, just as there are different types of cancer. In any one person there may be one or more types active.

There is more to healthy brain aging, however, than preventing or reversing cognitive decline. The goal is radiant brain health throughout your life span, well into old age. Get and stay sharp for as long as possible. The strategy of this book is to avoid the main causes of cognitive decline and Alzheimer's while you strengthen your brain and mental abilities.

Preventing and reversing cognitive decline

Since cognitive decline so often affects the hippocampus and reduces both neurogenesis and synaptogenesis, having the brain's growth and remodeling in an optimal range is mission critical. A study in the *Journal of Neuroscience* in 2019 showed that in genetic forms of Alzheimer's, neurogenesis is disrupted. When neurogenesis was returned to normal, the mice were fine, didn't show any memory deficits or signs of anxiety. [14]

This chapter looks at the many different factors that bring about cognitive decline and works to: increase neurogenic slowing, enhance the brain's metabolic and energetic functioning, reduce inflammation, heal the gut and blood-brain barrier, detoxify and regenerate the brain, work on the many mental and psychological factors involved in order to reverse this trend.

What if you're experiencing cognitive decline and anxious or depressed?

If you're experiencing cognitive decline, it is likely that you are or soon will feel anxiety and depression. A weakened, damaged, or shrinking hippocampus is a common link between cognition and the regulation of anxiety and depression. Read all sections of the book that apply to you.

The Psychological Side of Cognitive Decline

So much of cognitive decline is talked about from the physical side that it's easy to overlook the great importance of the psychological side. Given the medical slant to much of the popular literature, this is understandable, for physicians are trained to look to physical causes for disease states.

Only in the past few decades has research shown just how important psychological factors are in fostering disease. The field of psychoneuroimmunology shows, for example, the ways stress affects the body and paves the way for so many diseases, including heart disease, type 2 diabetes, autoimmune disorders, and inflammation, which is behind most every major disease.

Yet as this book points out endlessly, the physical and psychological are two sides of a single whole. When it comes to the mind and cognitive health, psychological factors loom large. These bring about either cognitive decline or cognitive enhancement, and a complete understanding of cognition must include both the physical and the psychological.

First we look at psychological factors—emotional, mental, spiritual—that play a significant role in either eroding memory or keeping the mind sharp.

The Emotional Level

Feeling good is both a cause and effect of a healthy brain. When you feel good, the brain comes alive and the neurogenic rate rises. Conversely, when your brain is working at a high level, you feel good. Emotional health and brain health go together.

How you feel impacts your brain

Good feelings—of contentment, peace and calm, love and caring—produce coherent brain waves and increase both neurogenesis and neuroplasticity, as well as lowering inflammation and creating a better intestinal environment. The brain functions best in positive emotional states.

When you feel good, contented and excited to be alive, you think clearly and lucidly. Your immune system hums along nicely, you easily shrug off small upsets and bounce back fairly quickly from big ones. Emotional health doesn't mean always feeling good, rather it's feeling whatever life hands us with a certain optimism and resilience.

Emotional well-being allows your brain to operate at peak performance. Feeling good activates your higher brain centers so you can utilize all the creativity and higher executive functioning of the prefrontal cortex.

On the other hand, when you feel chronically stressed, anxious, ashamed, lonely, or depressed, such feelings degrade the brain and cognition. Negative feelings—of anxiety, stress, depression, shame, anger—have the opposite effect. The incoherent brain waves produced in chronic negative states lower thinking ability and neurogenic rates, while inflammation rises and gut permeability increases. The brain deadens.

These painful emotional states alter brain function so the lower neural circuits get activated, such as the more primitive centers of fight-flight-freeze in the lower reptilian brain, the amygdala, and emotional limbic system.

Glucocorticoids flood the nervous system, which are toxic to brain cells over time. Inflammatory levels rise and attack neurons, resulting in more oxidation and brain fog. Blood glucose and insulin levels rise, creating more inflammation, impairing thinking ability, and hastening cognitive decline. Blood flow shifts the mind to more reactive, repetitious loops of thinking and rumination. This leads to less skillful actions, which in turn increase stress and fear in a negative feedback loop that furthers the downward spiral. As the brain goes downhill, cognition follows.

On the emotional level, the two most important factors are:

- how you feel
- the quality of your relationships

There is a strong relationship between these two things, for how you feel is influenced by your relationships, just as your relationships are impacted by how you feel.

Stress shrinks your brain and impairs memory

Research confirms that stress causes cognitive impairment through a number of different neural mechanisms: Glutamate receptor expression is suppressed, glucocorticoids are neurotoxic and actually kill brain cells, inflammation rises, the brain shrinks, and hippocampal atrophy occurs as neurogenic capacity reduces. [15]

Chapter 4 explains more fully the effects of stress, anxiety, and fear on the brain, including research linking elevated cortisol levels to brain shrinkage, memory impairment, and early onset of Alzheimer's. Harvard Medical School's lead researcher, Dr. Echouffo-Tcheugui, noted his study found elevated cortisol levels produced "memory loss and brain shrinkage in middle-aged people before symptoms started to show in ordinary, daily activities." [16]

By now there is an enormous body of research showing how anxiety, stress, and fear bring about cognitive decline. One study shows people with mild cognitive impairment and high anxiety were 135% more likely to develop Alzheimer's. Another study in *JAMA Psychiatry* shows how anxiety combines with other changes in the brain to accelerate cognitive decline. [17, 18]

One of the most important things for your brain is to get a break from stress and allow your nervous system to reset. When the sympathetic nervous system is overactive, rapid cognitive decline follows. Discovering ways to find peace and calmness by activating your parasympathetic nervous system lets your body find its homeostatic balance once again. Your brain and body enter repair mode rather than continually wearing themselves out by always being on high alert.

It's important to read Chapter 4, "Holistic Healing of Anxiety," to learn just how to deal with stress in ways that optimize your brain rather than fry it. This involves finding the optimal degree of stress, the Goldilocks zone of stress, where you are optimally challenged, neither overstimulated nor understimulated.

Negative feeling states are signs you aren't getting what you need, that life is out of balance. Becoming bored and understimulated is just as great a danger to cognition as stressful overstimulation. Are there interests or life ambitions that aren't being fulfilled? Is your growth blocked in some way? Has life become too comfortable and you're no longer engaged? Are there old disappointments or losses that haven't been assimilated? This is an area where therapy can be of great benefit to discover what needs aren't being met.

The quality of your relationships

One of the most important elements of both feeling good and staying sharp is social engagement. We are relational beings. Social stimulation keeps the mind active and tuned in to a whole host of subtle emotional cues. Not only are nurturing relationships essential for feeling good, they're necessary for maintaining good cognitive function.

There are two types of relationship dangers related to cognitive decline:

- loneliness
- toxic relationships

Too little relationship degrades the brain. Without enough social stimulation, the brain loses mental capacity. What's important, however, is not just the quantity of relationships but their quality.

Beyond Loneliness to Aloneness

Aloneness is a state of being, being comfortable in your own skin. In aloneness you can connect with yourself more deeply. By contacting yourself more fully there is a psychic renewal that can't come any other way. Constant contact with others can block the inner channels of self-awareness by which the self is nourished through contacting its own deeper source.

One of the great gifts of meditation and spiritual practices is that they open up the interior spaces of the psyche and are a kind of training in how to be alone. In opening to the inner depths of your subjective awareness, you encounter new sources of peace, joy, love, inspiration, creativity, and contentment.

Such a state of aloneness is very different from the more common experience of loneliness. Loneliness is a deficiency state, an inner sense of deprivation that comes with insufficient contact or not fitting in with people around you. All human beings require a good deal of loving, nourishing interaction with others, continually, throughout the life span. Loneliness is a sign your interpersonal needs aren't being met.

It's the subjective experience of feeling lonely that's key. This means it's the quality of your relationships that's important, not the quantity. A person can have many social contacts yet still feel lonely, just as it's possible to feel nourished by a few, high-quality relationships and feel alone, not lonely.

Isolation and loneliness bring cognitive decline. Loneliness is associated with a 40% increase in dementia risk in one study. [19] Another study followed participants over a twelve-year period and showed those who were lonely experienced 20% faster cognitive decline than other participants. [20]

Forty-six percent of Americans say they feel lonely sometimes or always. In older adults the figure is higher. More than one-third of Americans over fifty live by themselves. Loneliness affects cardiovascular health equivalent to smoking fifteen cigarettes a day and is associated with premature death. The toll on the brain and mind is equally strong.

An earlier study showed that people who felt lonely had more than double the risk of developing Alzheimer's compared to those who didn't. [21] Loneliness was connected to lower cognitive scores and more rapid cognitive decline. Feeling lonely is also associated with other unhealthy behaviors linked to dementia, such as excessive drinking and not exercising.

A strong social network of good friends is protective against memory loss. One study revealed having a good support system of friends had significant benefits on memory later in life, much more so than networks that consisted only of children or relatives. [22] As the researchers noted:

> "Social networks are the basis of social engagement, which is cognitively stimulating and may enhance neural plasticity in aging, thereby maintaining cognitive reserve. Thus, better social networks might lead to continued psychological stimulation, delaying cognitive decline or impairment."

So strong is the relationship between loneliness and cognitive decline that one study declared loneliness to be one of the precursors of dementia. The study's authors say, "Feelings of loneliness may signal a prodromal stage of dementia." [23]

Strong social networks are one of the very few constants in studies of so-called Blue Zones, that is, areas or cultures that have an unusually large number of centenarians, people who live over a hundred years. Centenarians in these cultures are embedded in a web of relationships with family and neighbors. They are viewed as important, contributing members of their communities, shown respect and given recognition for their contributions. How can such mirroring and affirmation fail to enhance health and cognition?

The other thing people in these areas have in common is ongoing exercise. Many of these people walk three to five miles daily as part of their normal life. Or they have daily chores of working in the garden, washing, cooking, and other forms of physical activity. None of them are sedentary. Physical activity together with active social engagement are two keys to keeping your brain sharp.

No matter what your age, though particularly if you're older, finding ways to reach out and establish ongoing, satisfying relationships is essential. As a person ages, it becomes more difficult to meet new people or make new friends, since these relationships most often are formed through work or school. It takes an active effort.

Exploring your interests takes you to events, places, and situations where you can find like-minded others. Try new things; accept social invitations, learn new skills by taking a class, or join a sports team, a hiking or nature or church group—wherever your interests lie, there are potential friends to be found.

This is another area where psychotherapy can help. Oftentimes the resistances to relationship are invisible. You don't see or even feel the anxiety that comes in opening up to others because it all operates unconsciously. Because of past wounding in relationships, a person erects barriers to protect against future hurts. It's very difficult to override these inner protections alone. Whereas with a trusted guide, these old wounds can be healed and the inner barriers lowered. The wounding that occurred in relationship can only be healed in relationship, with a therapeutic relationship providing the space for new emotional learning.

Toxic relationships are toxic to your brain

While the lack of relationships is one side of the relational aspect of cognitive decline, the wrong kind of relationships is the other. Being in relationships that are angry, scary, bullying, demeaning, shaming, or coercive is toxic to the brain. There is a large body of research to show that each of these kinds of relationships produce stress hormones such as glucocorticoids that shrink the brain, slow neurogenic activity, increase inflammation, and reduce memory.

Even having relationships that aren't bad but merely chronically superficial is toxic, for everyone needs deep intimacy, love, confirmation, and affirmation. Genuine intimacy means deeply sharing true, emotional sides of yourself with people who love and value you for who you authentically are (not just the role you play or the image you project). When you aren't seen and affirmed for you are, the self fragments, generally into anxiety, shame, and inadequacy.

Toxic relationships abound in this society. Overbearing bosses on power trips, angry co-workers, scary relatives, bullying classmates or teammates or colleagues, hostile so-called friends, rage-aholic in-laws, emotional vampires that feed on your good feelings, narcissistic clients, the list is endless. They all produce stress, but not the good kind.

One way to reliably produce anxiety, stress, depression, and cognitive decline in a mouse is to put it in a cage with a big bully mouse that bites it, pins it down, and dominates it. After an initial period of freaking out, the subordinate mouse becomes deeply depressed and slumps over, unresponsive to other stimuli. It's called a "social defeat" model of depression. And depression leads directly to brain shrinkage and cognitive decline. The longer the depression, the greater the cortical loss.

One of the goals of therapy is increase nourishing relationships and let go of toxic relationships. Cutting off toxic relationships and surrounding yourself with loving, supportive people is one of the surest ways to feeling better. Here again therapy can help navigate this process.

Unfortunately, no one can live entirely free of annoying people. Sometimes a person marries into a dysfunctional, toxic family that must be tolerated at times. A person can't always quit a job due to a boss who delights in demeaning subordinates. A bullying team member can't always be avoided.

In these cases, it's important to get a break from such relationships, just as with stress. It's necessary to spend time with other people who do care about you and can empathize with your difficulty. Nourishing relationships are the antidote to toxic relationships. Just as toxic relationships reduce neurogenic capacity and increase inflammation, positive relationships stimulate neurogenesis and neuroplasticity and reduce inflammation.

Love is neurogenic

One of the greatest discoveries of neuroscience is that love is neurogenic. Love produces oxytocin in the brain, which stimulates neurogenesis and neuroplasticity. [24] Love also is calming and anti-stress. When stress goes down, neurogenesis, neuroplasticity, and cognition go up. Neuroscience confirms what spiritual traditions, poets, and philosophers have said for millennia: We thrive in love. The brain thrives in love, too.

Emotional health and brain health are linked. Chronically feeling bad damages brain function and cognition. Conversely, poor brain health produces negative, painful emotional states. Improving one helps the other, though this doesn't necessarily fix the problem with the other.

Generally, life and relationships run on automatic. Paying attention to how you feel and the quality of your relationships brings the power to change. Changing your emotional and relationship patterns is an essential part of the holistic healing of cognitive decline.

The Mental Level

When your brain is sharp, you think well—lucidly, logically, creatively. There is a clarity that comes when your mind and brain function well. Your thinking is flexible and dynamic, not rigid or narrow. You remember what you need to remember, problem-solving comes easily, and you perceive situations and people without distortion.

The program of preventing and reversing cognitive decline in this book is about more than just stopping a downhill slide. Rather, it's about cognitive enhancement, bringing your mind up to its highest level.

Remember, measurable cognitive decline appears at two points in life, after graduation from college and after retirement. That's due to lack of cognitive stimulation. Before despairing, remember the other part of the study that showed with mental stimulation at these two points, cognitive decline didn't occur. It was the lack of mental stimulation that brought about cognitive decline,

One of the most insidious things about retirement is having nothing to do. A senior who spends the day watching TV and little else will experience cognitive decline quite rapidly. Just like a muscle that atrophies when not used, the brain needs ongoing stimulation to thrive. However, even after protracted neglect, mental stimulation picks the brain up again.

> *Hal had looked forward to retiring for ten years before he was eligible. After he did retire, he spent the next five years watching TV and playing golf with some buddies. Although he enjoyed golf, he found himself getting bored with his life. In addition, he found his memory was deteriorating much faster than he thought it should. This worried him.*
>
> *Hal hadn't enjoyed being a student in school. His mind would wander, and he never seemed to have the aptitude for book learning. He worked in construction his whole life, eventually becoming a manager in a large company.*
>
> *The idea that "mental stimulation" was important was a foreign idea to Hal, for the last thing he wanted was to go to school. But he perked up when he realized that mental stimulation comes in many forms aside from school. When I asked him about his interests he replied he'd had a fairly "normal" life of raising kids and doing a few things like gardening with his wife but hadn't explored much beyond this. As he thought about it more, he realized he actually had a number of interests that he'd never pursued.*
>
> *Hal had always harbored a secret desire to play the flute. Afraid he'd be laughed at by friends, he never learned. But in talking about stimulating the brain from different sides, he wondered if he could actually take flute lessons. To his surprise, he found he loved it.*
>
> *This was the beginning of Hal using his retirement to pursue his interests. He'd wanted to travel but never had. Soon he and his wife were doing eco-tours to places he'd only heard about. He took a cooking class to develop his foodie side. Not everything happened overnight or all at once. Over the next few years, he expanded his interests and his world widened.*
>
> *He checked back in five years later for an update. "My life is anything but boring," he said with a smile. "My mind feels like it's back online once again. My diet is better, but*

> *most of all I love my life. I'm doing so many exciting things I hardly have enough time in the day. I didn't know 'mental stimulation' could feel so good!"*

Mental stimulation, however, doesn't just mean doing some crossword puzzles. It's necessary to exercise your mind in different ways in order to keep all your mental faculties operating at a high level. There are a number of mental functions neuroscience has mapped that everyone uses daily.

Memory underpins most all of the brain's functions. Not only is memory the basis of the self, it's the foundation for almost everything you do, from getting dressed to eating, talking, walking, working, and going home. Memory is what makes you human. When memory goes, this foundation collapses, and soon all of the activities a normal person does go along with it. Even getting out of bed requires memory, and in advanced Alzheimer's the person can't even do this.

This again points to the central role of the hippocampus, for the hippocampus is the control center of memory, the central processing center that creates and organizes new memory. When the hippocampus is robust and healthy, with low inflammation and high neurogenic capacity, new memory is formed easily and quickly. Cognitive health, brain health, and hippocampal health go together. When hippocampal health declines, so does cognition.

This is a quick overview of the mental functions you want to preserve and improve:

Short-term memory, long-term memory, and working memory. Short-term memory is like a scratch pad that holds information for about twenty to thirty seconds. Most people can hold seven items in short-term memory, plus or minus two. Long-term memory can hold vast amounts of information for a long period of time. Working memory lets you act mentally on several things together. For example, having in mind a list of errands and crossing them off the list mentally as you accomplish them during the day.

Attention and focus. Attention can be broad and global, or it can be tight and focused like a spotlight. We need both functions, but complex tasks need more attention and focus to accomplish.

Emotion regulation. This requires good mental ability and memory as well as emotional integration. It's the ability to self-soothe when ashamed, to self-calm when scared, to stand back from powerful emotions and witness them, as well as to remind yourself you've survived worse in the past and will be okay, among other things.

Fluid and crystallized intelligence. Fluid intelligence is flexible and relates to how quickly and fully you take in new information. Crystallized intelligence is accumulated knowledge, experience, and vocabulary. The mind of the average person shows a very gradual decline in fluid intelligence from age twenty onward, whereas crystallized intelligence increases until age sixty, when it plateaus until age eighty, then begins a gradual descent. [25]

Executive function. This highest capacity comes from the most developed part of the brain, the prefrontal cortex. The prefrontal cortex holds the crown jewels of the brain, the highest human capacities: planning, will, empathy, compassion, intellect, creativity, the abilities to be self-reflective and have self-awareness.

Executive function runs the show. It uses working memory to hold several possibilities in mind at once, to plan ahead, to inhibit the desire for immediate gratification for the sake of future gratification, to be flexible and change directions midstream when obstacles arise, to make decisions and carry them out despite distractions. When memory declines, so does executive function.

Athletes are in peak form in their twenties and thirties, but philosophers flower in their fifties and above. However, with what we now know about brain health, these trends will need to be rewritten. No one knows what is possible at each age with optimal care.

All of these mental functions work together. They allow people to manage highly complex lives that involve juggling many different things and levels throughout the day.

The Key to Ongoing Mental Stimulation: Lifelong Learning

Your most precious asset is your mind. To keep it operating at its highest capacity, you need to use it. When you don't exercise your mind, it slows down, memory falters, and all the rest of the problems in this book ensue.

To have a mind that is interested in people and the world, curious to learn new things, and enjoys using what it knows is to be mentally engaged. Your brain and mind want to engage the world and bring forth their hidden abilities. The brain and mind thrive on active engagement and stimulation.

Unfortunately, because of the educational wounding too many people experience at school, it's easy to get turned off to mental stimulation or learning. But learning comes in many forms, not just school learning.

It's important to cross-train your mind, to use it in different ways. Research now shows that single activities such as crossword puzzles do not generalize to improve overall brain function. Doing crossword puzzles only increases your ability to do more crossword puzzles (although even here only up to about fifty before it plateaus and rises very slowly after this). To have a bright, high-functioning mind you need to use it in a variety of ways.

Mental stimulation comes in many forms:

- **Reading.** Books, articles, papers, blogs, poems, short stories, interviews, sports stories, fashion advice—it doesn't matter as long as you read.
- **Writing**. Emailing or journaling, tweeting or blogging, Instagram or Facebook posts, letters or articles, the longer the better.
- **Problem-solving.** Whether at work or home, a crossword puzzle or sudoku, a board game or card game, creating a budget, cooking a new meal, or doing a construction project—the more different kinds or problem-solving, the better.
- **Attention and concentration practice.** With the internet, attention spans have gone down to six seconds or less. Sticking with a task, immersing yourself in an activity without getting interrupted by texts, email, calls, or distractions allows your concentration "muscle" to build. Meditation is a proven way to increase attention and concentration. (See next section.)

- **Executive function tasks.** This means coordinating several mental abilities together. A project at work or even running errands at home involves organizing, planning, executing, keeping track of progress, following through, and completing the tasks. Retirement and a life of leisure erode this capacity, so staying active after retirement with ongoing practice is important.
- **Discussion groups.** This can be a formal group or simply talking and exploring a subject with a friend or two, whether you discuss a movie, a book, current events, sports, or anything else. Delving into a subject, having a back-and-forth discussion with another mind, exercises language, thinking, logic, memory, vocabulary, and attention. Talk about whatever interests you, don't keep it all inside.
- **Musical training**. Learning a musical instrument, singing, listening to music and singing along in your head—this exercises the right hemisphere especially.
- **Travel and exploring new environments.** New environments are highly neurogenic, both in stimulating new neural growth and keeping new neurons alive. Travel is a wonderful way to enrich the brain. Try taking a different route home or venture into a new neighborhood. It doesn't have to be exotic or around the world, though if you can afford it, go for it.
- **Video and computer games.** The research is very mixed here. Most so-called brain games produce zero cognitive improvement. Others produce only very small gains which don't generalize to other parts of the brain. Some research, however, shows a slight growth in certain specific kinds of spatial relations and visual acuity specifically related to the particular game.

The central secret to keeping your mind sharp is mental engagement and stimulation, that is, lifelong learning. You need to learn new things throughout your life. Remember, learning isn't just about memorizing facts and figures or attending college. Learning happens in many ways. You can take a class or workshop or online seminar or webinar, you can read a book on a subject of interest, hear a podcast or watch a YouTube video, attend a conference or go to a meet-up gathering. Even something like going home a different way or brushing your teeth with your left hand activates your brain and gets it out of its habitual routines.

Lifelong learning is key to keeping your brain alive, active, bright, and strong. It's about finding your unique genius, which often has nothing to do with formal education. Everyone has a unique brain and unique mental abilities. The wounding in school so many suffer is an immense tragedy, for intelligence comes in many forms and flavors.

No one can be good at everything, but everyone is good at certain things. Finding your brain's natural gifts and talents allows you to develop your brain to fulfill your potential. Then lifelong learning reinforces itself, because it feels good to use your brain's natural ability.

The brain weakens when deprived of this and gets stronger when exercising its gifts. You feel more alive when you use and stretch yourself and your brain.

Mental detoxification: passive media consumption assessment

One of the fastest ways to ensure your brain goes downhill quickly is to watch a lot of TV. Watching several hours each day is associated with more rapid cognitive decline, whereas playing board games for this amount of time is associated with a reduced risk of cognitive impairment. [26]

This doesn't just apply to older adults. It applies to younger adults and probably kids. A 2016 study showed that participants who watched more than three hours of TV daily in their mid-20s and were sedentary, showed cognitive decline in middle age. [27] That's not old age but middle age.

Passively watching TV an hour or two most days appears to be fine. But when a person spends three or more hours daily watching TV, the brain is understimulated. The brain needs active engagement to thrive. High amounts of passive TV watching numbs the brain over time.

The exception to this may be when you are confined to bed in a hospital for a few weeks. Watching some more TV may be better than just staring at the walls. But even here, mixing it up with reading, listening to music, writing emails, and talking or video-calling with friends is better for your brain.

Do an honest self-assessment of how much time you spend each day passively consuming media, such a watching TV or Netflix. Don't fudge. If you are regularly watching three hours or more daily, you are actively dulling your brain. It's a sign you need to find other ways to participate in life.

Should you do a cognitive test to see how your mind is doing? Unless a person is already noticeably impaired cognitively, you may or may not want to do either a professional cognitive assessment or one of the free online assessments. It can be useful to establish a baseline of cognitive performance, but generally most people recognize when they're slipping. Sometimes it's helpful to find out you aren't as far gone as you may think.

One study with older adults compared three types of leisure activities: mental stimulation (such as reading, playing cards, or board games), physical activity, and socializing. The authors of the study reported that,

> "… those who did not engage in any of the three activities experienced a significant global cognitive decline, those who engaged in any one of the activities maintained their cognition, and those who engaged in two or three activities improved their cognition." [28]

Every brain is unique, with a unique blend of talents, interests, and skills. It's necessary to see what kind of mental activities you thrive on and enjoy. Trying to force yourself to do crossword puzzles when you don't like crossword puzzles is worse than useless.

When something is too hard, it gets frustrating; when it's too easy, it gets boring. You need to find ways of using your mind that hit the sweet spot of optimal challenge and interest. Then you enter into the "flow state." That keeps you going and keeps your mind stimulated and alive.

The Spiritual Level

Two key questions this book asks are: Is your brain growing? Is your self growing? That's what this book seeks to facilitate. When your brain and self are growing, you thrive.

An even more fundamental question then arises: Is your soul growing? Is your spiritual growth moving forward? There is an outer growth of the brain and self as well as an inner growth of the soul or spirit. Both inner and outer powerfully affect the brain.

It's been a shock to many brain scientists that spirituality has a profound effect on the brain and cognition. After all, most neuroscientists look for material causes to produce brain effects, so dismissed spirituality out of hand. But the past couple of decades have produced hundreds of studies that show a powerful impact on brain health from a person's spiritual life.

Not only do people's spiritual lives affect their brains, spiritual practice has a greater impact on brain health than almost anything else. There are two distinct types of spiritual practice that have very dramatic, powerful effects on neurogenic rates, hippocampal health, and memory and mood. There are other spiritual factors that strongly impact how your brain engages the world that also carry significant neurogenic benefits.

Throughout the ages, the wise of all cultures have declared that spirit is the source of existence. Our most essential identity is spiritual. At the deepest level we are not this surface body, heart, and mind, but a soul or spiritual being.

As detailed more fully in Chapter 3, "Holistic Healing of Anxiety," the soul is viewed as our deepest identity in traditions of the Personal Divine (Christianity, Judaism, Islam, and the bhakti traditions of Hinduism), whereas spirit is how this deepest spiritual identity is viewed in traditions of the Impersonal Divine (Buddhism, Taoism, Advaita Vedanta).

Both traditions see that the foundation of human consciousness is soul or spirit, a self-existent bliss, love, light, and peace that far exceeds any sensory or ego pleasure. Spiritual practice brings this inner light to the surface so the outer ego or self becomes more purified, calm, silent. The more this inner peace, joy, and love infuse the ego or self, the better you feel and the greater the inner resilience against outer storms and suffering.

All the world's spiritual traditions affirm that this universe is fundamentally a spiritual creation. Happiness and fulfillment come as a person aligns with this larger spiritual reality. The realization of your spiritual center of love, peace, and light is the goal of spiritual practice and, for most people, a lifetime endeavor (at least). Spiritual practice allows the experience of soul or spirit to be more and more a part of daily life.

Spiritual Practices to Help with Cognitive Decline

Mindfulness practices and heart-opening practices have been the focus of concerted neuroscience research. Both show profound effects on the brain. Both are highly neurogenic.

Neuroscientific studies of meditation took time to appear. For a long period, meditation held no interest for neuroscience researchers because to someone observing a person meditating, it looks like nothing is happening. The person is just sitting there. But if you meditate, you understand that a great deal is happening inwardly. Meditation is a highly dynamic state.

It finally took neuroscientists who were also meditators to start investigating the effects of meditation. When they published their findings, they showed such astonishing results that brain research on meditation took off. There are now thousands of studies showing powerful effects of meditation on the brain. [29, 30]

Among the most surprising findings is that these meditation practices rapidly increase neurogenic rates along the entire length of the hippocampus. Most interventions will increase neurogenesis and synaptogenesis along one side or the other. Antidepressants, for example, work by increasing neurogenesis along the side of the hippocampus that regulates emotion but not the side involved in cognition. But meditation has a robust effect on the entire hippocampus. [31]

Further, these practices have been shown to be helpful for many kinds of disorders, ranging from anxiety, depression, PTSD, and autism to memory problems, creativity, focus, and attention problems like ADD and ADHD. Further, research documents measurable new brain growth in as little as eight weeks of meditating twenty minutes, twice a day. This rapid effect was not expected. Scientists anticipated that it would take years of meditation practice to show up on brain scans. Eight weeks was a complete surprise.

The two practices, mindfulness and heart opening, are detailed in Appendix B. These practices are helpful for all three problems this book discusses, and the directions are the same for each issue. Both practices need to be part of a holistic approach to brain and cognitive health. Try on different practices, then continue with one or two that work for you for a time. See what happens.

The Importance of Meaning

A meaningless life is an empty life. An empty life weakens the self, for it has no ground. The quest for meaning is universal. All people need to find meaning in their lives. At some point everyone asks the universal questions: Who am I? Why am I here? What is the nature of existence? Does God or a greater Intelligence exist, or is this just a random, purely physical universe?

Everyone, whether an atheist or staunch existentialist, Christian or Buddhist, Hindu or Islamist, needs to find meaning, even if the conclusion is that life is meaningless and each person creates their own meaning. For everyone, finding or creating meaning is a crucial existential task.

Spiritual traditions make life comprehensible. They provide a narrative that explains the nature of existence and each person's relationship to the cosmos. In aligning with Spirit and feeling connected to something infinitely greater, life finds its meaning and purpose.

When life is meaningful, emotion regulation is enhanced so a person can bear immense suffering. Meaning is a deep inner, ultimately spiritual resource that upholds the psyche. The existential psychologist Viktor Frankl attributed his survival in a Nazi concentration camp to his finding meaning in his experience, which resulted in his classic work *Man's Search for Meaning.* This book is helpful to anyone grappling with how find meaning in life. He recognized in his own life that any pain can be borne when it's seen as meaningful.

Meaning is a powerful stress-reducer. A meaningful life allows the stresses and defeats of life to be put into perspective. When your life has meaning, then daily setbacks are taken in stride and larger upheavals have something to teach or a deeper significance that are sustaining during dark times.

It's easy to understand why optimists live longer than pessimists, since a pessimist is continually bracing for the worst and in so doing creates ongoing stress. In contrast, spirituality has been called "positive paranoia." Negative paranoia is usually thoughts such as, "The universe is out to get me." By contrast, positive paranoia from religion says, "The universe (the Divine) is out to enlighten and awaken me, and all these experiences are there to help me along." Such an optimistic attitude makes all the difference in dealing with life's struggles.

Later life is a good time to take stock of how well you've aligned your life with your inner values. Older adulthood gives some perspective on life that isn't there when young or middle-aged. Retirement brings another look at your life's purpose. How does having more time affect your life mission? Are there new areas of meaning that open up with this time? This is also an area where therapy can be helpful.

A meaningful life brings a glow of enthusiasm and joy to tasks that might otherwise be considered mundane or routine. Meaning is a powerful dimension of mental health.

Spiritual Community

The Hindu sage Ramana Maharshi once said that the easiest way to support your spiritual practice is to hang out with other people who are also on a spiritual path. Every religion stresses the need for spiritual community—a congregation, sangha, satsang, or fellowship.

Many people find spiritual community within a tradition, through a local church or temple, meditation center or yoga studio. Other people find it outside a tradition, through groups or classes or informal collection of friends who are unaffiliated with a particular religious tradition. Since the self is relational, other people help to bring forth its own deeper possibilities.

Finding a spiritual community of fellow seekers, whether formal or informal, similar or disparate, reinforces your aspiration for a higher life and makes the dry periods more bearable. The Christian tradition emphasizes over and over again the importance of the congregation, the fellowship of seekers. Buddhism speaks of the three Refuges on the path: the Buddha, the Dharma (teaching), and the Sangha. Of these, according to the Buddha, the most important is sangha, or spiritual community.

Aside from meeting needs for interpersonal contact and strengthening the self in this way, spiritual community fortifies your sense of purpose and aspiration for a higher life. Community reinforces spiritual practice, and supportive relationships help a weakened brain become more sturdy by increasing neurogenic rates.

If you are not in any kind of spiritual community, try to find one (or several). It works on different levels: supporting your spiritual practice; meeting new people and socializing; learning new things; trying new practices; reading, discussing, and learning new perspectives on your tradition. All of these help strengthen cognition.

Spiritual Detoxification

Most people received so much junk along with the religion they grew up with that they need to detox from it to discover the pure gold of truth mixed with impure, polluted elements. Whether entering a religious tradition as a child or an adult, it usually comes with added superstition, beliefs, rituals, and models of behavior that no longer make sense or are inappropriate for the modern world. Many Christians, for example, find it important to work through the repressive anti-sexual, patriarchal, anti-body messages that are a holdover from past centuries.

It is important to question, to deconstruct the religion or traditions you are drawn to in order to make it truly your own instead of an introjected, off-the-shelf belief system you merely adopt. This process of deconstruction takes time and thought. Yet by ridding yourself of the toxic elements that accompany any organized religion, you bring forth the underlying bounty of spiritual nourishment at the core of every religion.

When a person finds spirituality in their religion of birth, that's wonderful, nothing else is needed. But increasingly more people find value in using practices and ideas from other traditions. At this time, when we have the riches of the world's spiritual traditions to draw from, more and more people find resonance with traditions from across the globe, taking them on in part or whole.

Some will look elsewhere and then return to discover their birth religion has insight and power they never saw before. Others will leave their birth religion altogether and find themselves in another tradition. Still others will find their spirituality with several traditions or even outside any tradition. However you find it, it is important to make your spiritual path fully your own with values you can embrace.

Such discernment also protects against absorbing new toxic elements in the future. Letting go of unnecessary guilt, fear, and shame that toxic religious values produce will enhance your brain.

The Physical Side of Cognitive Decline

There are a great many nutrients and natural supplements that directly affect cognitive decline which are virtually unknown to the wider public. Appendices are routinely skipped in most books, and usually this makes little difference. But for this book that would be an error.

The Healthy Brain Diet explained in Chapter 2, The Solution, has so many modifications and additions that you will miss critically important information unless you read Appendix E, The Physical Side of Cognitive Decline.

Most of these compounds are being studied by pharmaceutical companies in order to slightly tweak their structure so they can be patented. But why wait for this? Since Mother Nature already has the patent on these natural substances, why not avail yourself of the best that a billion years of evolution has developed for brain health?

There is an important book by Dale Bredesen, M.D., called *The End of Alzheimer's.* It distinguishes between four types of Alzheimer's, depending upon the cause: inflammation, high blood sugar, neurotoxins (mold, heavy metals), and hormonal imbalance. These categories are helpful both in reversing the disease (for which he's had some important success) and identifying strategies to prevent it. His work shows that reversing and preventing Alzheimer's is possible. It is a pioneering work that deserves wide recognition.

Like all first steps, it provides a foundation on which those that come after will build. While its research into certain interventions is excellent, together with lab tests to help identify the type of Alzheimer's, it neglects key areas. First, it fails to address the extensive dietary dimension offered here in this book. To Bredesen's credit he does recommend a ketogenic diet and some common-sense dietary suggestions like avoid gluten and dairy and eat more vegetables, but the minimal supplement recommendations leave out a great deal, namely the other three nutritional pillars of the Healthy Brain Diet in this book. Hundreds of nutritional studies have shown how powerfully diet affects the brain. To leave these nutritional studies aside is to ignore a major way to reverse cognitive decline.

Second, Bredesen gives short shrift to the immense importance of the psychological side of the equation. Like almost all medical approaches, it downplays the immense role that emotional, mental, and spiritual factors have on the health of the brain. Further, it only mentions but doesn't focus on the central role the hippocampus plays in memory processing, together with the need to restore and rejuvenate the hippocampus. Nevertheless, his program is a good starting point.

These case studies that inform this current book are one form of research, and although not the gold standard of clinical trials, they are usually how new discoveries come into the field. The recommendations in this book come from observations gleaned from decades of clinical practice.

Patty came in with a diagnosis of cognitive decline. In her early seventies, she wanted to do everything she could to recover her previous mental acuity. When we looked at her diet, it was apparent her lifetime of eating poorly had a big effect. High sugar, high carbohydrate intake, a love of fried and processed foods—her diet was a formula for cognitive decline.

Patty's inflammatory markers were high, her hemoglobin A1c was in the prediabetic range, and she'd had many rounds of antibiotics a few years before. While there was much to fix, Patty charged ahead and made all the recommended changes in her diet. She struggled at first with going ketogenic, but after three months, she was amazed at how good she felt. She thought she could remember better also.

After a year on the Healthy Brain Diet, Patty's inflammatory markers were way down. Her blood sugar level had also come down significantly, and she'd made good strides toward healing her gut and increasing her microbial diversity.

Additionally, she'd become more social again, no longer afraid that others would see her as cognitively impaired. Indeed, as her quick-witted self returned, she thrived on social contact, which made her feel better about herself and reinforced her dedication to her diet.

After two years, Patty felt twenty years younger. "My mind is sharp again. I feel better than I have since I was forty or fifty. I was terrified I was losing everything. I'm so grateful to be getting my mind back!"

In previous chapters this book has emphasized the importance of reducing inflammation, blood sugar levels, and neurotoxic exposure, and Appendix E continues this focus together with other nutritional strategies to prevent and reverse cognitive decline. The role of hormonal imbalance will also be considered, with attention to other factors such as exercise and sleep.

Go to Appendix E, The Physical Side of Cognitive Decline, to learn of powerful, natural ways to prevent and reverse cognitive decline, prevent amyloid plaque and tau build-up, and clear out excess amyloid and tau that have already accumulated.

Conclusion

Preventing and reversing cognitive decline requires a whole brain approach—physical, emotional, mental, spiritual levels. When the brain and self detox from their psychological and neurological toxins, and further, when both are healed and strengthened with optimal nourishment, cognition improves. This is true whether you begin in your thirties in relatively good shape or begin in your sixties or later, after decline has set in.

Cognitive decline and Alzheimer's are now seen as lifestyle diseases. Repairing the brain, healing the self, engaging at all levels with the world is vivifying. Your mind wakes up. You see more, feel more, remember more, think lucidly, and experience the clarity that is the hallmark of cognitive health.

Becoming and staying sharp is possible. It just takes attention and care. Investing the time and energy to develop a radiant brain and self allows aging to become a fulfillment of one's life, not just a downhill slide. The best is yet to come.

CHAPTER 6

BRAIN HEALTH AS A WAY OF LIFE

This book is about what's most important in this world: *your brain and self.*

This is a complex story that is simple at its core. Like most stories it's about a fight between the good guys and the bad guys. But here, instead of the villains being people, the characters include brain-damaging foods, environmental toxins, emotionally destructive forces and ignorant, inaccurate theories. And when they are expressed through people, they're characters who think they're good guys doing good in the world, who believe that pesticides are helpful or that certain chemicals help people (and there is a grain of truth in it, to thicken the plot further,)

There are a lot of moving parts in this tale, many plot twists and turns, and it's still incomplete. At this moment it looks like the bad guys are winning. The brain is under a sustained assault from many directions. The modern brain and self are weakening.

Make no mistake. This is an epic battle that is being waged. It's being fought every day in every part of the globe. You and everyone you know encounter a daily battlefield of destructive possibilities that will gradually erode your brain and emotional balance if you don't learn how to protect yourself and navigate this terrain with skill and grace.

The neurotoxic forces that are currently arrayed against everyone on the planet are powerful, well-funded and well-defended. But emerging knowledge in many fields provides the necessary arms to win this fight. I feel profoundly optimistic about the future and the brain's possibilities for healing and growth. Even though it looks bad right now, truth and health will eventually win out, I believe. The only question is how long it will take and how much worse it will get before turning the corner. I hope this book will be of some assistance to help turn the tide against entrenched forces that create so much emotional pain when the brain deteriorates.

Radiant Health

A vision of brain and psychological health shows most everyone is capable of operating at a higher level than at present. However, in aspiring for radiant health, it's important not to make this an unattainable ideal that you feel bad about if you fall short. Everybody starts from where they are, working on what they can, accepting the conditions of their life and the world as they are. The path of healing leads us to ever richer living, and it's this upward movement of growth that's essential, not a static image of perfection.

Brain health and mental health go together. Better brain health improves mental health, just as better mental health improves brain health. Neither can be reduced to the other, and both are needed for living fully and optimally.

A helpful analogy (which can also be misleading and overly simplistic) is to see the brain as the hardware and the self as software. With a weakened brain, the software will be "buggy," unable to perform well. Similarly, a well-developed physical brain won't reach its capacities without good software in place (an integrated, cohesive self). For such software not only brings out the brain's fullest potentials but actually adds to those potentials by increasing resilience.

The best brain needs the best software to bring out what it can do. And the best software (self) needs the best hardware (brain) to show what it's capable of.

The possibilities for radiant health that emerge from the latest research reveal an extraordinary picture: A brain and self that are joyously alive, vitally engaged, and excited to greet each new day's challenges, lovingly connected to others in personal life and work, confident, positive, able to handle adversity and to bounce back from setbacks. Feeling really good springs naturally from simply being alive.

This intrinsic vitality is a call to actively engage the world, to unfold our latent inner possibilities. Such a person is drawn to discover what's possible, to learn about other people, to appreciate the beauty that nature reveals and the intimate connections life offers. This brain and self have an emotional stability that allows painful, negative feelings to be felt, their meaning processed and moved through rather than avoided.

When the brain is continually attacked, when the brain's integrity is constantly being eroded, and when this happens in such small amounts that no one source is noticed, the world does indeed seem like a scary place. When leaky gut and leaky brain let in toxins that need to be continuously beaten back, the brain and self naturally feel under threat. And when the threat is unknown, the world appears to be very dangerous. Fear can then attach itself to anything.

When the brain and self are radiantly healthy, the world appears quite different. The joy of being alive vastly outweighs life's challenges. Dangers still exist but can be dealt with without thinking the sky is falling. What this means, however, is the brain's and self's capacities are engaged on every level: body, heart, mind, spirit.

In simpler times, when the world was less developed, all food was organic, there were hardly any neurotoxins in the environment, and the brain wasn't under siege like it is now. Dangers were easier to see. Nowadays, however, it a toxic jungle out there. Traveling without a map is hazardous to your health.

Just as a map was needed in times past to get through a jungle full of unexplored dangers, so modern life requires a whole other kind of map to avoid the predators and dangers in a techno-toxic environment. The map that's needed now is a multi-dimensional map, for the hazards are not just physical but emotional, mental, and spiritual.

Such a map needs to show not only what's dangerous and to be avoided or minimized, but also where to find succor and nourishment. Such a multi-dimensional map will point out the minefield that is daily life and show the way to safety, health, love, and peace.

This book lays out a map for brain health. It shows how neurotoxins abound, even in what should be the safest of places (who knew that handling receipts or cotton balls could expose you to endocrine-disrupting chemicals that could alter your brain chemistry?). Further, a multi-dimensional map is important not only to avoid neurotoxic influences but to nourish your brain and self.

After healing comes maintenance. Brain health is a way of life, not just a temporary fix. Live as if the brain and psyche matter. Nourish your body, brain, and self. As the reader knows well by now, this means to actively engage your full consciousness.

Yes, eat well and intelligently, exercise and rest your body, but nourish your self and spirit as well. Life is so much more than what's on the news or your screen. To enter into the deeper realms of living requires a brain and self that aren't in continual disintegration. It requires physical and psycho-spiritual practices that begin with your inherent aspiration for a greater, fuller life. The teachers, tools, practices, and people to assist then begin to show up, so you can choose those best suited for your unique path of unfolding.

The promise of psychological flourishing is more easily fulfilled when the brain is radiantly healthy. The inverse is also true, psychological integration assists the brain in becoming all it can be. The two go together to create new possibilities for human functioning. Unfolding the self's vast inner riches with a brain that actively engages the world, that only reaches its own highest possibilities when the psyche is engaged on all levels, this is true brain health and mental health.

Just as the greater possibilities for psychological growth weren't discovered until the 1960s and '70s, so the higher possibilities for radiant brain health didn't get discovered until a mere decade or so ago. Now it's clear psychological health and brain health go together, complete each other, and find their highest fulfillment only when both are realized.

Because of the current neurotoxic environment that most brains are subjected to, "normal" is considered healthy. But the absence of disease is a low bar for health, physical or mental. Health, healing, wholeness, holy—all come from the same root word. The human journey goes from fragmentation to wholeness, from less neural complexity to greater neural complexity, from just living to flourishing.

Then, everything opens up. When rooted in our deeper being, with a healthy brain and self, life is seen for the miracle it is.

APPENDIX A

SUMMARY OF THE HEALTHY BRAIN DIET

This is summary of the foods and nutrients included in Healing Phase of the Healthy Brain Diet. This includes all four principles:

- neurogenic
- ketogenic
- anti-inflammatory
- gut friendly

The Maintenance Phase modifies this based on each person's unique metabolic profile and blood test results.

Neurogenic

- omega-3s, 3–4 grams daily
- green tea extract, caffeine-free, 45% catechins, 300–725 mg daily
- curcumin, 200–1,200 mg daily depending on formulation
- blueberries, a cup a day or, better, extract equivalent
- hesperidin, 500 mg, 1–2 times daily
- luteolin, 50–100 mg, 1–2 times daily
- taurine, 1,000 mg, 1–2 times daily
- rosmarinic acid, 500–1,000 mg, 1–2 times daily
- whole soy and extracts containing daidzein and genistein
- ginseng extract, standardized extract, 200 mg, 1–3 times daily

- ginkgo biloba, 120 mg daily of standardized extract
- quercetin, 500 mg, 1–2 times daily
- vitamin E, gamma form, 200–400 mg, 1–2 times daily
- piperine, 10 mg, 1–2 times daily
- bacopa, 200–800 mg daily, spread over 1–3 times throughout the day
- DHEA and pregnenolone, 10–100 mg daily
- tryptophan and 5-HTP, 500–2,000 mg and 50–300 mg respectively, 1–2 times daily
- rhodiola, 200–700 mg, 1–2 times daily
- melatonin, .2 mg–10 mg at night
- huperzine A, 200–800 mcg daily
- mulberry, 500 mg daily
- red sage (salvia), 1,000 mg, 1–2 times daily
- goji berry (wolfberry), 500 mg, 1–2 times daily
- grape seed extract, 100 mg, 1–2 times daily
- St. John's wort, standardized extract 300–1,800 mg, 1–3 times daily
- apigenin, 50 mg, 1–2 times daily
- lithium (aspartate), 300 mcg–30 mg daily
- icariin (horny goat weed extract), depending upon extract concentration, 300–500 mg, 1–2 times daily
- berberine, 400 mg, 1–3 times daily
- baicalin (Chinese skullcap extract), 100–400 mg, 1–2 times daily

Other Nutrients that Increase BDNF

- magnesium-L-threonate, 2,000 mg daily (or more)
- L-carnosine and beta-alanine, 500 mg, 1–2 times daily and 1,000 mg. daily respectively
- vitamin D, 5,000–10,000 i.u. daily, as determined by blood test
- magnolol, 200 mg, 1-2 times daily
- alpha lipoic acid, 50–300 mg daily
- ashwagandha, dose depends upon extract concentration, 1–2 times daily

- resveratrol, 20–400 mg daily
- cocoa flavonoids and chocolate
- milk thistle extract (silymarin), 300 mg, 1–2 times daily
- lion's mane, 300–3,000 mg daily
- pantethine, 50–500 mg daily
- phosphatidylserine, 100 mg daily (or 300 mg for depression)
- cinnamon, depends upon extract

Ketogenic

Instead, a ketogenic diet consists of non-starchy, high-fiber vegetables and low-sugar fruit that provide the bulk of food. These include:

Non-starchy vegetables and low-sugar fruit:

asparagus
avocados
bell peppers
berries
bok choy
broccoli
brussels sprouts
cabbage
cauliflower
celery
chard
collards
cucumbers
eggplant
grapefruit
green beans
jicama
kale
leeks
lemons
limes

mushrooms
onions
parsley
radishes
salad greens
scallions
spinach
sprouts
summer squash
tomatoes (except cherry tomatoes, which can have excess carbs)
zucchini

The bulk of calories, however, come from healthy fats. These include:

Healthy fats:

almond milk
avocado oil
butter (organic and grass-fed or pastured)
cheese (except blue cheese)
coconut
coconut milk
coconut oil
pastured eggs
extra-virgin olive oil
ghee (grass-fed)
grass-fed meat
MCT oil (medium-chain triglycerides)
nuts and nut butters (especially macadamia, almonds, pecans)
olives
pastured, organic chicken
seeds (pumpkin, sunflower, flax, chia, sesame)
sour cream (organic, grass-fed)
wild-caught, low-mercury fish

Protein:

eggs (pastured, organic)
grass-fed cheese
grass-fed, organic meats
Greek yogurt
nuts
pastured, organic chicken
wild-caught, low-mercury fish

As you can see, this is quite a wide range of foods to enjoy. The internet is now full of keto-friendly desserts that are sweetened with stevia and/or monk fruit, so a sweet tooth can be happily indulged.

Anti-inflammatory

Extracts that decrease inflammation and are worth inviting into your daily diet, depending upon the degree of chronic inflammation in your body, include:

- apigenin, 50 mg, 1–2 times daily
- benfotiamine (a form of B-1 or thiamine), 150–600 mg daily
- berberine, 400 mg, 1–3 times daily
- borage oil or evening primrose oil, 1 gram, 1–2 times daily, contains GLA
- boswellia extract, 100 mg daily or more if in pain
- black cumin seed oil, 500 mg, 1–2 times daily
- blueberries and blueberry extract (highly anti-inflammatory)
- carnosine, 500–1,000 mg, 1–2 times daily
- cat's claw, 500 mg, 1–3 times daily
- Chinese skullcap (baicalin), 4:1 concentrate, 400 mg, 1–2 times daily
- curcumin, depends upon extract
- fisetin, 50–100 mg daily
- ginger, daily as an extract, amount depends on concentration
- green tea extract, 98% catechins, decaffeinated, 300–725 mg daily

- nettle root extract, 500 mg, 1–2 times daily
- omega-3 fatty acids, 3–4 grams daily
- P-5-P (most bioavailable form of B-6), 50–100 mg, 1–2 times daily
- piperine (pepper extract), 10 mg, 1–2 times daily
- pycnogenol (maritime pine bark extract), 50–100 mg, 1–2 times daily
- rosmarinic acid, 500–1,000 mg, 1–2 times daily, extract most available as Origanox
- sulforaphane (from broccoli sprouts extract, best with myrosinase), dosage depends upon extraction process
- tart cherry extract, 500 mg, 1–2 times daily

Antioxidants:

- vitamin A, 10,000 i.u. daily
- vitamin C, 500–1,000 mg, 1–2 times daily
- vitamin E (preferred as gamma tocopherol), 200–400 mg, 1–2 times daily
- lipoic acid, 100–300 mg, 1–3 times daily
- cysteine or NAC (precursors to glutathione), 600 mg, 1–2 times daily
- ubiquinol (Co-Q10), 30–100 mg,1–3 times daily

Gut friendly

Lactobacillus plantarum and Lactobacillus reuteri reduces gut wall permeability, according to Swedish researchers. [1] Bacillus spore strains increase tight junction integrity, and spores have greater survival rates through the harsh stomach acid that can kill many probiotics. [2]

In animal and cell studies the following bacterial strains have helped heal a leaky intestinal membrane. [3, 4] These include: Lactobacillus rhamnosus, L. paracasei, L. gasseri, L. helveticus, L. plantarum, Bifidobacterium infantis, B. longum. The plantarum strain has been shown to be especially helpful in repairing tight junction integrity. Eating fermented foods like unsweetened yogurt and kefir, sauerkraut, kimchi, and pickles builds new strains.

Common forms of prebiotics include organic psyllium husks (4–5 capsules daily with a glass of water), FOS (fructooligosaccharides), GOS (galactooligosaccharides), XOS (xylooligosaccharides) as well as resistant starch.

A product called ION Gut Health has been shown to repair and heal the tight junctions.

APPENDIX B:

MEDITATION PRACTICES

There are a number of meditation practices that have been well-researched, have been shown to be neurogenic, and show strong anti-anxiety, antidepressant and cognitive benefits. Before jumping in, however, it's helpful to understand the larger spiritual landscape.

A Brief Note on the Spiritual Context

The Perennial Philosophy consists of those core areas of agreement between all the world's traditions, first described by Aldous Huxley and developed by other philosophers such as Huston Smith. It points out that over the past few thousand years, two great streams of spirituality have emerged, which can be referred to as traditions of the Personal Divine and traditions of the Impersonal Divine.

The West has been most influenced by traditions of the Personal Divine. The traditions of Christianity, Judaism, and Islam view the Divine as a Personal Being. Much of the East, on the other hand, has been influenced by traditions of the Impersonal Divine: Buddhism, Advaita Vedanta, Taoism (although in India the Personal Divine traditions also hold powerful sway). These traditions view the Divine not as *a* Being but as pure Being itself, an infinite Impersonal consciousness. There are also traditions that hold both aspects of the Divine equally and declare the Divine to be both Personal and Impersonal, two sides of a single coin.

Traditions of the Personal Divine view our deepest identity to be a soul that is utterly unique and, in non-dual understandings, a portion of the Divine Being. In these traditions the soul exists in a relationship of love to the Divine, and spiritual practices center on opening the heart so the soul's aspiration, love, devotion, and longing for the Divine can pour forth and lift the soul Godward.

Traditions of the Impersonal Divine, on the other hand, see our deepest identity as spirit (atman or Buddha-nature) that is one with the infinite, impersonal consciousness. In these traditions, the spirit's identity is with the Divine, universal in all. Spiritual practices in these traditions center on mindfulness and using consciousness to discriminate between the real and the unreal.

Both the traditions of the Personal Divine and Impersonal Divine declare the secret of life is not to be found on the surface level of this outer material world but at the most profound levels of inner consciousness, in union with the Divine or Spirit, the ground and source of this universe.

Peace, love, light, joy flow from Spirit, the Divine. To the degree you are open to your inner being, peace and these other soul qualities can permeate the ego. When a person is cut off from this inner source, anxiety and suffering result. Or, if the inner being is able to pour its abundance into the surface being but the ego is so poorly organized that its inadequate self-soothing structures leak the peace like a sieve leaks water, then again anxiety and pain result. In this case, psychological work needs to complement spiritual practice.

Spiritual deepening is not a mere belief or idea but a dynamic experiential reality. Just reading about this doesn't go very far. It's necessary to jump into the pool and swim in these waters of spirit to feel the effects.

There are a great number of spiritual strategies to purify, quiet, and open the ego or surface self. Each major tradition has special practices within its tradition, and many of these practices are shared across multiple traditions.

Experiment with these practices to see what their effects are. It's not necessary to buy into any particular belief system to try these on. These are consciousness practices that can be utilized by any human being from any culture.

Heart-opening practices. Traditions of the Personal Divine place particular emphasis upon love, devotion, and opening the heart. In many of these traditions, the soul is located in the heart or behind the heart chakra. The density of the ego, with its layers of defenses, acts to constrict and harden the heart, preventing the flow of love, gratitude, compassion, and other spiritual feelings. Heart-opening practices involve amplifying love, compassion, gratitude, aspiration, devotion, surrender, and other feelings that purify the ego's hard outer shell. This brings forth the deeper soul's light, love, peace, and joy as it calls on the Divine for union.

There are different kinds of heart-opening practices:

- Devotional prayer. The seeker calls to the Divine in whatever form the person conceives of the Divine and offers up devotion, love, and bhakti. The Divine can be seen as Divine Father (how Jesus viewed the Divine), Divine Mother (as in Vedanta and Tantra as surrender to the Divine Shakti), Divine Child (the baby Krishna or baby Jesus), the Divine Friend (cow herder Krishna playing with the gopis or Jesus as friend of all), the Divine Lover (in Christian, Sufi, Vedantic, and Tantric traditions). The Divine assumes the form appropriate to the seeker and answers the soul's call through increasing union over time as the purification of the outer nature proceeds. Love shifts from impure to increasingly pure love for the Divine.

  Calling on Spirit for help, for succor, for soothing, and reassurance in the hour of need is a time-honored tradition that invites Divine grace.
- Heart-centered meditation. The seeker centers consciousness in the heart area and focuses on a feeling of love, devotion, surrender, or, since these feelings often may not be present, aspiration (for the Divine, for the true consciousness, for the soul's emergence). All other thoughts, feelings, and sensations are passively disregarded as this central feeling intensifies. By following or riding this wave of aspiration or love inward, the gates of the heart gradually open and the soul shines forth, its light and joy dispelling the egoic emptiness.

- Compassion practices. The seeker sends lovingkindness first to oneself, then to people close, then people less close, then to people far away, and then again to oneself. "May I [or loved ones, family, friends, co-workers, all beings] be happy. May I be healthy. May I have ease of being." All three phrases are spoken aloud or silently, first to oneself, then to each category, and ending with oneself again.

  This practice is a way to give solace and comfort to yourself. It has a soothing effect that can strengthen the self when it falters.

There are other heart-opening practices, but these are the most common. Here again there are many online sources that go into greater detail with instructions. You need to experiment to find what works best for you.

Aside from inner deepening, heart-opening practices are helpful in emotion regulation. Heart-opening practices bring a more loving gaze to the self, so the person can become more compassionate toward themselves rather than critical and judgmental. They allow the person to feel reassured and strengthened amidst emotional storms.

Mindfulness practices. Most traditions of the Impersonal Divine emphasize different varieties of mindfulness practice. It is best to experiment with several to find what works best for you. All mindfulness practices are designed to bring a person into the present moment. Over time, mindfulness practices "wake up" consciousness from the half-sleep of daily life. Most people don't realize the degree of their sleepwalking until they begin to wake up.

Mindfulness is often defined as "paying attention on purpose." In mindfulness there is an increasing awareness of everything happening internally as well as outside. As you pay attention to your own consciousness, the first thing most everyone notices is "monkey mind," that is, just how noisy and out of control your ordinary mental life is. By continuing to pay attention, however, this noise begins to settle down.

As thoughts and feelings calm down, the mind wakes up, the senses come alive, and the present moment opens into greater fullness. You begin to see how your normal life is a kind of half-conscious trance, a haze of images, memories, thoughts about the past and future, that is rarely centered in the actual moment that is right now. After all, the present is all that exists. The past is merely remembrance, regret, historical narrative or some other form of thinking. The future exists as anticipation, dread, hope, or some other form of thinking. Only the present moment truly exists, everything else is thought and fantasy. Coming into the present allows you to be fully alive.

There are numerous forms of mindfulness practice, and they are of two main kinds: focused, concentration practices and open awareness practices. Each is helpful for different reasons. Try each practice initially for fifteen to twenty minutes, then gradually increase to thirty to sixty minutes or however long you decide.

Most common forms of focused concentration practices include:

- Breath meditation. This is the usual starting point for most people. It involves focusing on the sensations of breathing, usually centered in a particular part of the body such as the abdomen, and simply observing the body sensation as the breath comes in and goes out. All other thoughts or feelings or sensations are simply noticed as they come but attention then returns to the sensations in the of the breath abdomen. Gradually other thoughts, feelings, and images recede and subtler and subtler sensations of breathing predominate. Consciousness calms down and opens up.

  By giving the person something to focus on other than painful feelings like anxiety or depression, this helps to tolerate the painful feelings and to see they are impermanent.
- Listening. Here the person focuses upon whatever sounds are present. Your consciousness becomes like a giant ear, taking in sounds all around you, above, below, everywhere. Know that nothing will ever sound exactly like this ever again, that these sounds are unique to this particular moment in time. Notice how each sound arises and then ends, giving way to new sounds that are ever changing.

- Progressive, focused attention. Here the focus begins with the breath, then after some months or years moves to other sensations, such as hearing or seeing. Then after focusing on each sense, attention shifts to feelings for months or years. Then thinking is the focus. Then everything together—body, emotions, thoughts. This shifts the process to more of an open awareness practice after concentration has been well developed.
- Sweeping. This form, popularized by Goenka, sweeps consciousness throughout the body, noticing various sensations in each area but not getting stuck anywhere. Beginning from the top of the head and scanning down through the neck, chest, abdomen, pelvis, legs, feet, then either returning to sweep down again from the top of the head or going from bottom back to top. This practice also leads to finer and finer perception which opens up the now.
- Mantra meditation. The inward repetition of a word or phrase over and over again is a technique found in most religious traditions. In India this is called "mantra meditation," and research shows that this silent repetition is calming to the mind and relaxing to the body. Some traditions believe both the meaning and the sound itself work to produce the effects on consciousness. Western research has shown that even the repetition of nonsense syllables will produce relaxation and calming effects.

Common forms of open awareness practice include:

- Bare attention. Here there are no steps or any particular focus, just become aware of whatever arises in consciousness. Krishnamurti referred to this as "choiceless awareness." It consists of pure observation, only watching the variety of mental, emotional, and physical stimuli without judging or justifying, and over time the dust settles and wakefulness increases. There is no effort to calm or still the mind, as such effort is simply more noise that stirs up more dust.

Here all painful or difficult feelings simply arise and pass away. They are seen as temporary, fleeting feelings and thoughts, and as the capacity to observe them increases, the person's reactivity diminishes. Pure awareness is an action that doesn't increase the noise and dust of ordinary consciousness but allows it to settle. As it settles, consciousness wakes up from its half-slumber of everyday life.

- Witnessing. This is from the Vedantic tradition and involves stepping back into your own consciousness to find a silent witness deep inside. It is similar to bare attention except this locates attention inside in a pure observer or witness soul that is utterly silent and without thought. Most people can find this for a second or two, but practice is needed to stay there for extended periods.

  As you can hold anxiety or depressive feelings in consciousness and separate from them, there comes a freedom by loosening your tight identification with these feelings. You see you are separate and different from them. The content of your emotions is like an outer skin but is not you or your deeper consciousness. This freedom makes painful feelings easier to tolerate.

There are still other forms of mindfulness meditation, but these are the most widely used. Anyone can begin a mindfulness practice easily. There are many free online resources, YouTube instructional videos, and a great many classes in most cities where mindfulness practices are taught.

Focused concentration practices are used to support emotion regulation by helping to tolerate painful or difficult feelings. Focusing on the breath or the bottom of your feet or some other object helps to anchor attention so that the sadness or depressive feelings come and go, rather than getting lost in painful affect. Strong feelings are easier to bear while concentrating on something else. Watching the breath, for example, breaks up the obsessive focus on depressive or anxious thoughts and feelings while bringing the person into the present moment.

Open awareness practices are used to open the person up and to bring the person into the present moment, rather than ruminating about the past or future. Opening the person up to new sensory stimuli or a greater range of thoughts and feelings can help break the cycle of rumination.

There is an intimate relationship between mindfulness and heart-opening practices. Each tradition uses both practices while emphasizing one over the other. Compassion practices are considered preliminary practices to mindfulness in many Buddhist traditions (for you can only be as mindful as your heart is open). Similarly, mindfulness or practices that increase peace are often preliminary in Personal Divine traditions, bringing peace and calmness in which the soul's feeling of aspiration or love can be more easily tuned in to.

Experiment with different meditations and see what you resonate with. Then stick to that practice to allow it to deepen and reveal the riches of your inner being.

APPENDIX C

THE PHYSICAL SIDE OF ANXIETY

Nutrition

This anti-anxiety part of the Healthy Brain Diet has the same two phases: the Healing Phase and the Maintenance Phase. To heal and regenerate the brain means to bring it up to its full neurogenic potential. The more intensive Healing Phase is highly neurogenic and follows the four principles discussed in Chapter 2:

- neurogenic
- ketogenic
- anti-inflammatory
- gut friendly

The Maintenance Phase can be started six to twenty-four months after symptoms have receded, and it consists of modifying the diet based on individual needs, for example going to low carb rather than strictly ketogenic. However, this chapter presents modifications of the diet outlined in Chapter 2 that are specifically designed to help with anxiety.

Healing Phase of Diet

Neurogenic

A general guideline is that something will lower anxiety to the degree to it increases neurogenic activity. Conversely, a weakened brain with low rates of neurogenesis and neuroplasticity exposes the brain to higher levels of anxiety, stress, and fear. This section highlights those nutrients that have been shown to exert anti-anxiety effects, but further research will no doubt show that others from Chapter 2 also are in this category.

Again, don't try to do everything, just as much as feels right for you.

Ashwagandha. This Indian herb has been used for centuries in traditional Ayurveda as a brain tonic. Ashwagandha increases BDNF levels in the brain, reduces cortisol and anxiety levels. After taking 300 mg of ashwagandha extract for two months, study participants had reductions in anxiety scores of 75.6% and reduction in cortisol levels of almost 28% from baseline. [1] Since reducing cortisol is so important for reducing anxiety, and with so few compounds that can do this, these dramatic results make ashwagandha worth trying for most people. It appears to work on the GABA system along very different neural pathways than benzodiazepines, producing calmness but not the numbness and deadness associated with benzodiazepines. [2] Usual dosages are 5–8% extract, 300 mg, 1–2 times daily.

Berberine. This plant extract improves blood glucose levels, increases BDNF levels, reduces inflammation and blood sugar levels, and it has demonstrated anti-anxiety effects. [3] Usual doses are 400 –500 mg, 1–3 times daily.

Omega-3s. A 2018 systematic review and meta-analysis of nineteen clinical trials concluded that omega-3s significantly reduce anxiety. The researchers noted that doses higher than 2 grams daily were associated with significantly higher anti-anxiety effects than lower doses. They also found that supplements containing less than 60% EPA were associated with reduced anxiety. [4]

If you have high levels of inflammation, however, or a blood test shows your high-sensitivity C-reactive protein level to be greater than

.55 for men and 1.0 for women, then a ratio of DHA to EPA of 1:2 may be better to help reduce inflammation. The U.S. government recommends a minimum of 3 grams daily. Most people can use 3–4 grams daily of omega-3.

Bacopa. This herb increases BDNF, neurogenesis, and neuroplasticity, and has been shown to be an effective anti-anxiety agent, as well as having strong antidepressant and cognitive-enhancing properties. [5, 6] Daily use depends on the strength of the extract. With 20% bacosides, doses vary between 200–800 mg daily, spread over 2–3 doses. Some people sleep better with it, some worse, depending on your metabolism.

Magnolol. This extract from magnolia bark is strongly neurogenic and has relaxing properties as well. There is evidence it is one of the few things that reduces cortisol. Cortisol levels increase with age and are very hard to bring down. Simply reducing cortisol levels alone increases neurogenesis, but magnolol additionally raises BDNF levels. [7] It comes as a patented product called Relora but is also available as a 90% extract. It can be taken daily in the amount that feels right or at night to aid sleep.

Magnesium L-threonate. This form of magnesium crosses the blood-brain barrier and calms excited neurons. It is both neurogenic and calming, as well as raising BDNF levels. Usual dose is 2 grams (three capsules), but as mentioned earlier, some people take as many as 12 daily to reach optimal blood magnesium levels.

Resveratrol. A July 2019 study showed resveratrol has anti-anxiety and antidepressant effects by blocking an enzyme called PDE4, which is involved in cortisol release. [8] Typical doses range from 30 mg to 400 mg daily.

Chinese skullcap. The extract baicalin comes from Chinese skullcap, not to be confused with American skullcap, which has different flavonoids. Four of Chinese skullcap's flavonoids have strong anti-anxiety effects through binding with the GABA sites in the brain, as well as neuroprotective effects on neurons through different mechanisms, including neurogenic, antioxidant, anti-excitotoxicity, anti-inflammatory actions. [9, 10] It's commonly available as a 400 mg extract taken daily, however each person may need more or less than this amount. As with anything, experiment to see what's right for you.

Curcumin. One of the superstars of brain health, this extract of turmeric has potent neurogenic, anti-inflammatory effects and demonstrated anti-anxiety effects. [11, 12] Since it is poorly absorbed, it's best taken with piperine, phospholipids, or in the form of micronized nanoparticles which studies show can increase absorption by between eight and fifty times.

Green tea. Another brain health superstar, the EGCG polyphenols in green tea are powerfully neurogenic, anti-inflammatory, and have a calming effect via the GABA system in the brain. Research shows strong anti-anxiety effects. [13] If taken in green tea or in an extract that contains caffeine, however, the anti-anxiety effects are negated. Best to take as a caffeine-free extract. The maximum daily amount of EGCG is 400 mg. More than this has been associated with a rare risk of liver toxicity.

Carnosine and beta-alanine. These amino acids have anti-glycation, anti-inflammatory, and antioxidant effects in addition to increasing BDNF and neurogenesis. Beta-alanine is a precursor to carnosine, and both have been shown to have anti-anxiety effects. [14, 15] Suggested amounts are 500 mg and 1,000 mg respectively, 1–2 times daily.

Tryptophan. This precursor to serotonin has been shown to increase neurogenesis and reduce anxiety. [16] Raising levels of serotonin (or dopamine or norepinephrine and epinephrine) increases the brain's rate of neurogenesis, and it is this heightened neurogenic activity that appears responsible for the antidepressant and anti-anxiety effects of SSRIs, SDRIs, and NRIs. Taking tryptophan, especially on a short-term basis, may have a similar neurogenic action but without the side effects of prescribed medication. Typical doses range from 500–2,000 mg daily. A dose of 2.5 grams at bed has been shown to increase sleep quality and length.

Ketogenic

The state of nutritional ketosis is strongly calming for most people. When the brain is using the preferred fuel of ketone bodies, rather than relying solely on the dirty fuel of glucose, the heightened metabolic efficiency of ketosis produces a stabilizing effect on the brain. As the brain stabilizes, the self feels more peaceful. Anxiety recedes.

The anti-anxiety effects of ketosis are one of its greatest benefits. When a person is well into nutritional ketosis, this high octane–fueled brain performs better, more smoothly, and with less "noise" in the form of stress, anxiety, or depression. The brain has greater inner metabolic resource to draw on. As a consequence, the person feels better, functions better, and is less easily disrupted by negative affect.

Unfortunately, many people on a ketogenic diet also ingest high amounts of coffee or caffeine, which can partially or entirely cancel out its anxiety-reducing effects. Another confounding variable is that oftentimes people think they are in ketosis but are not. Indeed, when people who believe they are in ketosis do not notice less anxiety, it's often a sign that they are not actually in the state of nutritional ketosis (as discussed earlier, this is defined as 0.5–3.0 mM/dLor above).

It is no accident that the striking eight-fold increase in childhood anxiety rates coincides with the change in the Standard American Diet (SAD) from moderate fat, moderate carb to low fat and high carb. A diet high that is low in good fats and fiber, and high in bad fats and carbohydrates, especially simple carbohydrates like sugar, is a formula for creating an anxious brain.

While there is greater metabolic benefit from producing your own ketones via a ketogenic diet (endogenous ketones), you can also take a number of ketone supplements to boost your body's supply (called "exogenous ketones"). One study with mice showed reduced anxiety simply from taking exogenous ketones. [17] Since some people find it hard to get into and maintain a state of nutritional ketosis, supplementing with exogenous ketones may help achieve the ketogenic part of the Brain Healthy Diet.

Anti-inflammatory

Chronic inflammation helps produce a state of anxiety. And chronic stress and anxiety result in increased inflammation. It's another vicious cycle that spirals downward as the person feels worse and worse.

People who are anxious often have gastro-intestinal (GI) disorders. After migraines, GI disorders are the most common disorders that people with anxiety report. Further, those who have inflammatory disorders of the gut very often also report anxiety. [18] Given all the glyphosate, pesticides, antibiotics, and other gut-disrupting elements in the environment that lead to inflammation, leaky gut and intestinal problems are hardly surprising.

A confusing element in the relationship between anxiety and chronic inflammation is that glucocorticoid stress hormones such as cortisol initially reduce inflammation. This is why cortisone and other synthetic hormones are used to lower inflammation. Over time, however, chronically high levels of stress hormones cause the opposite effect and raise inflammation levels. The body's immune cells become resistant to cortisol's regulatory effect on inflammation, and inflammation rises. [19]

This may explain why most but not all studies have shown higher inflammation levels are associated with anxiety. [20,] Some studies have shown this is a greater factor in older adults rather than younger adults, as the inflammatory marker hs-CRP rises with age, although other studies have found no age-related differences. [21]

Given what's known about brain mechanisms involved in anxiety, reducing inflammation is an important pathway toward healing. A key blood test for everyone is the high-sensitivity C-reactive protein (hs-CRP) blood test to find out your general inflammation level. If your hs-CRP blood level is above .55 for a male or 1.0 for a female, getting your inflammation level down is crucial. Even if your numbers are below this, keeping your inflammation levels low is extremely important for overall physical and mental health.

The ketogenic diet helps as it's strongly anti-inflammatory. Ketogenic medical researcher Stephen Phinney, M.D., published a study that measured seventeen separate inflammatory markers and showed they all went down on a ketogenic diet. [22]

In addition, there are powerful, natural anti-inflammatory nutrients that act quickly and directly to reduce inflammation, listed in Chapter 2 and summarized in Appendix A. Take as many as you need to lower your inflammation and hs-CRP levels to below .55 for men and 1.0 for women.

Gut Friendly

It's no accident that anxiety and fear often feel like a sinking in the pit of your stomach. When you're anxious it feels like the bottom drops out as your gut contracts and bowels loosen. Even as the chest may also tighten, the overall feeling of anxiety is generally rooted in the gut.

The role of intestinal health and the microbiome in anxiety is immense. The epidemic of leaky gut and sub-clinical cases of leaky gut, common to the point of including almost everyone, sensitizes people so they are "spring-loaded" for anxiety. Add to this the decimation of the microbiome and lack of healthy bacteria that produce calming effects in the gut and brain, and you have a recipe for anxiety and chronic stress.

As Chapter 2, "The Solution," details, the overuse of antibiotics in the developed world has wiped out crucial elements of the microbiome for virtually everyone. The loss of critical bacterial strains also disrupts the tight junctions of the protective intestinal lining. Opening these gates lets dangerous toxins, bacteria, and particles into the body. The foreign invaders wreak as much damage as they can before the body mounts a defense through releasing inflammatory cytokines.

To briefly review, the rising inflammation works as well as it can to neutralize the invaders, But when the doors are always open, this becomes chronic inflammation that then attacks the body's own cells, endangering all systems of the body and leading to anxiety, depression, and cognitive decline, as well as a host of other illnesses.

On top of this, the ubiquitous pesticide (and antibiotic) glyphosate not only kills intestinal bacteria but dramatically opens up the floodgates of the semi-porous membrane at the intestinal barrier. The lack of a good boundary allows poisons, pesticides, small particles, molds, and harmful bacteria to stream into the body.

As the tight junctions of the intestinal lining open, so do the tight junctions of the blood-brain barrier. Even greater damage occurs to the delicate neurons as toxins and invaders pour into the now unprotected brain. The brain also launches an inflammatory cascade to defend itself. But here again, with the gates always somewhat open, the temporary defense of high inflammation becomes chronic, and the inflammatory defense attacks the neurons of the brain. The body's defenses are turned on themselves as brain cells become the target. Anxiety follows (as can depression and cognitive decline).

Remember, glyphosate has been detected in the blood of 93% of Americans, in all samples of oats (including organic oats), commercial wheat, many other crops, and in very high amounts of GMO foods like corn, soy, and cottonseed oil. Commercial meats are loaded with it, as animals are fed GMO corn and soy, and the dust and rain in the Midwest, the South, and central California contain glyphosate. Exposure also comes from feminine hygiene products containing cotton, since cotton, as a GMO, is so heavily contaminated with it.

Generalized anxiety disorder involves a free-floating fear that something bad is about happen or may already be happening. With leaky brain and gut, something bad *is* happening. It's happening on a level where the person has no idea what the real issue is, but the body knows something is terribly wrong. The brain is literally under assault. It makes sense that the feeling of alarm, of anxiety, is the body's signal to alert the person that something is horribly off. But since this occurs at such a deep physiological level below awareness, the person cannot fathom what the actual danger is. The resulting anxiety, however, is all too real.

Re-read the section in Chapter 2, The Solution, for further information on restoring the integrity of the tight junctions. Additionally, increasing the number of healthy bacterial strains involves using certain probiotics to install the particular strains that have been shown to have anti-anxiety effects. Recall the study reported earlier in which mice that were genetically bred to be anxious had their microbiome replaced with the microbiome of mice genetically bred to be fearless. At the same time, the fearless mice had their microbial strains replaced with those from the anxious mice. The results were nothing short of startling. The anxious mice became fearless explorers, while the genetically fearless mice became scared and anxious. Thus, the microbiome changed epigenetic expression.

Certain gut bacteria reduce anxiety via several mechanisms:

- In the intestine, bacteria produce 90% of the body's serotonin, and they produce and consume other neurotransmitters such as GABA, dopamine, and norepinephrine.
- Bacteria interact with the nervous system to alter the body's own production of neurotransmitters.
- Certain strains of bacteria increase the body's production of BDNF, thereby increasing the rate of neurogenesis and neuroplasticity.
- Some strains lower cortisol and other stress hormones.
- Certain bacteria stimulate the vagus nerve, which promotes relaxation and anxiety relief.
- Some strains increase GABA receptors in the brain and increase GABA levels, thereby increasing feelings of calm and relaxation.
- Other strains reduce enteric excitability and inflammation, further decreasing anxiety.
- Certain strains influence gene expression in the amygdala and prefrontal cortex. Without these, the amygdala and prefrontal cortex are anxious and dysregulated, but with them anxiety-like behaviors decrease. [22]

Even if the bacterial strains consumed in a probiotic do not take up residence and colonize the intestinal tract, research shows that these strains have an effect just by passing through. This is why taking certain strains for longer periods or ongoing may be necessary, so these strains can exert their anti-anxiety influence over time.

Some of the key strains that have been shown to be effective in anxiety are:

- **Lactobacillus rhamnosus.** A study of seventy people showed L. rhamnosus lowered anxiety; in mice it reduced anxiety and altered GABA gene expression. [23, 24] Researcher Dr. John

Cryan at University College in Cork, Ireland commented, "The mice [given rhamnosus] were more chilled out."

- **Bifidobacterium longum.** This strain lowers anxiety and increases BDNF levels, promoting neuroplasticity and neurogenesis. [25, 26]
- In humans and mice, one study found it more effective than an SSRI medication (citalopram) used to treat anxiety. [27, 28]
- **Lactobacillus plantarum.** Several studies have shown this strain to be effective in reducing anxiety, lowering inflammatory cytokines, and increasing anti-inflammatory cytokines, as well as increasing neurotransmitter levels, especially dopamine and serotonin. [29]
- **Lactobacillus reuteri**. Although most people have this strain, some do not and many have very low levels. The lack of it caused social deficits in animals, but adding it back in reversed these deficits, which were similar to symptoms of social anxiety. It reduces stress hormone levels, is anti-inflammatory, and alters gene expression of GABA receptors. Neuroscience researcher Shelly Buffington, at Baylor College of Medicine, said, "We found that treatment with this single bacterial strain was able to rescue their social behaviors." [30, 31]
- **Bifidobacterium breve**. This strain lowered anxiety in mice and also improved cognitive performance. [26] It's present in breast milk, and the amount in your gut declines as you age.
- **Lactobacillus casei**.
- **Lactobacillus fermentum**.

The most research has been done on the top six strains, less on the bottom two. The results with both animals and humans are quite convincing. Mood is profoundly influenced by the microbiome. Without certain strains, anxiety rises dramatically. When certain strains are present, anxiety goes down, replaced by feelings of calm, relaxation, and inner peace.

Remember to feed the microbiome well with a high fiber diet of low carb vegetables. Healing the gut is a major priority in healing anxiety and stress.

Micromanage Your Anxiety: A Note on Micronutrients

As with depression and cognitive decline, the absence of certain micronutrients can cause or exacerbate anxiety. Taking supplemental amounts of the following may help reduce anxiety.

Magnesium. One of the most helpful nutrients for anxiety is magnesium. Involved in more than three hundred metabolic functions in the body, magnesium is central to health, especially brain health. For some people anxiety regulation is simply a matter of magnesium regulation. When they have adequate magnesium, their anxiety level drops. Given that the great majority of people are deficient in magnesium due to magnesium-depleted soil and food, together with living in a magnesium-depleting, high EMF world, most people need supplemental magnesium.

There are three forms recommended: magnesium glycinate, magnesium taurate, and magnesium-L-threonate. The first helps relax the body without loose stools that can come from other forms of magnesium, while the second, discussed above, more readily crosses the blood-brain barrier to calm neurons directly and, as already discussed, is neurogenic. Magnesium research shows it activates GABA receptors and reduces anxiety in humans and animals.

Each person needs to experiment to see what dosage level helps. Although more may be necessary depending upon an individual's unique metabolism, a good place to start is two 400 mg magnesium glycinate 1–2 times a day and 3 666-mg magnesium-L-threonate capsules daily. Some people take up to 12 capsules of L-threonate.

Vitamin D. Vitamin D levels are closely tied to both anxiety and depression. [32] As already discussed, recent calculations reveal that standard measures for sufficiency were miscalculated by a factor of ten, so that the great majority of people are well below optimal vitamin D levels. Seventy-five percent of Americans are deficient in vitamin D, and when sufficiency cutoff is changed to 40 or 60 ng/mL, deficiency rates are estimated at 90%. Even at the 30ng/mL level, 97% of African-Americans and 90% of Mexican-Americans are deficient in this nutrient. Optimal blood levels are 60–100 ng/ml.

Most people need to take 5,000–10,000 i.u. daily until optimal levels are achieved. Since blood levels rise slowly, yearly testing is sufficient. Remember to also take vitamin K as well to ensure that calcium reaches your bones.

Niacin. This B vitamin has been used to treat anxiety for decades, beginning with Dr. Abram Hoffer in the 1950s. Because the flush is annoying for some people, taking the non-flush form of niacinamide works just as well (for anxiety, not for cholesterol). Common suggested dosage is 500 mg, 3 times daily.

Thiamine (B-1). Supplemental B-1 at 500 mg twice daily can help with anxiety.

B-6 (pyridoxine). This vitamin, especially the P-5-P form, is one of the precursors of GABA and other calming neurotransmitters. Some people take this before bed to help with sleep. Usual doses are 50–100 mg, 1–2 times daily.

B-12. A deficiency in this vitamin can cause anxiety, but also too much B-12 can cause anxiety. This is a stimulating vitamin, so exercise caution when experimenting with it. It's an essential micronutrient important for brain, cognitive, and emotional functioning. Some people are very sensitive to it and can't tolerate it while others need it. Doses range from 15—5,000 mcg daily, a very wide range.

Zinc. This is essential for mental health. In both humans and animals zinc supplementation reduced anxiety. [33, 34] Zinc is essential for GABA production. Usual doses are up to 40 mg daily.

Vitamin C. This old favorite has been shown to limit cortisol levels and significantly reduce anxiety. While 500 mg daily is enough for general health, anxiety and stress reduction studies used larger doses. It's good to use a buffered version to prevent gastrointestinal distress. Take 3 grams daily, time-release preferred since it's metabolized quickly. [35]

Choline. Just like folate, choline is involved in the methylation cycle. Some people have difficulty with this process, particularly those with the MTHFR gene mutation. One study showed that participants with the lowest choline levels experienced high anxiety levels. [36] One of the best sources of choline is grass-fed meat. It can also be taken as a supplement, and Alpha-GPC is a recommended form, 300 mg, 1–2 times daily.

Immediate relief from anxiety

Anxiety feels really, really terrible. When feeling strong or overwhelming anxiety, you want relief—as soon as possible. With intense anxiety, long-term solutions go out the window. Stopping the anxious feeling NOW is the only priority.

This is when people turn to anti-anxiety medication like Klonopin, Ativan, Valium, or other benzodiazepines. Or else they self-medicate with alcohol or marijuana. There is certainly a place for medications that provide immediate relief from overpowering anxiety. At times benzodiazepines can be just what's needed to calm down. However, just like alcohol or marijuana, all these drugs have serious problems when it comes to the brain.

As discussed earlier, benzodiazepines dull the brain and consciousness. They do numb the anxiety but at the cost of alertness and awareness. Long-term brain changes, addiction, and dependency are among the hazards when used for longer than a few days or weeks.

Alcohol's problems are well-known by now. Aside from being toxic to neurons, alcohol slows neurogenesis and neuroplasticity, thus producing more problems in the long run. Marijuana has its own hazards, from interfering with short-term memory to numbness and mental fog. CBD oil, theoretically devoid of the high from marijuana, may stimulate neurogenesis in lower doses but impairs neurogenesis in higher doses. [37] Initial research indicates it may interfere with memory reconsolidation but further study is needed. Many people find CBD helpful, and the current wave of enthusiasm for CBD oil may prove its usefulness as an anti-inflammatory, pain reliever, and stress reducer. Further studies and time will tell if there are other effects not yet known.

There are a number of brain-healthy supplements, however, that can provide quick relief from anxiety. Aside from producing calmness and relaxation rapidly, many of these herbal extracts and nutrients promote brain plasticity and neurogenesis, which are integral for long-term healing.

Magnesium. As discussed earlier, magnesium is heavily involved in regulating anxiety. For some people this is the only supplement they need. For immediate relief, a common starting point is two 400 mg tablets of magnesium glycinate in the morning and two in the evening. At the same time, take one or two capsules of magnesium-L-threonate morning and evening. Often more is needed. Dr. Joseph Mercola said he needs 10–12 capsules of the L-threonate form daily to experience beneficial effects.

The L-threonate form of magnesium readily crosses the blood-brain barrier and calms the nerves as well as muscles and body. Magnesium is very safe, and excess magnesium is simply eliminated from the body. Neither of these forms of magnesium have the side effect of diarrhea, so experiment and see. Adjust up or down based what you experience.

GABA. Gamma-aminobutyric acid (GABA) is the primary inhibitory (calming) neurotransmitter that counterbalances the excitatory neurotransmitter glutamate. GABA levels in the brain appear to diminish with age, perhaps contributing to the increase in sleep disturbances and cognitive decline in aging. Anti-anxiety medication such as benzodiazepines bind to the GABA receptors to produce their effects. Unfortunately, they downregulate the production of GABA and GABA receptors, perhaps permanently.

The idea is to increase GABA temporarily in the brain to produce relaxation. Taking GABA directly can do this, although reports are mixed about how bioavailable it is. Theoretical objections have been raised which note the size of the GABA molecule makes it difficult to pass the blood-brain barrier. Clinical practice, on the other hand, shows people report feeling a strong relaxing, calming effect when taking GABA.

This is something to try yourself and see the results. Common dosages range from 500–1,000 mg for strong anxiety or for sleep an hour before bed. The minimum effective dose is 250 mg, and this can be taken 3 times throughout the day for anxiety and stress relief. Some people report better absorption when combined with other things such as 150 mg of L-theanine or 20–50 mg of taurine, glycine, and tyrosine.

For many people, I've found that the most effective way to take GABA is the sublingual form, which crosses the blood-brain barrier more efficiently. Start with a 125 mg lozenge and then add another if needed. This route also produces the quickest absorption and can quickly lead to sleep.

The P-5-P form of B-6 is a precursor to GABA and helps the body synthesize it. Taking 100 mg or more of P-5-P can help anxiety and sleep.

I do not recommend phenibut or picamilon, two compounds developed in the Soviet Union that allow GABA to cross the blood-brain barrier. They can produce dependence quickly, much like benzodiazepines.

Lithium orotate. Small amounts of the orotate form of lithium are neurogenic and reduce anxiety. As a mineral, it's freely available in amounts from 1 mg to 30 mg.

Most people recognize lithium as a medication to treat bipolar disorder. This psychiatric medication uses the form of lithium carbonate. Since lithium carbonate has difficulty crossing the blood-brain barrier, massive amounts are used, which eventually become toxic, just as a hundred tons of salt would be toxic. However, lithium orotate does not have these toxic effects and, in fact, appears to be neuroprotective. It is recommended by some as a way to fight cognitive decline in small doses. Finding the right dose for you that reduces anxiety but doesn't cause lethargy means experimenting. Usual doses are 5–25 mg daily.

Magnolia extract. Two extracts of magnolia bark are honokiol and magnolol. These modulate GABA receptors, reduce cortisol levels, and alleviate anxiety by promoting relaxation. [38] Magnolia extract can be used throughout the day and at night as a sleep aid. A common patented form called Relora is widely available, and magnolia extracts are available over the internet. Dosages vary depending on the person, 1–2 or more 300 mg capsules of Relora or 1–2 capsules of 200 mg 90% magnolia bark extract.

Tryptophan and 5-HTP. Tryptophan is a precursor to serotonin. Along the way to becoming serotonin, it becomes 5-HTP, a more immediate precursor. While both are neurogenic, tryptophan causes a more immediate relaxation response in most people. Taking up to 4 grams of tryptophan is fine for most people. Numerous studies have shown taking 2.5 grams before bedtime helps sleep. Other people respond better to 5-HTP, 100–200 mg before bed.

L-theanine. This is the primary amino acid in green tea that produces calming effects and blocks the stimulating effects of caffeine. It increases GABA, serotonin, and dopamine. It is used in China and other Asian countries to treat anxiety and depression, and it's added to soft drinks and chewing gum in Japan as a relaxation aid. It appears to increase EEG alpha waves, much as meditation does, which is why it's known for being relaxing without being sedating. Usual doses range from 100–200 mg, up to 400 mg, both for anxiety as well as a sleep aid.

Lemon balm. This herb has been used for thousands of years to help with anxiety and sleep. Taking 600 mg protected against stress in one study, and taking 300 mg twice daily improved anxiety in another. Sleep improved with this dose as well. It activates GABA receptors in the brain. Clinical trials have used doses from 300 –1,600 mg daily.

Chinese skullcap and American skullcap. These different but related species have somewhat different effects. Chinese skullcap contains baicalin, which as mentioned earlier is neurogenic and works on the GABA system. American skullcap can be more sedating, so be careful not to overdo. Sometimes people report a hangover effect from American skullcap.

L-Ornithine. This amino acid is being used as a sleep aide and anxiolytic supplement. Standard dose is 500 mg, 1–2 times daily or just before sleep.

Melatonin. This hormone produced by the pineal gland is essential for good immunity, good sleep, neurogenesis, and neuroplasticity, and a great many other metabolic and brain functions. The brain produces it at night, in darkness. Unfortunately, less and less of it is produced as a person ages. Taking supplemental melatonin helps many people sleep better and longer. Taking too much can produce drowsiness, so be sure to take only as much as works for you. Some evidence indicates that over time it may cause the body to downregulate its own production of melatonin, so taking breaks is advised. Dose varies from .2 mg to 10 mg before bed, though some people do more.

Apigenin. The use of chamomile tea to calm nerves and reduce anxiety led researchers to investigate its active constituents. Apigenin is a major one. This polyphenol is neurogenic and reduces cortisol in humans. Try 50–100 mg, 1–2 times daily.

More sedating supplements

Valerian. This is the herbal supplement most widely used to help sleep and produce relaxation. Many people find it produces a dulling hangover effect the next day when used as a sleep aid, while others do not report this. Doses vary widely depending upon the concentration.

Kava. This South Pacific plant is used throughout Polynesia, Micronesia, and Hawaii for its sedating effects. There are kava bars in some places. It has been shown to alleviate anxiety in studies. Extracts of kava from organic solvents have been linked to liver toxicity, but most water-based extractions are safe. While it can be too strong for some, it depends upon the concentration and dosage.

Bioactive milk peptides (casein decapeptides). These have been used in Europe to help sleep and promote relaxation and are now available in the U.S. under the brand name Lactium. Take 150 mg at night for sleep or during the day for relaxation.

To decrease anxiety, stop consuming these

The first thing I ask when a new patient consults me about anxiety is, "Do you drink coffee?" Coffee, tea, and energy drinks are so common that they're often viewed as just part of life. Most people consume caffeine in large or small amounts. But your nervous system doesn't differentiate between caffeine and adrenaline. If you suffer from anxiety, the first thing to consider doing is stopping or cutting down on caffeine. Coffee is liquid anxiety.

Caffeine drinks, pills, even caffeine-infused gummy bears are everywhere. As Chapter 2 mentioned, caffeine is problematic for two key reasons. First, caffeine in any amount slows neurogenesis and neuroplasticity. Second, caffeine constricts the blood vessels of the brain, which isn't desirable, as you want more blood to the brain, not less. Despite some short-term gains of muscle performance and short-term memory recall, caffeine is not a long-term friend for your brain.

The polyphenols in coffee are terrific for the brain. If you want to drink decaf or take a supplement that has the neurogenic ingredient in coffee berry fruit (preferably also in a decaffeinated form) go ahead. These are brain healthy. But caffeine itself, despite its omnipresence in society, can cause and exacerbate anxiety. Stop or cut way down.

Many people are so habituated to coffee or caffeine that cutting down and weaning off it seems impossibly hard. However, this too is simply a habit. It just takes a little time for your body to learn to wake itself up again naturally.

To help this shift, make sure you have enough B-5 and B-12. Both are psychic energizers, but be careful here as well, for too much of these B's can cause anxiety. Aerobic exercise also helps your body learn to wake itself up. It can take a week of feeling more subdued before your body learns to wake itself up without a stimulant. After you've made this transition and your body naturally comes alive when you wake up, you'll wonder why you were so attached to caffeine.

Other stimulants can cause anxiety as well. These include: theobromine (the stimulant in dark chocolate), Ritalin, Adderall, crystal meth and cocaine. Trying to reduce anxiety while taking caffeine or any stimulant is like trying to put out a fire by pouring gasoline on it.

Maintenance Phase of Diet

After being on the healing phase of this diet for six to twenty-four months and experiencing reduced anxiety, you can shift into the maintenance phase. Staying healthy doesn't require the same rigorous diet that healing does.

For most people this involves reducing the number of neurogenic supplements, gradually adding in more carbs, reducing the anti-inflammatory supplements but continuing along the general lines of the diet, i.e., low carb and high good fat and fiber. It's a process of experimentation. You have to discover what your unique body needs.

Some people will continue with the healing phase of the diet permanently. It can feel so good that people report they don't want to interrupt it. Others switch to cyclical keto (six days of keto, then cycling off for a carb day of 100–150 grams). Still others leave the zone of nutritional ketosis entirely but remain relatively low carb. Only you can know what feels right.

> *Debbie entered therapy suffering from anxiety and eating issues. A vegan for the past five years, she was a bright, idealistic person who genuinely tried to do the right thing in her life. Coming from a family that had many common problems, it quickly became clear that her diet was the immediate danger to her brain and sense of well-being.*
>
> *She was initially resistant to the idea of eating animal products but changed her mind when she learned about the research on the dangers of a vegan diet. She started taking 4 grams daily of omega-3s, eating pastured chicken and dairy, with occasionally some grass-fed meat or wild fish. She loved all veggies she could eat. Having avoided fat for most of her life, she was shocked to find how much better she soon felt when she got most of her calories from fat.*
>
> *She experimented slowly with different neurogenic and anti-inflammatory supplements. Soon she felt so much better that she decided to incorporate more of them into her daily regimen. Some she continued and a few didn't feel right. She stopped drinking coffee and caffeine tea, and immediately she started sleeping better, which also had a calming effect.*
>
> *After two months of going full ketogenic, she bounced into the office astounded at how much better she felt. "I feel more solid and grounded but at the same time calm and clear. I can think better, but most of all I feel calm and steady. It's amazing!"*
>
> *Six months later she felt so good she decided to take a break and check back in once a month. These monthly check-ins occurred over the next year. At that point she was "feeling better than I've ever felt. I had no idea how much my diet influences my mood. It's a crime more people don't know about this."*

Taking responsibility for your health means letting yourself experiment, try new things and combinations. Even if an experiment seems like a failure, usually you learn something in the process. Trial and error is how most important things in life are learned.

Other Physical Factors

Exercise. Aerobic exercise can be a way to "burn off" the excess energy of anxiety. Your body revs up while exercising, then cools down and returns to homeostatic balance when you rest afterward. Doing aerobic exercise three to five days a week is optimal. Since aerobic exercise increases the rate of neurogenesis and neuroplasticity, this reduces anxiety. Further, the new neurons produced during aerobic exercise appear to be resistant to stress and show less gene expression related to stress. Researchers who discovered this said the new neurons were "specifically buffered from exposure to stressful experience." Aerobic exercise created brains that seemed biochemically and molecularly calm. [39]

One problem I've seen with a few patients is overtraining. They run every day and don't take a break. As a result, their anxiety increases, sometimes even breaking out in hives from running too consistently. Take at least a day or two off per week to let your body slow down.

Whereas aerobic exercise seems better for the brain in depression and cognitive decline, other forms of exercise work just as well if not better for anxiety. Yoga, Pilates, qigong, tai chi, and other gentle forms produce muscular relaxation and feelings of calm. These forms of exercise stimulate the parasympathetic nervous system so the body and brain can unhook from the "fight-flight-or-freeze" mode of the sympathetic system. When your muscles relax, anxiety eases.

Yoga is probably the ideal form of exercise for anxiety. The stretching brings a relaxation response to the muscles afterward, and in many yoga classes a short meditation at the end of class deepens the relaxation. Whether it's a form of restorative yoga or a more athletic form, the stillness and alive calm after a yoga session is hard to beat. Yoga nidra takes this further by bringing the mind into a deep state of relaxation.

Progressive relaxation. Fear and relaxation are mutually exclusive. If you are deeply relaxed, you don't feel anxious. Anxiety produces muscle tension throughout the body. It's noteworthy that many people do not even know what it's like to be profoundly relaxed. One way to bring awareness to tense muscles is to tense them even more and then to relax them. Progressive relaxation involves tensing and then relaxing each major muscle group of your body to produce a relaxed state.

Originally used in psychotherapy and taught over eight weeks in hourly sessions, this has been modified so that most anyone can do it on their own. There are many sources that describe this online. The idea is to lie down comfortably, close your eyes, and then tense each major muscle group, hold the tension for five seconds, and then release. It makes no difference whether you begin from the head and work down or vice versa.

Tense the muscles of your head, tongue, eyes ... hold for five seconds, and then relax. Then tense the muscles of your neck ... hold for five seconds, and then release. Work your way down your body. When you finish, tense your entire body ... hold for five seconds, and then relax. Let the muscle tension fade away and sink into a deeper and deeper state of relaxation.

Practicing this brings progressively greater results. The body learns the relaxation response as you repeat this over days and weeks. Allowing your body to enter a profound state of relaxation is an antidote to stress and anxiety. When you have this as a reference point, you can see how much tension accompanies anxiety.

Breathing. One of the first orders of business in treating panic disorders is to teach the person how to breathe. It may sound strange to teach someone how to breathe, since clearly the person is breathing if they're alive. However, most people don't know how to breathe properly.

In a state of panic or anxiety, many people have rapid but very shallow breath. They may take short, rapid breaths from their upper chest and with a tight belly. Not only is shallow breathing very inefficient, but the body isn't getting the oxygen it needs. The trick is to bring the air deep into your lower lungs, because the lower lungs are full of alveoli. This happens through belly breathing, called "diaphragmatic breathing," which more fully oxygenates your body and brain.

Learning diaphragmatic breathing is simple. Put one hand on your chest and one hand on your belly. Breathe so your lower hand moves and your upper hand hardly moves at all. To breathe this way, you need to activate your diaphragm, which pulls the air deep into your lower lungs. Try to take one breath about every five or six seconds or so. Whenever you feel panicky or anxious, breathe from your belly, not too fast or too slow. This will calm your system.

Another important aspect is breathing through your nose. Nose breathing also pulls air into your lower lungs. The lower lungs are full of parasympathetic nerve receptors to bring relaxation, whereas the upper lungs prompt us to hyperventilate and activate the sympathetic, fight-flight-or-freeze response. When you take regular, slow breaths through your nose, this activates your parasympathetic nervous system, producing calmness.

Sleep. Sleep is essential to feeling calm and lowering anxiety. When you get enough sleep, the brain has greater resources to deal with life's stresses. But when you don't get enough sleep, you wake up feeling more "on edge," with higher amounts of circulating stress hormones such as cortisol, more toxic brain debris because it didn't get cleared out in sleep, reduced neurogenic activity, impaired memory and cognitive ability that reduces decision-making quality. In healthy adults, a single night of sleep deprivation will trigger anxiety the next morning, according to one study. [40]

Going from 7.5 to 6.5 hours of sleep at night increases expression of genes associated with stress, inflammation, diabetes, and cancer risk. Losing one hour of sleep during the spring shift to daylight savings time results in more car accidents, work injuries, and heart attacks over the next two to three days.

The amygdala, a key brain system that triggers fear and anxiety, is 60% more reactive with sleep deprivation. It's believed this is due to the dampening down of the prefrontal cortex function. [41] A hyper aroused amygdala is the precursor for anxiety. Sleep refreshes and calms the body and all the brain's subsystems.

Unfortunately, anxiety and stress disrupt sleep. Insomnia and sleep disorders are prevalent in anxiety disorders. Getting seven or eight hours of sleep per night is one of the most important supports of brain health. Read the section on developing good sleep hygiene in Chapter 2, "The Solution." If need be, try some of the relaxing herbs or supplements just discussed above to help get to sleep and stay asleep.

Hormone imbalances and toxicity from heavy metals, mold, and EMFs. Too much or too little thyroid, testosterone, estrogen, progesterone, or other hormones can cause anxiety, depression, or cognitive decline. Birth control pills have been linked to anxiety and depression. Menopause is often accompanied by anxiety as estrogen levels plunge. Male "andropause," or reduced testosterone associated with aging, can cause anxiety or depression. Thyroid problems are a sure path to anxiety. So is glucocorticoid excess due to always-on adrenals from stress.

Getting hormone levels tested can lead to correcting the problem. Finding your optimal hormone level may take some time but can lead to dramatic results. Try to find a physician who is knowledgeable in this area and uses bioidentical hormones whenever possible.

Heavy metal toxicity or toxicity from mold can wreak havoc with your nervous system and mood. Anxiety is one of the most common symptoms.

Anxiety can be a side effect of 24/7 media culture, creating sympathetic overstimulation. For example, the stressful, often alarming content that websites use to pull in viewers jacks up the adrenaline. And as you watch the news, pay attention to the tone of voice, the background music, the urgency and crisis nature that are intended to keep you watching—all this stimulates the stress response and increases glucocorticoid levels. Online life is a life of images not real, physical human contact that provides touch, downtime, and a chance to reset your nervous system through parasympathetic balancing.

The electromagnetic fields (EMFs) from cell phones, Wi-Fi, smart meters, etc., have been shown to cause emotional disturbances, particularly anxiety and depression. Animal studies show diverse high impacts on the brain even with low-level EMFs. [42] See Chapter 2, "The Solution," for more on diagnosing and correcting these issues.

Anxiety as a side effect of medication. There are numerous medications that can cause anxiety. Some examples are:

- medications with caffeine (many aspirin brands have this)
- steroids like cortisone (to treat allergies, arthritis)
- ADHD drugs (such as Adderall, Ritalin)
- Decongestants (such as Sudafed)
- thyroid medication
- asthma medications
- some herbs or excess vitamins, such as ginseng, B-12 or B-6

Be sure to check what medications or stimulating herbs and supplements you're taking that might contribute to anxiety.

APPENDIX D

THE PHYSICAL SIDE OF DEPRESSION

Nutrition

This antidepressant diet has two phases: the Healing Phase and the Maintenance Phase. The more intensive Healing Phase is highly neurogenic and follows the four principles discussed in Chapter 2, "The Solution":

- neurogenic
- ketogenic
- anti-inflammatory
- gut friendly

The Maintenance Phase can be started six to twenty-four months after symptoms have receded, and it consists of modifying the diet based on individual needs, for example going to low carb rather than strictly ketogenic. However, this chapter presents modifications of the diet outlined in Chapter 2 that are specifically designed to resolve depression.

Healing Phase of Diet

Neurogenic

This section highlights the antidepressant power of certain key nutrients. The more neurogenic nutrients listed in Chapter 2 you can include in your diet, the greater the impact against depression. Remember, almost no one can do all of them, so don't try to be totalistic, just do what feels right for your system.

Curcumin or turmeric. This is particularly important for depression, not only for its powerful effects on neurogenesis and neuroplasticity but for its anti-inflammatory properties. One of the most important brain discoveries is that depression is an inflammatory process for most people. It is important to take as many of the anti-inflammatory nutrients as possible, and curcumin is one of the most powerful.

Additionally, curcumin alone has been shown to be an effective antidepressant. [1, 2] A meta-analysis of six studies showed it to be "safe, well-tolerated and efficacious" against depression, and three of the studies showed significant anti-anxiety effects. [3] An Australian study showed doses of 250 mg of curcumin were just as effective as 500 mg daily for depression and anxiety. [4]

Since it is poorly absorbed, be sure to take it either with phospholipids (e.g., eggs or lecithin), piperine, or in micronized form, as this will increase bioavailability by eight to fifty times.

Omega-3s. Countries with high rates of omega-3 consumption have low rates of depression. [5] In an interview, Joseph Hibbeln, M.D., from the National Institute on Alcohol Abuse and Alcoholism (NIAAA) said, "The strongest evidence was found for managing major depressive symptoms, with the effect of omega-3s being at least as great if not greater than antidepressant medications." [6, 7]

For most conditions, a balance between DHA and EPA is optimal. However, in depression, given that this is often an inflammatory condition, taking more EPA may be a better strategy for most. A two to one ratio of EPA to DHA is a preferable balance in this case. Three to four grams of this mixture daily works for most people, but in depression it may be better to begin with a slightly higher amount, at least for the first few months. If your hs-CRP blood test is below .55 for men or 1.0 for women, then a one to one ratio of EPA to DHA is preferable. (See discussion below.)

Again, make sure your source is molecularly distilled to avoid any mercury or other contaminants. Store it in a cool place in a dark container so it doesn't oxidize through heat or light. For vegetarians this nutrient is especially important, as blood levels of omega-3s generally run low, so use an algae form.

Green tea extract. Here again, the EGCGs in green tea powerfully stimulate neurogenesis and neuroplasticity. Additionally, its strong anti-inflammatory and antioxidant properties make it three times as effective against depression. Best to use decaffeinated extracts, 725 mg of 45% EGCG once daily.

Melatonin. Getting enough sleep is critical in depression. There is a tendency to sleep either too much or too little. Melatonin can help you sleep more and better if you're sleeping too little. Some time-release forms allow melatonin to be absorbed in the later hours of the night when it's most needed. Dosage varies by person, from .2 mg to 10 mg.

St. John's wort. This herb requires a prescription in Europe but not in the U.S. It's been shown to be more effective than SSRIs for mild to moderate depression. A recent study shows it not only has powerful neurotrophic effects (it increased neuroplasticity by 25% and neurogenesis by 25–50% in just a few days), it is also neuroprotective against toxins with strong anti-inflammatory powers. [8]

Vitamin D. The "sunshine vitamin," aka "happiness vitamin," is very important in healing depression. [9] Vitamin D has been shown to be helpful in depression not linked to seasonal pattern (SAD). It increases BDNF and neuroplasticity, is anti-inflammatory, antioxidant, and neuroprotective.

A 2014 paper noted that the original recommendations for vitamin D were based on a mathematical error that was never corrected, underestimating daily need by a factor of ten. The early medical belief that it's easy to overdose on vitamin D has been shown to be untrue; it's actually rather difficult to take too much. While the American Medical Association believes 20 ng/mL are sufficient, recent research puts over 60 ng/mL as best for disease prevention. [10] Optimal blood levels are 60–100 ng/ml.

The great majority of people are well below optimal vitamin D levels. Seventy-five percent of Americans are deficient in vitamin D, and when sufficiency cutoff is changed to 40 or 60 ng/mL, deficiency rates are estimated at 90%. Even at the 30ng/mL level,

97% of African Americans and 90% of Mexican-Americans are deficient in this nutrient.

Most people need to take 5,000–10,000 i.u. daily until optimal levels are achieved. Since blood levels rise slowly, yearly testing is sufficient. Remember to also take vitamin K to ensure calcium reaches your bones.

Ginkgo biloba. By raising BDNF levels and increasing neurogenesis, this compound is helpful not only for memory but depression.

Taurine. This amino acid has been shown to have an antidepressant effect. [11] It also increases BDNF levels and neurogenesis. Take 500–1,000 mg daily.

DHEA. This naturally occurring hormone can have strong antidepressant effects in some people. For a few this works like a miracle, especially if they are over fifty. For most others, however, it has little effect, so experimentation is necessary. Aside from being the so-called youth hormone, it's a precursor to testosterone, estrogen, and other androgens. Usual dosages range from 25–100 mg daily. Sometimes after a few weeks or months the person adapts to the new level and the dosage is needs to be increased.

Berberine. This yellow compound increases BDNF, is anti-inflammatory, and improves blood glucose levels. On its own, it is also an effective anti-depressant agent. [12, 13] Usual doses are 400 mg, 2–3 times daily.

Blueberries. The anthocyanin dye in blueberries is highly neuroprotective and neurogenic. Blueberries and other berries have the lowest sugar content of fruits, but they still do contain sugar, so be careful how much you consume. Too much can knock you out of ketosis. Blueberry extract with 25% anthocyanin content is an excellent alternative.

Quercetin. This neurogenic flavonoid is also highly anti-inflammatory, antioxidant, and neuroprotective. It is also senolytic, meaning it cleans up old, senescent cells that impair performance. Take 500 mg, 1–2 times daily.

Bacopa. This extract increases BDNF and has been shown to be antidepressant in mouse models of depression. [14] Dosage depends on strength of extract.

Carnosine. This amino acid has been shown to have antidepressant, anti-inflammatory, antioxidant, and antiglycation effects. [15] It rejuvenates old pre-senescent cells and mitochondria. It helps reduce the effects of cortisol and helps with stress. Take 500 mg, 1–2 times daily.

Ketogenic

The ketogenic diet may be the most powerful antidepressant diet there is. Most people who were raised on or continue to eat the standard American diet (SAD) set themselves up for depression, as well as anxiety and cognitive decline. There's a reason it's called the SAD diet—it's depressogenic. The SAD diet is high carb, low good fat and high bad fat, low fiber, highly inflammatory, and more and more research points to it leading directly to depression, anxiety, Alzheimer's, diabetes, obesity, cancers, heart disease, and other inflammatory diseases.

One of the tenets of this book is that sooner or later, sugar becomes neurotoxic. Excess sugar intake eventuates in insulin resistance, and an estimated 80% of Americans have some degree of insulin resistance. As mentioned previously, a high sugar diet cuts the rate of neurogenesis by 50%.

Sugar sets the stage for depression in several ways: by being inflammatory, through increasing glycation, slowing neurogenesis and neuroplasticity and through increased oxidation. A 2016 study showed a strong link between high-sugar diets and depression in post-menopausal women. A 2017 study found men consuming 67 grams of sugar a day were 23% more likely to become depressed than those who consumed 40 grams or less. [16, 17]

The ketogenic diet changes all that. It has a mood-stabilizing effect and is neurogenic, neuroprotective, and anti-inflammatory. When combined with high fiber intake (low carb vegetables), it is very gut friendly. Additionally, the more efficient brain metabolism in ketosis has a mood elevating effect in most people. There are two controlled studies showing antidepressant effects of a ketogenic diet in mice but as of this writing not yet any studies with humans. [18,19] One study even showed greater resistance to depression in adult offspring when pregnant female mice were fed a ketogenic diet, with 4.8% greater brain volume in the cerebellum.

My clinical experience with patients provides case study evidence that many people who've been depressed for decades emerge from it after adopting a ketogenic diet.

Vegetarians have double the rate of depression and anxiety in some studies. [20, 21] This is probably due to a lack of omega-3s, B-12, and healthy fats, as well as increased intake of grains and unhealthy vegetable oils and fats. Adapting the Healthy Brain Diet to exclude meat takes some extra thought to get the proper neural nutrients.

Some people find it hard to give up most carbohydrates and decide to supplement with exogenous ketones. Though the full metabolic benefits of ketosis do not accrue with exogenous ketones, many do. There is one study on mice that shows anti-anxiety effects from exogenous ketones alone. Since anxiety and depression are so closely linked, it is a good bet that exogenous ketones also work to reduce depression. A full-on ketogenic diet is preferable to low carb and supplementing with dietary ketones, but here again, do as much as you can.

Anti-inflammatory

Chronic inflammation is behind most chronic diseases the developed world faces: cancer, heart disease, diabetes, obesity, cancer, Alzheimer's, and depression. Although not everyone who is depressed has higher inflammatory blood markers, most do. That's why this section is critically important, to learn how to incorporate natural, powerful anti-inflammatory nutrients to lower inflammation and heal depression.

The "cytokine model of cognitive function" shows how the cytokine signaling behind inflammation has powerful neurological effects on cognition and mood, particularly depression and anxiety. Inflammatory cytokines trigger a cascade of neural events that interfere with neurotransmitters, slow neurogenesis and neuroplasticity, decrease BDNF levels, attack neurons, and produce behavioral changes called "sickness behavior" that includes anhedonia, sleep changes, decreased social interaction, and fever. [22, 23]

To find out your general inflammatory level, everyone should get the high sensitivity c-reactive protein (hs-CRP) blood test. If your hs-CRP blood level is above .55 for a male or 1.0 for a female, getting your inflammation level down is crucial. Even if your numbers are below this, keeping your inflammation levels low is extremely important for overall physical and mental health.

The ketogenic diet is a good starting point as it's strongly anti-inflammatory. Ketogenic medical researcher Stephen Phinney, M.D. published a study measuring seventeen separate inflammatory markers. All seventeen markers went down on a ketogenic diet. [24]

In addition, there are powerful, natural anti-inflammatory nutrients that act quickly and directly to reduce inflammation, listed in Chapter 2. For depression especially, the more of these you can include in your daily regimen, the better. Of particular importance are:

- omega-3s
- curcumin (be sure to take with something to increase bioavailability, such as piperine, phospholipids, or micronized curcumin)
- green tea extract
- carnosine (at least 500 mg, 2 times daily)
- berberine (400 mg, 2–3 times daily) has strong antidepressant effects [25]
- ginger extract
- rosmarinic acid
- Gamma linoleic acid (GLA), found in borage oil, evening primrose oil; depressed patients have lower levels [26] (1,000 mg, 1–2 times daily)

Gut friendly

The importance of intestinal health and a diverse microbiome can hardly be overstated. A healthy intestinal and microbial environment is key to feeling good.

The "gut-brain axis" referred to earlier has given way to a sub-specialty called "neurogastroenterology." Research in this field reveals direct biochemical signaling between the intestinal tract and the brain. This communication is bi-directional, and it occurs by way of the enteric nervous system, the immune system, the neuroendocrine system, and the autonomic nervous system.

Depression and anxiety have now been linked to reductions in the diversity of the intestinal microbiome, a deficiency in certain strains, and an overgrowth of unhealthy strains of bacteria. European research published in 2019 was the first population-level study to link gut bacteria to depression. There are two different strains of gut bacteria that are depleted in people with depression, regardless of antidepressant treatments. [27]

Even emotional stress, apart from antibiotics or pesticides, can reduce microbial diversity and disrupt the tight junctions, increasing the permeability of the intestinal lining. Since depression and anxiety are related to stress, researchers have begun exploring how manipulating the microbiome and increasing intestinal health can help depression. [28]

Certain probiotics have been found to be helpful for depression. A number of studies have been done with mice as well as humans showing a strong influence on mood from particular strains of bacteria.

The first three strains have been researched the most extensively and show significant reduction in depression in humans. [29] Studies in mice show the first two probiotics work in several ways to reduce depression, anxiety, and stress. Epinephrine (adrenaline) and norepinephrine levels fell 28% and 51%, while the stress hormone corticosterone fell 68%. Intestinal permeability dropped by 57%, which indicates a tightening of the "leaky gut" induced by stress. BDNF increased as well as doublecortin, both indicating increased neurogenesis and neuroplasticity. [30]

A study done with Bifidobacterium longum at McMaster University showed 64% of participants had significant reduction in depression, along with an increase in quality of life scores. Brain scans showed that brain areas associated with depression, including the amygdala and fronto-limbic regions, were less active and reduced their reaction to "negative emotional stimuli," so they weren't as reactive to sad experiences or images. [31]

Because certain probiotics have been shown to have such a profound effect on mood, they have been dubbed "psychobiotics." Most of these are available commercially:

- Lactobacillus helveticus
- Lactobacillus rhamnosus
- Lactobacillus acidophilus
- Lactobacillus casei
- Lactobacillus brevis
- Bifidobacterium bifidum
- Bifidobacterium longum
- Bifidobacterium infantis

It should also be noted that taking probiotics has been shown to reduce systemic inflammation, so often elevated in depression, making probiotics another part of the anti-inflammatory strategy for reducing depression. [28]

Micromanage Your Depression: A Note on Micronutrients

There are a number of micronutrient deficiencies that can cause depression or depression-like symptoms. These vitamins, minerals, and natural molecules are essential to the brain's proper functioning. Most people are deficient in many of these.

Vitamin D. This has already been discussed as a powerful neurogenic vitamin. Most people have levels below the optimal 60–100 mmol. You can still be depressed when your level is in this range, but it's harder.

B vitamins, especially folate (B-9), B-5, and B-12. The family of B vitamins are responsible for numerous metabolic and neurological functions. Low levels are common in depression, with low levels of dietary folate raising the risk of depression by 300%. [32] Vitamin B supplements have been shown to improve depression outcomes. [33] Most people can get enough with a simple B complex vitamin, either 50 or 100. Some people who are very deficient will need higher doses, especially of B-5 (pantothenic acid) and B-12, both of which are psychic energizers.

Folate metabolism is impaired in some people with the MTHFR gene mutations. Only 7% of people with low folate respond to antidepressant, whereas 44% of those with normal levels do. The most bioavailable form is methylfolate. Usual doses are 400–800 mg daily.

B-5 can be taken in daily doses from 50–500 mg.

B-12 is often deficient in vegetarians and vegans since it isn't generally present in plant foods. Dairy, eggs, and meat are the main sources. The most bioavailable form is methylcobalamin. Doses range from 20 mcg to 5,000 mcg. If you get overstimulated or have difficulty sleeping when taking this, cut back.

Zinc. This mineral is used by more enzymes than any other mineral. It helps control inflammation, immunity, and mood. Research has shown beneficial effects of zinc supplementation on depression, and it boosts the effectiveness of antidepressants. [34] Typical doses are 25–50 mg daily.

Iodine. Iodine deficiency can be a major problem since it's so crucial for the thyroid. When the thyroid slows down, it looks exactly like depression. If you don't eat fish or sea algae or commercial table salt that is fortified with iodine, you may be deficient. Recommended dose is about 150 mcg daily.

Iron. Depression can result from too little iron (anemia), most common among premenopausal women. Depression can also result from too much iron, at least in men. [35] See Chapter 2 for how to increase or decrease iron levels to reach optimal ferritin blood levels.

SAMe. This naturally occurring molecule is present throughout the body. Some people respond well to it, but most of the people I've seen find it turns off their feelings, leaving them feeling a neutral gray rather than more alive. Many complain they can't cry when taking this. Nevertheless, for some it works well, and it usually works within days, rather than the four to eight weeks for SSRIs. Doses are 400–1,600 mg daily.

Alpha lipoic acid. The body makes this anti-oxidant which boosts energy, assists in regulating blood sugar, and helps stabilize mood. [36] Doses range from 50–400 mg daily, with higher ranges of 600–1,200 mg for diabetic neuropathy.

Acetyl-L-carnitine. How depressed a person is has been linked to the level of acetyl-L-carnitine (ALCAR), and ALCAR has been shown to be effective in its treatment. [37] It is also neuroprotective. Some people find it too stimulating, so experiment. Doses range from 1–3 grams daily.

Coenzyme Q10 (CoQ10). Lower CoQ10 levels are present in depressed patients. Supplementation with CoQ10 can help with depression, especially when inflammation is involved. [38] Those who take statins are at particular risk of low CoQ10 levels. Doses range from 50–1,200 mg daily, with 100–200 mg typical.

Selenium. This mineral is also key for proper thyroid function and making the body's most important antioxidant glutathione. Daily dose is usually 55 mcg.

Ursolic acid. This supplement increases the production of irisin, a brain messenger that has been shown to have antidepressant effects by regulating energy metabolism. It also increases BDNF and neuroplasticity. [39, 40] Usual doses are 150–300 mg daily.

Magnesium. The majority of people are deficient in this key mineral. In a randomized clinical trial, magnesium supplementation improved mild to moderate depression within two weeks—quite a rapid response. [41] Low magnesium levels are significantly associated with depression, especially in younger adults. [42] Given that younger adults are most exposed to EMF contamination, which is rampant, as discussed earlier, and that EMF exposure depletes magnesium, most everyone with a cell phone can benefit from magnesium.

Magnesium stimulates the calming neurotransmitter GABA, and so is useful in anxiety as well, and it inhibits NMDA receptors, which are involved in depression and is how ketamine appears to work, though magnesium is without ketamine's side effects. Usual range is 200–800 mg daily, both from traditional forms of magnesium such as magnesium glycinate as well as magnesium-L-threonate, which crosses the blood-brain barrier.

Maintenance Phase of Diet

After the depression has lifted and you've been symptom free for six to twenty-four months, you can switch into the Maintenance Phase of the Healthy Brain Diet, as it's best to give the necessary time for the brain to heal and grow into this new, symptom-free state. The brain needs to heal, to make new connections and re-wire itself in its non-depressed state, to make the new non-depressed state normal. This takes some time. Don't rush it. Allow your brain to develop a solid foundation of health and well-being.

When this is well established, the Maintenance Phase begins. This is necessarily experimental, since for each person it will look quite different. Some people will need to remain very close to the Healing Phase, while others can make more changes.

The key elements of change in the Maintenance Phase are backing off from the strict ketogenic diet, reducing the number of neurogenic, probiotic, and anti-inflammatory supplements.

Bringing more carbohydrates into the diet is the biggest change, and this very much depends upon each individual's blood glucose level and hemoglobin A1c test. If you can tolerate higher carbs as evidenced by these tests and you feel fine with a higher carbohydrate load, then go ahead. If not, back up and shift to a lower carb intake.

A low carbohydrate, higher fat and high fiber diet is preferable for most people but not all. A few people can return to a high carb diet, though at some point this will need to change when insulin resistance sets in. A cyclical ketogenic diet that has higher carb intake one or two days a week works for many people. Some will need or want to remain ketogenic for life. It depends upon the person.

Since inflammation is behind most diseases and usually involved in depression, continuing to monitor your high-sensitivity CRP blood test is important. If this goes very low, you can have more flexibility in this area, although even then I'd suggest maintaining as much of the anti-inflammatory diet as possible as a preventative against future disease or depression.

It's similar with probiotics, prebiotics, and a high fiber diet. Keeping your gut healthy is an ongoing process.

Bobbie had been on antidepressants for over twenty years, yet he was still depressed. His diet, not surprisingly, was the SAD diet. Although physically active as a construction worker, he had problems with sleep.

He was so desperate to get off the SSRIs he'd been on that he jumped into the Healthy Brain Diet eagerly. Giving up carbs and processed foods was a challenge for the first month, but then it got easier as he felt better and better. His initial resistance to doing so many neurogenic and anti-inflammatory supplements gave way to understanding that he couldn't get everything from food alone.

After two months, he was fully keto-adapted. "I feel like my brain is turbo-charged," he said one day. "My mood is better than it's been any time in my adult life." After six months of feeling good, he decided to slowly cut down his SSRI and then go off it entirely. His physician warned him against this, telling him he had a biological disease that required antidepressants for the rest of his life. Undaunted, he wanted to see for himself if he could live without medication.

The next six months were difficult at times, as his brain slowly needed to upregulate its production of serotonin and key signaling molecules. But at the end of six and then twelve months, he felt better than he could have imagined.

"I know I have psychological issues to deal with, but changing my diet has done more for my mental health than all the therapy I've ever tried. I feel like my brain is humming at a high level rather than just sputtering along. This feels like nothing short of a miracle!"

The entire Maintenance Phase becomes a way of lifelong eating rather than a special diet. Of course, as with any lifestyle, it requires continual tweaking and modifications as you age. What works at one stage stops working later on. Life becomes an ongoing experiment, a flexible movement of adjustment and readjustment rather than a set plan forever.

Other physical factors

Exercise. Together with diet, exercise exerts a profound effect on the health of the brain as well as other bodily systems. It helps DNA repair and protects against genetic damage, improves epigenetic expression to increase health, reduces inflammation, improves glucose sensitivity and mitochondrial function, improves intracellular communication and stem cell migration, clears senescent cells, increases brain size and heart function as well as overall vitality.

Exercise has a powerful effect on depression, but exercising may be the last thing in the world a depressed person wants to do. Nevertheless, if you can get yourself to exercise, it will pay off in significantly improved mood.

There are two types of exercise that have been shown to be helpful in depression: aerobic exercise and strength training.

Aerobic exercise. The "runner's high" is one of the best antidepressants known. For a while it was believed that those who ran marathons were immune from depression, but this was later shown to be false. Nevertheless, it is more difficult to be depressed if you have an aerobic exercise regimen—running, biking, swimming, fast dancing, walking, or anything that gets you breathing hard.

The powerful brain and body changes that come with running or any other kind of aerobic exercise work against depression from several angles. Aerobic exercise is strongly neurogenic, increasing neurogenesis and neuroplasticity. It increases BDNF, endorphins, anandamide, and the neurotransmitters serotonin, dopamine, and noradrenaline, lowers insulin resistance, reduces inflammation, improves mitochondrial metabolism, vascularization, and heart health—all of which improve brain health. [43]

There is an important caveat to this, however. What has been most effective is sustained aerobic exercise, not the currently popular high intensity interval training (HIIT). The aerobic exercise should last for at least twenty minutes or longer, at least three to five times per week. HIIT is good for many things such as insulin resistance and heart health, but it does not appear to affect neurogenesis or neuroplasticity. Probably doing HIIT once or twice a week is also a good idea for general fitness but sustained aerobic training for half an hour appears better for fighting depression.

Start easy and build up gradually. For someone who hasn't exercised, it takes time to work up to higher intensity workouts. This can be hard to imagine while depressed, yet moving even a little will result in feeling better immediately. And this positive reinforcement can be the encouragement to continue. Begin with walking, then walk more and faster. See where your body wants to take it.

Aside from diet, aerobic exercise is probably the most effective antidepressant known. It's called "the exercise prescription." It's free, and the side effects of improved health add to its benefits.

Strength training. Lifting weights or exercise that builds muscle has been shown to significantly reduce depressive symptoms. A meta-analysis that appeared in the *Journal of the American Medical Association* of thirty-thre trials involving nearly two thousand people revealed that strength training improves mood so strongly it is as effective as medication and is a viable alternative. [44] The greatest improvements in mood were with those with mild to moderate depression rather than those without depression.

Twice a week strength training is suggested. Another review showed other impressive mood benefits including reduction in anxiety, improvements with cognition and sleep in older depressed adults, and improvement in self-esteem. [45]

Sleep. A good night's sleep refreshes the brain and self. Even one night of less than six hours sleep results in measurable cognitive decline and impaired emotion regulation. Getting insufficient sleep over time gradually wears down your emotional resilience, making you more cranky, anxious, and depressed.

Depression can cause a person to sleep either more or less. Sleeping too much can be almost as detrimental as sleeping too little. Ensuring you get a good night's sleep is an important part of recovery from depression. Practicing the good sleep hygiene mentioned in Chapter 2 will ensure your brain gets the rest it needs for renewal.

Detoxification from heavy metals, mold, and EMFs. Some people are so poisoned by such things as having lead pipes growing up, having parents who cooked with aluminum pans, high fish intake, moldy environments, and exposure to high levels of EMFs that until they detox, they will continue to be depressed.

Microwave EMFs activate voltage-gated calcium channels that are concentrated in the brain. [46] Studies have EMF exposure associated with at least thirteen psychiatric effects, especially depression and anxiety. [47] See the section on Physical Detoxification in Chapter 2.

Depression as a side effect of medication. A recent study in the *Journal of the American Medical Association* shows that over one-third of Americans take a medication that has depression as a known side effect. Users of these drugs have higher rates of depression. Further, many people are taking more than one of these drugs, and the risk of depression increases for each additional drug taken. [48]

The drugs are commonly used medications such as: anti-acid proton pump inhibitors for acid reflux, beta blockers for high blood pressure, common antibiotics, birth control pills, antidepressants (ironically), and even prescription-strength ibuprofen. Many of these do not require a prescription and are sold over-the-counter. Another study links statins with depression, which shows the importance of cholesterol for healthy brain function and the cognitive impairment that can come when cholesterol levels fall too low. [49] Statins are taken by more Americans than any other medication, with antidepressants a close second.

If you are taking one or more of these medications, don't stop but consult with your healthcare professional to see if other options exist that don't carry the side effect of depression.

APPENDIX E

THE PHYSICAL SIDE OF COGNITIVE DECLINE

Nutrition

The brain is always "under construction." It is in constant movement, creating new connections and growing new neurons, pruning old neurons and cleaning up toxic residue, always modeling and remodeling itself in an ongoing cycle of slow-motion repair-heal-regenerate.

To ensure this cycle works optimally means having the capacity to build new neurons and new connections between neurons, to carry out the garbage (autophagy, pruning, disposal of waste) and repair damaged neurons. High-quality building materials are needed to grow new neural cellular tissue and to repair damage. The brain's blood-brain barrier needs to be intact in order to protect it from neurotoxins. Cleaning out the toxic residues means the brain's natural cleansing mechanisms must function at a high level.

Diet has a major impact on all of this.

Healing Phase of Diet

The brain changes associated with cognitive decline, Alzheimer's, and other forms of dementia begin decades before symptoms appear. Once you experience symptoms of cognitive decline, it's important to act quickly. There's no time to waste. Even better is prevention starting in your thirties, forties, or fifties, which is when the brain changes associated with Alzheimer's begin.

If you do have signs of cognitive decline, implement as much of the Healing Phase of the diet as you can manage, and shift to the Maintenance Phase after symptoms recede. Again, do as much as you can, don't try to do it all or beat yourself up when you fall short.

Neurogenic

For the hippocampus to organize and consolidate new memories, it's critical that neurogenesis and neuroplasticity function at a high level. Increasing neurogenesis and neuroplasticity increases memory and cognitive function. Mice that have boosted neurogenic capacity show strong cognitive and memory gains over those without this neurogenic boost.

Increasing neurogenic capacity by raising levels of BDNF and other brain growth compounds is central to this approach. Higher levels of BDNF are associated with lower levels of Alzheimer's and protection against amyloid and tau neurodegeneration. [1] Higher BDNF levels also are associated with greater cognitive reserve and protection against Alzheimer's pathology. [2]

Increasing your neurogenic capacity is key to preventing and reversing cognitive decline. The neurogenic nutrients and natural substances detailed in Chapter 2 should all be considered here. They all raise levels of neurotrophic factors, particularly BDNF. This section only highlights a few that have been shown to be especially helpful because they do double or triple duty, clearing amyloid or tau or something else.

EGCG (green tea extract). The polyphenols in green tea have powerful healing effects on the brain. The most active ingredient is epigallocatechin gallate (EGCG). This catechin stimulates neurogenesis, neuroplasticity, and alpha secretase (thus inhibiting amyloid), while suppressing beta secretase by an astounding 38% (another pathway to inhibit amyloid), and suppressing the phosphorylation of tau. [3] Best formulations are caffeine-free and 98% polyphenols, 75% catechins and 45% EGCG. Standard doses are 300–725 mg, once daily. More than this can, in rare cases, be toxic to the liver.

Curcumin. This extract of turmeric has properties that both prevent and reverse cognitive decline. Strongly neurogenic, it also is anti-inflammatory, antioxidant, chelates heavy metals, inhibits amyloid from accumulating, and promotes clearing of amyloid plaques after they have formed. On top of this, curcumin and curcuminoids attenuate the hyperphosphorylation of tau and enhance the clearance of tau.

Additional properties of curcumin include enhancing insulin sensitivity, delaying degradation of neurons and inhibiting acetylcholinesterase. [4] As one research paper put it, "curcumin has the potential to be more efficacious than current treatments. However, its usefulness as a therapeutic agent may be hindered by its low bioavailability. If the challenge of low bioavailability is overcome, curcumin-based medications for AD may be on the horizon."

The issue of low bioavailability of curcuminoids has been previously discussed. Taking the pepper extract piperine enhances bioavailability by eight to ten times, as does micronizing it or taking it with phospholipids such as egg yolks or lecithin. Other processes make it water-soluble and even more bioavailable. Depending upon the type, usually taken 1–2 times daily.

Berberine. This plant extract improves neurogenesis and synaptogenesis, blood sugar, and insulin sensitivity; is anti-inflammatory, antidepressant, and anxiolytic; and it both inhibits amyloid production and prevents tau hyperphosphorylation. [5] All this makes it one of the stars of brain health. Usual dose is 400–500 mg standardized extract, 1–3 times daily.

Quercetin. Another heavy hitter, quercetin is anti-inflammatory, antioxidant, and promotes neurogenesis and neuroplasticity. It finds and destroys senescent cells throughout the body and brain, which adds to its anti-inflammatory effect as senescent cells produce inflammatory cytokines. Further, it inhibits beta secretase by a remarkable 20–30%, thus reducing the buildup of amyloid plaques. [6] Usual doses range from 250–500 mg, 1–2 times daily.

Omega-3s. Omega-3s are not only the single most important building block of the brain, they are anti-inflammatory, antioxidant, and help clear amyloid buildup. They also prevent cortical shrinkage. One study found that higher blood levels of omega-3s preserves brain size and cognitive function, plus it corresponds to larger total brain and hippocampal volume. [7, 8] Another study found that lower DHA levels are associated with smaller brain volumes. [9] Omega-3s also remove amyloid plaque. [10]

This book has stressed that omega-3s are the single most important nutrient for brain health. Most people need 3–4 grams daily, evenly distributed between EPA and DHA. DHA, remember, is the basic building block of the brain. A recent Chinese study showed that 2 grams daily of DHA for 12 months improved IQ among older people with mild cognitive impairment. This study of adults sixty-five and older showed a 10% higher IQ after a year in the DHA group, with significant increase in two IQ subtests, Information and Digit Span. These subtests are indicators of long-term and short-term memory respectively. [11]

If your high-sensitivity C-reactive protein blood test is over .55 for men or 1.0 for women, however, which is indicative of higher inflammation, then a 2:1 ratio of EPA to DHA is better to reduce inflammation. Always make sure the omega-3 source is molecularly distilled to remove mercury. It's also helpful to get an omega-3 index blood test to find out if you are deficient (90% of Americans are). Ideal levels are between 8–12%.

Ashwagandha. This Indian herb increases BDNF levels, promotes neurite growth, has anti-anxiety and antidepressant properties, and it leads to increased clearance of amyloid. Researchers at India's National Brain Research Centre reversed memory loss in mice. After receiving ashwagandha for twenty days, cognition improved significantly, and after thirty days behavior returned to normal. Ashwagandha boosted a liver protein that helped clear amyloid from the brain. [12] Dosage depends upon the extract, 1–2 times daily.

Luteolin. In addition to being neurogenic and anti-inflammatory, luteolin reduces tau hyperphosphorylation. Most formulations are insufficient, better is 50–100 mg. taken 1–2 times daily.

Icariin. This flavonoid extract from horny goat weed has been shown to reverse cognitive deficits in rats. It increases neurogenesis and neuroplasticity as well as BDNF levels. [13] It is neuroprotective, antidepressant, anti-inflammatory, and promotes heart health. Depending upon the concentration, 300–500 mg, 1–2 times daily.

Taurine. This amino acid has been shown to increase neurogenesis and neuroplasticity, reduce inflammation and excitotoxicity from glutamate, and it binds to amyloid in animal models. [14] Take 1 gram, 1–2 times daily.

BDNF. Brain-derived neurotrophic factor is a central player throughout this book. Research shows that reduced levels of BDNF have a crucial role in Alzheimer's disease. A growing body of evidence indicates protective effects of BDNF against the neurotoxicity of tau-related degeneration. Raising BDNF levels in one study, "attenuated behavioral deficits, prevented neuron loss, alleviated synaptic degeneration and reduced neuronal abnormality." [15] Everything in this section and the corresponding section in Chapter 2, "The Solution," raises BDNF levels, including a ketogenic diet.

Ketogenic

Alzheimer's disease has been called "type 3 diabetes." Impaired glucose metabolism is a common factor in Alzheimer's, and switching to ketone bodies for fuel, instead of solely relying on glucose, is becoming a key pillar of Alzheimer's treatment. Dramatic improvement to cognitive function can come when faulty glucose metabolism is replaced by ketones for energy in the brain. Numerous studies have demonstrated this. [16, 17, 18]

For a fuller explanation of why a ketogenic or low carbohydrate diet is good for your brain, please read Chapter 2, "The Solution." It details how elevated blood sugar levels are directly tied to cognitive decline and inflammation. In short, with age, blood glucose levels rise. This produces glycation in neurons, or misfolded proteins that make cells dysfunctional. Inflammation follows, and amyloid follows inflammation.

The link between high blood sugar (insulin resistance) and cognitive decline was first noticed in diabetics. Those with higher blood glucose levels experienced cognitive decline faster than those with lower glucose levels. [19] Further research extended this to non-diabetics, such as those with metabolic syndrome. Higher HbA1c levels resulted in faster brain atrophy. [20]

Then more recent research showed that this was true for everyone. A 2013 study title says it all, "Higher Glucose Levels Associated with Lower Memory and Reduced Hippocampal Microstructure." It showed a direct link between hemoglobin A1c levels (a three-month average of blood sugar levels) and the size of the hippocampus and memory. Even so-called normal HbA1c levels that most physicians treat as healthy were shown to impair memory, and cognition, and to reduce brain size. [21] The evidence is clear: The higher your blood sugar level, the faster your cognition will deteriorate.

This is yet another reason why getting your HbA1c level measured is essential. Any value above 5.2 should be reduced immediately, and a ketogenic or low carbohydrate diet is the best way for most everyone to do this. In addition, a ketogenic diet provides the brain with super fuel rather than just sugar, which burns dirty. This is why it's so useful in Alzheimer's and cognitive decline.

When the husband of Mary Newport, M.D., was diagnosed with early-onset Alzheimer's, she tried many different treatments to no avail. She finally came upon coconut oil, and with 1–2 tablespoons daily, his condition significantly reversed. Later on, he came almost entirely back when switched to MCT oil. She was one of the first to extoll the virtues of ketone bodies to help with Alzheimer's.

Research done by the Mayo Clinic found that carbohydrate-rich diets are associated with an 89% increased risk for dementia. On the other hand, eating a diet high in healthy fats is associated with a 44% reduced risk. In another study, people who had diets high in unhealthy trans fats were 74% more likely to develop dementia. [22, 23]

The ketogenic diet is described by researchers as "neuroprotective" and is being used in clinical trials with Alzheimer's, Parkinson's, ALS, and other neurological disorders. It has been shown to be effective in reversing cognitive decline. [24] A 2019 study showed a low carb diet was helpful in older adults with cognitive impairment. [25] By using fat for fuel rather than just glucose, the brain operates at a higher level.

One of the problems with the ketogenic diet is that it's hard for many people to do or stick with. There is an addiction-like attachment to carbohydrates. Many people feel set in their dietary ways and resist eating in new ways. It's a surprise when people first go keto to discover that it's actually much easier than they thought it would be.

Dietary habits are simply what you've gotten used to. With a little effort, you can prepare different foods, and soon that becomes second-nature and habitual. The craving for carbs diminishes rather quickly after being in ketosis for a few months. The variety of fats impart satiety and the high fiber, moderate protein provide a wealth of taste delights.

Stevia, monk fruit, allulose, and erythritol serve as sugar alternatives to satisfy your sweet tooth that don't raise your blood sugar level. As paleo or keto-friendly products multiply, more and more desserts are becoming available.

Another way to enter into mild ketosis is intermittent fasting by restricting your eating to a six- or eight-hour window—say between ten a.m. and six p.m. or between noon and six p.m. Many authorities think that autophagy reaches its peak at sixteen hours of fasting, and this lets the body produce some ketones for fuel. This is best backed up by low carbohydrate eating, and this regimen was used in the Buck Foundation study that reversed cognitive decline.

In summary, a ketogenic diet improves cognition and brain health through several key pathways. It increases the cellular cleanup process (called "autophagy") and so improves removal of faltering neurons and brain debris, it lowers blood sugar levels and increases insulin sensitivity, it increases metabolic efficiency by improving mitochondrial health and the numbers of mitochondria, it reduces oxidative stress, and it activates genes that reduce inflammation and boost metabolism.

Anti-inflammatory

Chronic inflammation levels rise with age, this has been called "inflammaging." Earlier chapters detail the extensive damage inflammation causes in the body and the brain. As the mitochondria in neurons become inflamed, the neurons become less and less efficient, resulting in brain fog, an inability to think or concentrate.

Remember, when you have a head cold and are mentally foggy, that's due to the inflammation in your head and brain.

The brain attacks its own brain cells, as inflammation acts like a flamethrower on neurons and destroys the delicate connections between neurons at the synapses. Neurogenesis and neuroplasticity slow to a crawl. The blood vessels that supply the brain with its constant high needs for energy and oxygen are targeted, blood vessels burst or are damaged, and vascular dementia, the leading cause of cognitive decline and dementia after Alzheimer's, may ensue.

Further, it's well known that Alzheimer's disease is an inflammatory condition. Amyloid plaque levels are tied to inflammation levels. [26] Further, one study showed that high inflammatory diet was associated with higher inflammatory markers and, "accelerated cognitive decline at older ages." [27]

Another study looked at inflammation levels in over sixteen hundred people in their thirties and forties, then tested them again twenty-four years later. There was a direct correlation between inflammation levels, decline of brain volume, and cognition. Those with the highest inflammation levels at mid-life had the worst memory and the most shrunken brains later on. [28]

So, once again, the time is now. When someone complains of cognitive decline, inflammation and other factors have been operating for decades. It's never too late to lower your inflammation levels, and it's never too early.

The best time to monitor your inflammation level is when you are younger. How young? Given the toxic environment most people grow up in, the earlier the better. Your twenties or thirties are great, your teens are better, and while an infant is better still. Since the mother's level of inflammation shapes the baby's brain development and higher rates of mothers' neurogenesis and neuroplasticity correlate with higher infant neurogenic rates, brain health begins in the womb. The best time to begin is whenever you realize brain health is important.

For the brain to thrive, inflammation must be brought to healthy levels. Check your high-sensitivity C-reactive protein blood test results. If they are over .5 for a male or 1.0 for a female, it's important to lower inflammation immediately. Taking as many of the anti-inflammatory substances as you can targets multiple inflammatory pathways and signaling molecules.

A complete list is given in Chapter 2 and Appendix A. This short list below highlights only those anti-inflammatory compounds that do double duty to either prevent amyloid or tau accumulation or else work to clear amyloid deposits or tau once formed. [6]

- carnosine
- fisetin
- curcumin
- omega-3s
- EGCGs
- chinese skullcap (baicalin)
- blueberry polyphenols
- apigenin
- rosmarinic acid (found in rosemary, basil, and other herbs)

Gut friendly

The assault of the developed world on microbiome produces inflammation in the gut and problems with the intestinal filter (tight junctions). Inflammation in the intestinal lining produces inflammation in the brain. [29] A leaky gut probably indicates a leaky brain (and therefore a toxic and inflamed brain).

The overuse of antibiotics in developed countries has contributed to the decimation of the microbiome. Remember, indigenous cultures have 20,000– 30,000 strains of gut bacteria, whereas in the west the figure is closer to 5,000–10,000. This loss of diversity also means a major loss of immunity, since 70% of the immune system is comes from the gut and microbiome.

The loss of diversity in the microbiome affects cognition. Increased prevalence of Alzheimer's is correlated with the loss of diversity in gut bacteria as measured in populations in various countries. Additionally, the loss of gut organisms affects inflammation. Changes in gut bacteria increases inflammation. A recent study showed that taking certain probiotics not only reduced inflammation, it also produced a remarkable cognitive gain. [30]

Glyphosate has been found in 93% of Americans. This means that at least 93% of Americans have some degree of dysfunction in their protective intestinal barrier, disrupting the tight junctions that should keep out toxins and let in nutrients. To review what was discussed earlier, the same signaling system works in the tight junctions of the gut and the blood-brain barrier. When the tight junctions in the intestines open up and let in toxins, the tight junctions in the blood-brain barrier open up and let in toxins as well.

There is a need to increase microbial diversity in the gut, reduce intestinal inflammation, and repair the disrupted tight junctions. Repairing the intestinal barrier simultaneously helps repair the blood-brain barrier in order to maintain a healthy boundary between the outside world and the inside world.

The following probiotics have been shown to reduce inflammation and increase cognitive scores significantly in Alzheimer's patients. [30]

- Lactobacillus acidophilus
- Lactobacillus casei
- Lactobacillus fermentum
- Bifidobacterium bifidum

The integrity of the tight junctions in the gut parallel those of the blood-brain barrier. Recent research indicates that disruptions of the blood-brain barrier are a sign that cognitive decline is underway. In an article in the prestigious scientific journal *Nature* entitled, "Blood-Brain Barrier Breakdown Is an Early Biomarker for Cognitive Dysfunction," the researchers show that even before symptoms of cognitive decline or Alzheimer's have set in, breakdown of the blood-brain barrier in the hippocampus precedes the accumulation of amyloid and tau and/or Alzheimer's changes. [31]

Strains that have been shown to reduce intestinal permeability and heal the tight junctions include: Lactobacillus rhamnosus, L. paracasei, L. gasseri, L. helveticus, L. plantarum, Bifidobacterium infantis, B. longum. [32]

Additional strategies are to find out if you are lectin sensitive and avoid lectins if you are, consuming more omega-3s, eating fermented food, avoiding alcohol and medications that impair tight junctions such as proton pump inhibitors and NSAIDs such as ibuprofen. Chapter 2 goes into more specifics for repairing the compromised intestinal and blood-brain barrier.

Nutrients to help clear amyloid and tau

To prevent or reverse cognitive decline and Alzheimer's, several strategies are needed.

- First, prevent or reverse the brain conditions that stimulate excess amyloid and tau buildup (such as inflammation, high insulin and glucose levels, toxins).
- Second, turn down the signals that increase amyloid and tau formation.
- Third, clear the amyloid and tau that has already accumulated.

The first strategy works to lower your levels of inflammation, blood sugar and insulin to healthy low levels, prevent ingesting toxins, provide high amounts of nutrients for the brain, keep neurogenic factors high, and ensure a strong, protective blood-brain barrier to keep out toxins that do get into the body. That is exactly what the diet recommended by this book does.

The second strategy prevents amyloid and tau buildup by using specific nutrients and natural substances to turn down the signals that increase levels of amyloid and tau. To downregulate mechanisms that stimulate amyloid plaque formation, three signaling molecules need to be inhibited or increased, as discussed earlier: alpha secretase, beta secretase, and gamma secretase. After amyloid has aggregated, tau accumulates and becomes toxic in its hyperphosphorylated state. Therefore, it's important both to prevent amyloid from aggregating and inhibit signaling molecules that hyperphosphorylate tau.

The third strategy utilizes natural substances that have been shown to clear amyloid and tau.

There is solid research evidence to show that the substances below work to prevent the buildup or clearing of amyloid and/or tau, although some of the work has been done on animals rather than humans. Each is commercially available as a stand-alone extract or supplement.

This approach accords with research that recommends preventing the buildup and clearing of both amyloid and tau together. The authors note, "One implication of our work is that approaches combining anti-amyloid beta and anti-tau therapies might be more effective than either alone." [33]

Each of these compounds below are being considered as possible candidates for drug development. By changing one tiny part of the molecules in these substances, pharmaceutical companies are able to patent the new molecule and market it. However, it may be that Nature knows best. Utilizing a wide array of different compounds may maximize the prevention and reversal of amyloid and tau buildup as well as their clearance. [3, 4 5, 6, 10, 34, 35, 36]

Alpha Secretase Stimulators

Amyloid is formed from a protein called "amyloid precursor protein" (APP), which is found throughout the brain and is inactive. Alpha secretase prevents amyloid from forming by taking APP and changing the molecule in another direction, thereby reducing the raw material from which amyloid is made. These substances stimulate the activity of alpha secretase:

- green tea extract, caffeine-free, 45% catechins, 300–725 mg daily
- salvia (danshen, red sage) 1,000 mg, 1–2 times daily
- resveratrol, 20–400 mg daily
- magnesium glycinate, 200–400 mg, 1–2 times daily
- magnesium-L-threonate, 2,000 mg daily
- huperzine A, 200–800 mcg daily
- acetyl-L-carnitine, 600–2,500 mg daily
- wild celery or celery seeds

Beta Secretase Inhibitors

The brain's first step in producing amyloid is that beta secretase cleaves the APP molecule. By lowering the amount of beta secretase, amyloid production is inhibited. The following substances inhibit beta secretase:

- American or Korean ginseng, standardized extract, 200 mg, 1–3 times daily
- green tea extract, caffeine-free, 45% catechins, 300–725 mg daily
- DHEA, 10–100 mg daily
- licorice root (better to use deglycyrrhizinated form), 750 mg daily
- ginkgo biloba, 120 mg daily of standardized extract
- bovine cartilage
- myricetin (a 20–30% reduction), 100 mg, 1–2 times daily

Gamma Secretase Inhibitors

After beta secretase begins the transformation of APP into amyloid, gamma secretase then comes along to complete the process. The inhibition of gamma secretase has been considered a viable strategy in the fight against Alzheimer's, but currently there are only natural substances that do this, only one of which is commercially available:

- black cohosh, root and extract, 530 mg and 20 mg, 1–2 times daily
- Pterocarpus erinaceus extract (not available at time of writing)

These are the only two substances known at present to effectively inhibit gamma secretase. The ideal strategy is to inhibit both beta secretase and gamma secretase, but inhibiting either one helps.

Substances to Inhibit or Reduce Tau Formation

A number of compounds have been shown to either inhibit the production of tau or else clear tau that has already formed. Usual dosages are given but experiment and see what works for you.

- myricetin (current research shows this to be the most effective agent at clearing tau), 100 mg, 1–2 times daily
- rosmarinic acid (found in rosemary, basil, etc.), 500–1,000 mg, 1–2 times daily
- cinnamon extract, depends upon extract
- aged garlic extract, 600–1,200 mg daily
- ginseng, standardized extract, 200 mg, 1–3 times daily
- grape seed extract, 100 mg, 1–2 times daily
- salvia (red sage), 1,000 mg, 1–2 times daily
- ferulic acid, 250 mg, 1–2 times daily
- olive oil, 1–2 tablespoons daily
- curcumin, 200–1,200 mg daily depending on formulation
- resveratrol, 20–400 mg daily
- green tea extract (EGCG), caffeine-free, 45% catechins, 300–725 mg daily
- fulvic acid and humic acid (from shilajit), 250 mg standardized extract, 1–2 times daily
- BDNF (protects against tau-related Alzheimer's neurodegeneration)

Natural substances that clear amyloid or tau

Once amyloid has formed in the brain, the importance of clearing it can hardly be overstated. These natural nutrients and compounds clear amyloid from the brain, and some have dual action and also clear tau or reduce tau hyperphosphorylation. Typical doses are listed, but individualize to suit your body.

- Chinese skullcap or baicalin (not American skullcap), 100 –400 mg, 1–2 times daily
- kaempferol, 100 mg, 1-2 times daily

- fisetin, 100 mg daily
- ellegic acid (from pomegranate), 40% extract, 250 mg daily
- resveratrol, 20–400 mg daily
- olive oil (olive leaf extract or oleuropein), 1–2 tablespoons daily
- colostrinin (proline-rich peptides from colostrum)
- huperzine A, 200–800 mcg daily
- rosmarinic acid (from basil and rosemary), 500–1,000 mg, 1–2 times daily
- luteolin, 50–100 mg, 1–2 times daily
- apigenin, 50 mg, 1–2 times daily
- Ashwagandha, depends upon extract concentration, 1–2 times daily
- vitamin D, 5,000–10,000 i.u. daily (as determined by blood test)
- phosphatidylserine (together with ginkgo biloba), 100 mg daily
- rutin, 500 mg daily
- nattokinase, 20 mg (2,000 FU) daily
- blueberry polyphenols, 1 cup daily or equivalent extract
- lion's mane, 300–3,000 mg daily
- sulforaphane, 5–50 mg daily
- NAD+, (nicotinamide riboside, 100 mg daily, or NMN, 50 mg, 1–2 times daily)
- icariin, depending upon extract concentration, 300–500 mg, 1–2 times daily
- taurine, 1,000 mg, 1–2 times daily
- PQQ (pyrroloquinoline), 20 mg daily

Combining these three strategies of: (1) preventing or reversing the conditions that stimulate amyloid and tau, (2) reducing amyloid and tau formation and buildup after this has begun, and (3) clearing amyloid and tau once formed, may represent some of the most powerful measures to prevent or reverse cognitive decline. This is the first time all these strategies and natural substances have been published together in one place.

Micromanage Your Cognition: A Note on Micronutrients

A number of micronutrients and herbs have been shown to help cognition.

Vitamin D. This vitamin is involved in so many cellular functions it's no surprise it figures strongly into brain health. Vitamin D increases neurogenesis and neuroplasticity, protects against neuroinflammation, and helps clear the brain of amyloid before it can lead to Alzheimer's. Lower levels of vitamin D are associated with memory loss, "substantial cognitive decline," and increased risk for dementia. [37, 38, 39, 40]

While mainstream medical standards show 64% of Americans have too little vitamin D to keep cells functioning at peak capacity, other health practitioners put the figure at closer to 90%. Most people can use 5,000–10,000 i.u. daily until reaching optimum levels of 60–100 ng/mL. Blood testing is important to monitor your levels. Vitamin K-2 is also important to take along with vitamin D to ensure the bone health.

Magnesium. Here again the vast majority of Americans are deficient in this mineral. The forms of glycinate and L-threonate are recommended, with doses varying for each person. Most people can benefit from 1–3 tablets of 400 mg glycinate daily and 3 capsules of L-threonate daily.

Iron. Iron excess is linked to Alzheimer's. Iron overload, which is very common, causes a rusting effect in the brain. It interacts with amyloid to generate toxic free radicals, increasing oxidative stress on neurons. [41] Ideal blood levels of iron (called "ferritin" in blood tests) are 30–40 ng/mL. You don't want to be below 20 or above 80 (which is very common) if you are a male or non-menstruating woman. If over 80, donate blood as often as you can to bring your blood level down. (See Chapter 2, "The Solution," for more on iron levels.)

Wild green oat extract. Dopamine levels diminish as you age. Lower dopamine levels are mostly the result of an increase in the enzyme MAO-B. Wild green oat extract inhibits MAO-B and helps dopamine nerve transmission, which normally declines with age. Try 800 mg extract, 1–2 times daily.

Bacopa. This herb from India has antioxidant and anti-inflammatory properties, and several human trials have shown it has cognitive-enhancing effects as well as improves memory. Clinical trials showed improvements in working memory, visual processing speed, lower anxiety, and depression. [42, 43] Usual dose is 300 mg bacopa extract daily.

Ursolic acid. This compound stimulates the production of irisin, a brain chemical stimulated by exercise that protects against dementia and damage from amyloid. Irisin levels were found to be particularly high in brains of people who were free of dementia when they died but hardly could be detected in those who had Alzheimer's at death. Typical dosage range is 150–300 mg per day.

Beets and beet extract. Beets contain a substance called "betanin" that binds to metals and reduces the oxidative stress from amyloid by up to 90%. Unfortunately, beets are high in sugar, but two capsules of beet extract offer the benefits without the sugar. [44] Beet extract also increases the body's production of nitric oxide, thereby enhancing blood flow, which is particularly important for brain health.

Choline. Choline is an essential nutrient that the body uses to make acetylcholine, a neurotransmitter involved in cognition, memory, sleep, and muscle control. One widely held theory of cognitive decline ties this into declining levels of acetylcholine in the brain together with a decrease in the neurons that use it.

The most bioavailable form of choline is glyceryl phosphoryl choline (GPC or sometimes called alpha GPC). A review of thirteen studies involving over four thousand participants found that GPC groups showed neurological improvements and relief of symptoms of cerebral deterioration that was "superior or equivalent" to prescription drugs and superior to the forms of lecithin or pure choline. [45] Usual dosage is 300 mg, 1–2 times daily.

Vitamin E. A 2014 study in the *JAMA* showed that vitamin E in the form of alpha tocopherol slowed cognitive decline in mild to moderate Alzheimer's. [46] Most current research shows that the gamma tocopherol form of vitamin E is superior, so it raises the possibility of enhancing vitamin E's effect by using this form instead. Take 200–400 i.u. daily.

Maintenance Phase of Diet

Once you have reached your neurogenic potential and feel better, think better, and remember better, with no more brain fog or cognitive decline, it is helpful to stay on the diet for six to twenty-four months. This allows the brain to heal and regenerate itself. After this you can switch into maintenance mode, which means modifying the diet along the lines particular to your unique metabolism.

What this means for most people, is moving from ketogenic to low carbohydrate and easing up around supplements. Monitoring your blood work is the best way to determine how to modify your regimen. For example, if your high-sensitivity C-reactive protein (hs-CRP) test shows you to be under .55 for a male or 1.0 for a female, then you can consider reducing anti-inflammatory supplements. On the other hand, keeping chronic inflammation low is key to brain health, so you may want to stick with a winning game to make sure your levels stay down. It's up to you and depends upon your health goals. In the Maintenance Phase, you have more choice and can experiment to see what works and what doesn't.

It's similar in switching from ketogenic to low carbohydrate. How much carbohydrate you can tolerate before blood sugar rises (along with inflammation) or brain fog or memory problems set in, depends upon your individual metabolism. Continual experimentation is the only way to find out the best maintenance diet for you.

Other physical factors

For most people diet has an outsized role in brain health. However, the brain can be significantly affected by other factors as well, especially exercise, sleep, exposure to toxins, medication, and hormonal imbalances.

Exercise. The impact of exercise on the brain is immense. Exercise increases the production of BDNF (brain fertilizer) along with neurogenesis and neuroplasticity; reduces inflammation, free radicals, and stress; increases insulin sensitivity and glucose metabolism; helps clear away senescent cells; and on top of this it makes you feel better.

When you don't exercise, your body feels sluggish. Your brain becomes sluggish as well. Neurite growth slows, neurogenesis and neuroplasticity slow down, brain neurotropic growth factors decrease—the brain's whole neurogenic capacity diminishes.

While all exercise is good for you, two types are especially good for your brain: strength training and, even better, aerobic exercise. Strength training has been shown to have cognitive benefits, for cognition is tied to muscle strength, especially the strength of leg muscles. Strength training at least once per week and preferably twice is highly recommended for overall health and cognition.

The very best exercise for the brain, however, is aerobic exercise. Remember, aerobic exercise is anything that gets you breathing hard and your heart rate elevated. This includes: running, cycling, swimming, fast dancing or walking, hiking up hills.

Aerobic exercise improves cardiovascular fitness, which in itself is good for your brain, and further benefits accrue, such as dramatically increasing BDNF, neurogenesis, neuroplasticity, and insulin sensitivity while lowering inflammation. When researchers want to increase neurogenesis in mice, they simply put a running wheel into the cages (but remember, half of these new brain cells are pruned quickly unless other measures are taken, such as taking hesperidin or exposure to new environments).

Looking at the impact of fitness in mid-life, Swedish researchers at the University of Gothenburg found that forty-five years later, women with the best cardiovascular fitness had an 88% lower risk of dementia than those with even moderate fitness. The incidence of dementia in the low fitness group was 32%, those in the high fitness group just 5%. Even in the high fitness group, the average age of dementia was eleven years older than in the medium fitness group. [47] Reducing dementia risk by almost 90% shows just how dramatic cardiovascular fitness is for the brain.

Just because you haven't exercised doesn't mean it's too late to start. At whatever age you begin, your brain benefits. Research shows that aerobic exercise reverses cognitive decline in sedentary older adults. A study of 160 men and women over fifty-five with cognitive impairments showed that aerobic exercise three times a week for six months had significant improvements in memory, language, and executive function. [48]

Other research has confirmed that better heart and vascular health not only prevents the brain shrinkage that usually occurs with aging but actually increases brain volume of both gray and white matter, thus preventing cognitive decline. This did not occur in the control group that did yoga stretches and nonaerobic toning exercises. The study's authors said:

"These results suggest that cardiovascular fitness is associated with the sparing of brain tissue in aging humans. Furthermore, these results suggest a strong biological basis for the role of aerobic fitness in maintaining and enhancing central nervous system health and cognitive functioning in older adults." [49]

Yet another angle on the importance of cardiovascular fitness and cognitive health comes from research that ties blood-pressure levels to dementia. Higher blood-pressure levels lead to higher levels of both dementia and Alzheimer's. Vascular dementia is second only to Alzheimer's for types of dementia. What research has discovered, however, is that high blood pressure not only causes vascular dementia but Alzheimer's as well. Interestingly, high blood pressure seems more related to the more destructive tau tangles than amyloid plaque buildup. [50, 51]

Aerobic exercise is most effective for increasing neurogenic capacity when it lasts twenty minutes or longer. High intensity interval training (HIIT), while it improves cardiovascular fitness and has many metabolic benefits, barely moves the needle when it comes to increasing neurogenesis. [52]

Start slowly and build up gradually. If you've been sedentary, just try walking a little each day, and slowly, over weeks and months, walk farther and more briskly. Pretty soon you'll build your aerobic fitness to twenty to thirty minutes, three to five times a week. You'll not only feel better, you'll think better.

It doesn't take much. One study showed that seniors aged sixty to eighty who walked thirty to forty-five minutes three days per week for a year increased the size of their hippocampus by 2% (instead of the usual shrinkage). Higher levels of fitness were also associated with a bigger prefrontal cortex (the seat of executive function and higher brain abilities) and improved memory. [53]

If you're more active, try to get yourself breathing pretty hard for thirty to forty minutes three or four times weekly. Once a week interval training is good to throw into the mix for other reasons, as it improves such things as cardiovascular health along different lines than endurance type exercise. Aerobic training three to five times weekly plus strength training once or twice a week will provide a significant neurogenic boost to your brain.

Yet another reason to exercise comes from recent studies that show exercise increases the brain's production of irisin, a brain chemical that improves brain health and may lessen the damage from Alzheimer's. So aside from the positive effects exercise has on remodeling the brain through ramping up neuroplasticity and neurogenesis, improving thinking and emotional resilience, and increasing the health of synapses between neurons to allow for better communication between brain cells, the brain releases irisin during exercise.

Researchers found that increasing irisin levels in mice protected against amyloid damage and was neuroprotective. [54] When prevented from creating irisin during exercise, the mice did as poorly as sedentary mice with amyloid in their brains. As just noted above, taking the supplement ursolic acid stimulates the production of irisin, but it's unknown whether this pathway matches or possibly even exceeds levels that come from exercise.

Recent research has shown that prolonged sitting is also detrimental to your health, so getting up and walking around for a couple of minutes every hour or half hour is suggested to keep things flowing. Sustained physical activity is ideal, as the lifestyle of our caveperson ancestors did not include spending the day on couches.

Sleep. Most people don't know how good sleep is for the brain and so tend to minimize it. But sleep is one of the primary prevention strategies to keep the mind sharp. When you know why, you see how critical it is to get a good night's sleep, which means seven or eight hours for almost everyone. (See Chapter 2.)

Sleep, especially in the later hours, activates the glymphatic system, a recently discovered mechanism by which the brain cleans itself. Since the brain is protected by the blood-brain barrier, until recently no one understood how the brain cleared toxins out of its system. An aquarium needs a filter to clean itself, or else it becomes clogged with poisons that kill the fish. Similarly, the brain needs some way to eliminate the toxic by-products of metabolism that accumulate each day.

As discussed in Chapter 2, the glymphatic system is to the brain what the lymphatic system is to the body, a way of cleansing and detoxifying noxious residues of normal cellular processes. When you sleep, the neurons shrink by 30–50% while the brain is bathed in cerebrospinal fluid. This nighttime "shower" of cleansing fluid and glial cells flushes out the metabolic debris that accumulates each day. One of the most important things the glymphatic system clears out is amyloid.

By now the reader knows that the toxic buildup of amyloid in the brain is something to avoid as much as possible. Getting less than seven or eight hours of sleep each night prevents the clearance of this amyloid buildup. While poor sleep for a few nights won't immediately result in cognitive decline, if it becomes a pattern it sets the stage. A 2018 study showed that even a single night of sleep deprivation resulted in increased amyloid accumulation in the human brain. Remarkably, pulling an all-nighter increases amyloid in the hippocampus and in the cerebrospinal fluid by as much as 25–30%.[55, 56]

One strategy that is being actively pursued by Alzheimer's researchers and drug companies is to enhance the clearance of amyloid via the glymphatic system. The drainage of the glymphatic system occurs near the olfactory bulb and hippocampus, the two brain systems where neurogenesis occurs. When this drainage is blocked or prevented from happening, it's understandable the hippocampus would suffer, both in the form of amyloid accumulation and reduced neurogenic activity. A 2016 study showed that supplementing with omega-3s improves the function of the glymphatic system and improves clearance of amyloid from the brain.[57]

Good sleep hygiene improves your chances of getting a good night's sleep. This includes: going to bed around the same time every night so your body learns to fall asleep then; avoid eating three hours before sleep; avoid caffeine or stimulants from the afternoon on, unless you have a high tolerance; avoid blue light from computer, TV, cell phone, or tablet screens two or three hours before bed, by setting the night shift control; avoid stimulating content on movies or TV before bed; avoid alcohol before sleep as it prevents the deeper stages of sleep when the main cleansing occurs from happening; reduce stress and anxiety. (See Chapter 3, "Holistic Healing for Anxiety," for more complete practices.)

Detoxification from heavy metals, mold, and EMFs. Our modern environment is so polluted we hardly notice. Chapters 1 and 2 go into greater detail showing how heavy metals (especially mercury, lead, arsenic, aluminum, and cadmium) impair brain function. Heavy metal particles in smog, for example, that are smaller than 2.5 micrometers enter the bloodstream and cross the blood-brain barrier. Once inside the brain these tiny particles smash into the delicate neurons and devastate brain cells, creating inflammation and free radical damage, paving the way for amyloid and tau buildup. Some researchers estimate that 20–30% of Alzheimer's worldwide is due to smog.

Heavy metal contamination, such a mercury excess, and mycotoxins from mold exposure can cause cognitive decline and mimic Alzheimer's. Doing the tests in Chapter 2 can diagnose the degree to which the brain is impaired due to toxins. Detoxing from these toxins is one of the reversible types of Alzheimer's.

Exposure to high levels of electromagnetic fields (EMFs) has neurological consequences that are only just starting to be understood. EMF exposure from cell phones, Wi-Fi, computers, and other sources of electro-smog strongly affect the mitochondria of neurons. The resulting oxidation and inflammation can create brain fog, cognitive decline, and fatigue. See Chapter 2, "The Solution," for further discussion and how to reduce exposure.

Cognitive decline as a side effect of medication or hormone imbalance. There are an astonishingly high number of medications that impair cognition and produce symptoms of cognitive decline. Several studies have shown that commonly prescribed drugs as well as many over-the-counter medications produce cognitive impairment. [58, 59, 60] Such medications include statins and anticholinergic drugs.

It's important to check the list below to see if any of these drugs may be causing memory problems or brain fog. Very often alternative medication can be used that does not have the side effect of cognitive impairment, although this is not always the case. Statins, for example, used to treat high blood pressure, work by reducing cholesterol. But cholesterol is necessary for brain function, and reducing its level too much can produce memory problems and cognitive impairment. MIT researcher Stephanie Senoff, Ph.D., predicts a coming wave of Alzheimer's due to overuse of statins.

A partial list of these drugs that might induce cognitive decline includes:

- statins
- antidepressants
- beta blockers
- antibiotics
- antidiabetics (e.g., insulin)
- heartburn medication for GERD (e.g., proton pump inhibitors)
- laxatives
- pain medications
- steroids
- antihistamines
- tranquilizers (benzodiazepines such as Klonopin, Ativan, Xanax)
- sleep medication (Sonata, Lunesta, Ambien)
- anticholinergics (e.g., anticholinergic antidepressants, antiepileptic drugs, bladder antimuscarinic drugs, antipsychotics, Benadryl, Parkinson's drugs)

Another cause of cognitive decline can be hormonal imbalance. The most prevalent one is thyroid, which is low in many older adults. Getting a thyroid function test will either confirm this or rule it out. Since many people are deficient in iodine, taking supplemental kelp or iodine can often restore healthy thyroid levels.

The sex hormones of estradiol, progesterone, and testosterone can affect cognition when levels are low. It's important to work with a physician who is experienced in working with cognitive decline and uses bioidentical hormones, if augmentation is needed.

With testosterone, even supplemental testosterone may only be effective in the short-term due to the body's action of aromatizing testosterone and transforming it into estrogen compounds. Oftentimes taking something to block the aromatization of testosterone is sufficient, instead of taking supplemental testosterone.

Low levels of DHEA, pregnenolone, or cortisol can also produce cognitive impairment. Taking supplemental DHEA or pregnenolone, which are over-the-counter supplements, can work wonders for some people. Begin with 10 mg daily, then go up to 25 mg. Some people feel best at 50 or even 100 mg daily, so experimentation is necessary to reach ideal blood levels.

REFERENCES

Chapter 1: The Problem

1. Gray, P. (2010). "The decline of play and rise in children's mental disorders." *Psychology Today.* Jan 26.
2. Twenge, J., et al. (2010). "Birth cohort increases in psychopathology among young Americans, 1938–2007: A cross-temporal meta-analysis of the MMPI." *Clinical Psychology Review 30.* 145–154.
3. Healy, D. (2004). *Let them eat Prozac.* New York: NYU Press.
4. *Independent,* UK. (2016). "Teenage mental-health crisis: Rates of depression have soared in past 25 years. How has society managed to produce a generation of teenagers in which mental-health problems are so prevalent?" Feb 16.
5. Alzheimer's Association website (2018). alz.org
6. Whitaker, R. (2010). *Anatomy of an epidemic.* New York: Random House.
7. Khullar, D. (2018). "The largest health disparity we don't talk about." *New York Times.* May 31, p 1.
8. Sapolsky, R. (1994). *Why zebras don't get ulcers.* New York: W. H. Freeman and Company.
9. Sapolsky, R. (2001). "Depression, antidepressants, and the shrinking hippocampus." Proceedings of the National Academy of Science. Oct 23, Vol 98(22):12320–12322.
10. Siegel, D. (2015). *The developing mind, 2nd Edition.* New York: Guilford.
11. Masterson, J. (2015). *The personality disorders through the lens of attachment theory: A clinical integration.* Phoenix, AZ: Zeig, Tucker & Theison.
12. Lewis, T., et al. (2007). *A general theory of love.* New York: Vintage.
13. Costa, L., et al. (2008). "Neurotoxicity of pesticides: A brief review." *Frontiers in Bioscience.* Feb, 13:1240–9.
14. Hamblin, J. (2014). "The toxins that threaten our brains." *The Atlantic.* Mar 18.
15. *Environmental Health Perspectives.* (2010). May, 118(5):699–704.
16. Temkin, A. (2018). "Breakfast with a dose of Roundup?" *Environmental Working Group.* Aug 15. ewg.org
17. Chow, L. (2015). "85% of tampons contain Monsanto's 'cancer causing' gluphosate." EcoWatch.com. Oct 26.
18. Mercola, J. (2019). "Top tips to detoxify your body." Mercola.com. Jan 27, interview with Dietrich Klinghardt.
19. Centers for Disease Control and Prevention. (2014). "Chronic hazard advisory panel on phthalates." (PDF).
20. Heriot Watt University (2018). "Academic reveals more than 100 tiny plastics in every meal." *News.* Apr 3.
21. Barron, L. (2018). "Microplastic contamination is found in most bottled water, a new study says." *Time.* Mar 18.
22. Environmental Health Perspectives. (2012). Nov 15.
23. Brunst, K. J., et al. (2019). "Myo-inositol mediates the effects of traffic-related air pollution on generalized anxiety symptoms at age 12 years." *Environmental Research.* August, Vol 175: 71-78
24. Yolton, K., et al., (2019). "Lifetime exposure to traffic-related air pollution and symptoms of anxiety and depression at age 12 years." *Environ Res.* June;173:199-206
25. Zhang, X., et al. (2018). "The impact of exposure to air pollution on cognitive performance." Proceedings of the National Academy of Sciences. Aug 27.
26. Perlmutter, D. (2013). *Grain brain.* New York: Little, Brown and Co.
27. Mercola, J. (2017). "The harmful effects of electromagnetic fields explained." Interview with Marin Pall. Sep 3, articles.mercola.com
28. Pall, M. (2013). "Electromagnetic fields act via activation of voltage-gated calcium channels to produce beneficial or adverse effects." *Journal of Cellular and Molecular Medicine.* Aug, 17(8):958–65.
29. Pall, M. (2016). "Microwave frequency electromagnetic fields (EMFs) produce widespread neuropsychiatric effects including depression." *Journal of Chemical Neuroanatomy.* Sep, 75(Pt B):43–51.
30. Docety, J., Cacciopo, J. (eds.). (2011). *The oxford handbook of social neuroscience.* Oxford, England: Oxford University Press.
31. Felliti, V. J., et al. (1998). "Relationship of childhood abuse and household dysfunction to many of the leading causes of death in adults: The ACE study." *American Journal of Preventive Medicine.* May, Vol 14, Issue 4:245–58.
32. Pearce, J. C. (2004). "Nurturance: A biological imperative." *Shift Publication,* Institute of Noetic Sciences. June–Aug, No 3:16–19.
33. Dickerson, S. S., et al. (2004). "Immunological effects of induced shame and guilt." *Psychosomatic Medicine.* Jan–Feb, 66(1):124–131.

34. Frederickson, B., et al. (2013). "A functional genomic perspective on well-being." Proceedings of the National Academy of Sciences. Vol 110, No 33:13684–13689.
35. Frankl, V. (2006). *Man's search for meaning*. Boston: Beacon Press.
36. El-Mallakh, R. S., et al. (2011). "Tardive dysphoria: The role of long-term antidepressant use in inducing chronic depression." *Medical Hypothesis*. Vol 76:769–773.
37. Cortright, B. (2015). *The neurogenesis diet and lifestyle*. Mill Valley, CA: Psyche Media.
38. Lee, C. (2010). "Brain damage from benzodiazepines: The troubling facts, risks, and history of minor tranquilizers." *Psychology Today*. Nov 18.
39. Mercola, J. (2019). "What does the evidence say about antidepressants?" Mercola.com. Apr 4, interview with Peter Breggin.

Chapter 2: The Solution

1. Cortright, B. (2015). *The neurogenesis diet and lifestyle*. Mill Valley, CA: Psyche Media.
2. Bernard, R., et al. (2010). "Altered expression of glutamate signaling, growth factor, and glia genes in the locus coeruleus of patients with major depression." *Molecular Psychiatry*. 16:634–646.
3. Xing, Y., et al. (2013). "Injury of cortical neurons is caused by the advanced glycation end products-mediated pathway." *Neural Regeneration Research*. Apr 5, 8(10):909–915.
4. Maslow, A. (1976). *The farther reaches of human nature*. New York: Penguin Books.
5. Guo, L., et al. (2018). "Relationship between depression and inflammatory factors and brain-derived neurotrophic factor in patients with perimenopause syndrome." *Experimental and Therapeutic Medicine*. May, 15(5):44236–40.
6. Conklin, S. M., Gianaros, P. J., Brown, S. M., et al. (2007). "Long-chain omega-3 fatty acid intake is associated positively with corticolimbic gray matter volume in healthy adults." *Neuroscience Letters*. June 29, 421(3):209–12.
7. Beltz, B. S., Tlusty, M. F., Benton, J. L., Sandeman, D. C. (2007). "Omega-3 fatty acids upregulate adult neurogenesis." *Neuroscience Letters*.
8. Zainuddin, M. S. A., & Thuret, S. (2012). "Nutrition, adult hippocampal neurogenesis and mental health." *British Medical Bulletin*. 103, 1:89–114. DOI:10.1093/bmb/lds021.
9. Stangl, D., & Thuret, S. (2009). "Impact of diet on adult hippocampal neurogenesis." *Genes Nutr*. Dec, 4(4):271–282.
10. Beltz, B. S., Tlusty, M. F., Benton, J. L., and Sandeman, D. C. "Omega-3 fatty acids upregulate adult neurogenesis."
11. Heinrichs, S. C. (2010). "Dietary omega-3 fatty acid supplementation for optimizing neuronal structure and function." *Molecular Nutrition & Food Research*. Apr, 54(4):447–56.
12. Wurtman, R. J., Cansev, M., Sakamoto, T., Ulus, I. H. (2009). "Use of phosphatide precursors to promote synaptogenesis." *Annual Review of Nutrition*. 29:59–87.
13. Grayson, D., et al. (2014). "Dietary omega-3 fatty acids modulate large-scale systems organizations in the rhesus macaque brain." *Journal of Neuroscience*. Feb 5, 34(6):2065–2074.
14. Grayson, D., et al. (2014). "Dietary omega-3 fatty acids modulate large-scale systems organization in the rmacaque brain." *Journal of Neuroscience*. Feb 5, 34(6): 2065–2074.
15. Conklin, S. M., et al. (2007). "Long-chain omega-3 fatty acid intake is associated positively with corticolimbic gray matter volume in healthy adults." *Neurosci Lett*. Jun 29, 421(3):209–12.
16. Antya, N., et al. (2009). "Omega-3 fatty acids (fish oil) and depression-related cognition in healthy volunteers." *J Psychopharmacology*. Sep, 23(7):831–40.
17. Cole, G. M., et al. (2009). "Omega-3 fatty acids and dementia." *Prostaglandins Leukot Essent Fatty Acids*. Aug–Sep, 81(2–3):213–21.
18. Lewis, M. (2016). Interview with David Perlmutter. http://www.drperlmutter.com/empowering-neurologist-david-perlmutter-michael-lewis/
19. Lewis, M. (2016). *When brains collide*. New York: Lioncrest Publishing.
20. Lewis, M. (2016). When brains collide. New York: Lioncrest.
21. Osher, Y., Belmaker, R. H. (2009). "Omega-3 fatty acids in depression: A review of three studies." *CNS Neuroscience & Therapeutics. Summer*, 15(2):128–33.
22. Freemantle, E., Vandal, M., Tremblay-Mercier, J., Tremblay, S., Blachere, J. C., Begin, M. E., Brenna, J. T., Windust, A., Cunnane, S. C. (2006). "Omega-3 fatty acids, energy substrates, and brain function during aging." *Prostaglandins Leukotrienes and Essential Fatty Acids*. 75:213–220.
23. Gomez-Pinilla, F. (2008). "Brain foods: The effects of nutrients on brain function." *Nature Reviews Neuroscience*. 9:568–578.
24. Harper, C., et al. (2006). "Flax oil increases the plasma concentrations of cardioprotective (n-3) fatty acids in humans." *Journal of Nutrition*. Jan 1, Vol 136, Issue 1:83–87.
25. (2012). *Molecular Nutrition & Food Research*. Aug, 56(8):1292–303. doi: 10.1002/mnfr.201200035. Epub Jun 13, 2012.

26. Wang, Y., Li, M., Xu, X., Song, M., Tao, H., Bai, Y. "Green tea epigallocatechin-3-gallate (EGCG) promotes neural progenitor cell proliferation and sonic hedgehog pathway activation during adult hippocampal neurogenesis."
27. Goepp, J. (2008). "New research on the benefits of green tea." *Life Extension*. Apr.
28. Yoo, K. Y., Choi, J. H., Hwang, I. K., Lee, C. H., Lee, S. O., Han, S. M., Shin, H. C., Kang, I. J., Won, M. H. (2010). "Epigallocatechin-3-gallate increases cell proliferation and neuroblasts in the subgranular zone of the dentate gyrus in adult mice." *Phytotherapy Research*. July, 24(7):1065–70. doi: 10.1002/ptr.3083.
29. Borgwardt, S., Hammann, F., Scheffler, K., Kreuter, M., Drewe, J., Beglinger, C. (2012). "Neural effects of green tea extract on dorsolateral prefrontal cortex. *European Journal of Clinical Nutrition*. Nov, 66(11):1187–92.
30. Han, M. E., Park, K. H., Baek, S. Y., Kim, B. S., Kim, J. B., Kim, H. J., Oh, S. O. (2007). "Inhibitory effects of caffeine on hippocampal neurogenesis and function." *Biochemical and Biophysical Research Communications*. May 18, 356(4):976–80. Epub Mar 26, 2007.
31. Wentz, C. T., Magavi, S. S. (2009). "Caffeine alters proliferation of neuronal precursors in the adult hippocampus." *Neuropharmacology*. May–June, 56(6–7):994–1000. doi: 10.1016/j.neuropharm.2009.02.002. PMID: 19217915. Epub Feb 13, 2009.
32. Kim, S. J., Son, T. G., Park, H. R., Park, M., Kim, M. S., Kim, H. S., Chung, H. Y., Mattson, M. P., Lee, J. (2008). "Curcumin stimulates proliferation of embryonic neural progenitor cells and neurogenesis in the adult hippocampus." *Journal of Biological Chemistry*. May 23, 283(21):14497–505. doi: 10.1074/jbc.M708373200. Epub Mar 24, 2008.
33. Ng, T. P., Chiam, P. C., Lee, T., Chua, H. C., Lim, L., Kua, E. H. (2006). "Curry consumption and cognitive function in the elderly." *American Journal of Epidemiology*. Nov 1, 164(9):898–906. Epub Jul 26, 2006.
34. Bhutani, M. K., Bishnoi, M., Kulkarni, S. K. (2009). "Anti-depressant like effect of curcumin and its combination with piperine in unpredictable chronic stress-induced behavioral, biochemical and neurochemical changes." *Pharmacology Biochemistry and Behavior. Mar*, 92(1):39–43. doi: 10.1016/j.pbb.2008.10.007. Epub Oct 25, 2008.
35. Casadesus, G., Shukitt-Hale, B., Stellwagen, H. M., et al. (2004). "Modulation of hippocampal plasticity and cognitive behavior by short-term blueberry supplementation in aged rats." *Nutritional Neuroscience*. Oct, 7(5–6):309–16.
36. Acosta, S., Jernberg, J., Sanberg, C. D., Sanberg, P. R., Small, B. J., Gemma, C., Bickford, P. C. (2010). "Daily supplementation with GrandFusion improves memory and learning in aged rats." *Rejuvenation Res*. Oct, 13(5):581–8. doi: 10.1089/rej.2009.1011. Epub Jun 29, 2010.
37. Joseph, J. A., Shukitt-Hale, B., Lau, F. C. "Fruit polyphenols and their effects on neuronal signaling and behavior in senescence." *Annals of the New York Academy of Sciences*.
38. Joseph, J. A., Denisova, N. A., Arendash, G., et al. (2003). "Blueberry supplementation enhances signaling and prevents behavioral deficits in an Alzheimer disease model." *Nutritional Neuroscience*. June, 6(3):153–62.
39. Joseph, J. A., Carey, A., Brewer, G. J., Lau, F. C., Fisher, D. R. (2007). "Dopamine and abeta-induced stress signaling and decrements in Ca2+ buffering in primary neonatal hippocampal cells are antagonized by blueberry extract." *Journal of Alzheimer's Disease*. July, 11(4):433–46.
40. Devore, E. E., Kang, J. H., Breteler, M. M., Grodstein, F. A. (2012). "Dietary intakes of berries and flavonoids in relation to cognitive decline." *Neurology*. July, 72(1):135–43. doi: 10.1002/ana.23594. Epub Apr 26, 2012.
41. Joseph, J. A., Shukitt-Hale, B., Willis, L. M. (2009). "Grape juice, berries, and walnuts affect brain aging and behavior." *Journal of Nutrition*. Sep, 139(9):1813S–7S. doi: 10.3945/jn.109.108266. Epub Jul 29, 2009. Review.
42. Dai, Q., Borenstein, A. R., Wu, Y., Jackson, J. C., Larson, E.B. (2006). "Fruit and vegetable juices and Alzheimer's disease: The kame project." *American Journal of Medicine*. Sep, 119(9):751–9.
43. Lau, F. C., Shukitt-Hale, B., Joseph, J. A. (2007). "Nutritional intervention in brain aging: Reducing the effects of inflammation and oxidative stress." *Subcell Biochemistry*. Sep, 42:299–318.
44. McGeer, P. L., McGeer, E. G. (2004). "Inflammation and neurodegeneration in Parkinson's disease." *Parkinsonism Related Disorders*. May, 10 Suppl 1:S3–S7.
45. Joseph, J. A., Denisova, N. A., Arendash, G., et al. (2003). "Blueberry supplementation enhances signaling and prevents behavioral deficits in an Alzheimer disease model." *Nutritional Neuroscience*. June, 6(3):153–62.
46. Joseph, J. A., Carey, A., Brewer, G. J., Lau, F. C., Fisher, D. R. (2007). "Dopamine and abeta-induced stress signaling and decrements in Ca2+ buffering in primary neonatal hippocampal cells are antagonized by blueberry extract." *Journal of Alzheimer's Disease*. July, 11(4):433–46.
47. Shukitt-Hale, B., Carey, A. N., Jenkins, D., Rabin, B. M., Joseph, J. A. (2007). "Beneficial effects of fruit extracts on neuronal function and behavior in a rodent model of accelerated aging." *Neurobiological Aging*. Aug, 28(8):1187–94.
48. McGuire, S. O., Sortwell, C. E., Shukitt-Hale, B., et al. (2006). "Dietary supplementation with blueberry extract improves survival of transplanted dopamine neurons." *Nutritional Neuroscience*. Oct, 9(5–6):251–8.
49. Suh, N., Paul, S., Hao, X., et al. (2007). "Pterostilbene, an active constituent of blueberries, suppresses aberrant crypt foci formation in the azoxymethane-induced colon carcinogenesis model in rats." *Clinical Cancer Research*. Jan 1, 13(1):350–5.

50. Heinonen, M. (2007). "Antioxidant activity and antimicrobial effect of berry phenolics—a Finnish perspective." *Molecular Nutrition and Food Research.* June, 51(6):684–91.
51. Russell, W. R., Labat, A., Scobbie, L., Duncan, S. H. (2007). "Availability of blueberry phenolics for microbial metabolism in the colon and the potential inflammatory implications." *Molecular Nutrition and Food Research.* June, 51(6):726–31.
52. Zafra-Stone, S., Yasmin, T., Bagchi, M., et al. (2007). "Berry anthocyanins as novel antioxidants in human health and disease prevention." *Molecular Nutrition and Food Research.* June, 51(6):675–83.
53. Zafra-Stone, S., Yasmin, T., Bagchi, M., et al. (2007). "Berry anthocyanins as novel antioxidants in human health and disease prevention." *Molecular Nutrition & Food Research.* June, 51(6):675–83.
54. Nones, J., Leite de Sampaio, S., Gomes, F. (2012). "Effects of the flavonoid hesperidin in cerebral progenitors in rats: Indirect action through astrocytes." *International Journal of Developmental Neuroscience.* June, 30(4) 303–313.
55. Tchantchou, F., Lacor, P. N., Cao, Z., Lao, L., Hou, Y., Cui, C., Klein, W. L., Luo, Y. (2009). "Stimulation of neurogenesis and synaptogenesis by bilobalide and quercetin via common final pathway in hippocampal neurons." *Journal of Alzheimer's Disease.* 18(4):787–98. doi: 10.3233/JAD-2009-1189.
56. Yoo, D. Y., Nam, Y., Kim, W., Yoo, K. Y., Park, J., Lee, C. H., Choi, J. H., Yoon, Y. S., Kim, D. W., Won, M. H., Hwang, I. K. (2011). "Effects of ginkgo biloba extract on promotion of neurogenesis in the hippocampal dentate gyrus in C57BL/6 mice." *Journal of Veterinary Medical Science.* Jan, 73(1):71–6. Epub Aug 30, 2010.
57. Jang, S., Dilger, R. N., and Johnson, R. W.* (2010). "Luteolin inhibits microglia and alters hippocampal-dependent spatial working memory in aged mice1,2,3." *Journal of Nutrition.* Oct, 140(10):1892–1898. doi: 10.3945/jn.110.123273. PMCID: PMC2937579. Epub Aug 4, 2010.
58. Crupi, R., Paterniti, I., Ahmad, A., Campolo, M., Esposito, E., Cuzzocrea, S. (2013). "Effects of palmitoylethanolamide and luteolin in an animal model of anxiety/depression." *CNS & Neurological Disorders—Drug Targets.* Nov, 12(7):989–1001.
59. Xu, S. L., Bi, C. W. C., Choi, R. C. Y., Zhu, K. Y., Miernisha, A., Dong, T. T. X., and Tsim, K. W. K. (2013). "Flavonoids induce the synthesis and secretion of neurotrophic factors in cultured rat astrocytes: A signaling response mediated by estrogen receptor." *Evidence-Based Complementary and Alternative Medicine.* Vol 2013, Article 127075. http://dx.doi.org/10.1155/2013/127075
60. Taupin, P. (2009). "Apigenin and related compounds stimulate adult neurogenesis." Mars, Inc., the Salk Institute for Biological Studies: WO2008147483. Dublin City University, School of Biotechnology, Glasnevin, Dublin 9, Ireland. Expert Opinion on Therapeutic Patents (Impact Factor: 3.53). May 19(4):523–7. doi: 10.1517/13543770902721279.
61. Zainuddin, M. S. A., & Thuret, S. (2012). "Nutrition, adult hippocampal neurogenesis and mental health." *British Medical Bulletin.* 103 (1) 89–114. doi: 10.1093/bmb/lds021.
62. Moriguchi, S., Shinoda, Y., Yamamoto, Y., Sasaki, Y., Miyajima, K., Tagashira, H., Fukunaga, K. (2013). "Stimulation of the sigma-1 receptor by DHEA enhances synaptic efficacy and neurogenesis in the hippocampal dentate gyrus of olfactory bulbectomized mice." *PLoS One.* Apr 8, 8(4):e60863. doi: 10.1371/journal.pone.0060863.
63. (2006). "Therapeutic potential of neurogenesis for prevention and recovery from Alzheimer's disease: Allopregnanolone as a proof of concept neurogenic agent." *Current Alzheimer's Research.* July, 3(3):185–90.
64. Lai, P. L., et al. (2013). "Neurotrophic properties of the lion's mane medicinal mushroom, from Malaysia." *Int J Med Mushrooms.* 15(6) 539–54.
65. Zhuang, P. W., et al. (2013). "Baicalin regulates neuronal fate decision in neural. Progenitor cells and stimulates adult neurogenesis in adult rats." *CNS Neurosci Ther. Mar,* 19(3):154–62.
66. Wu, B., et al. (2012). "Icariin improves cognitive deficits and activates quiescent neural stem cells in aging rats." *J Ethnopharmacol.* Aug 1, 142(3):746–53.
67. Lee, C. H., Kim, J. M., Kim, D. H., Park, S. J., Liu, X., Cai, M., Hong, J. G., Park, J. H., Ryu, J. H. (2013). "Effects of sun ginseng on memory enhancement and hippocampal neurogenesis." *Phytotherapy Research.* Sep, 27(9):1293–9. doi: 10.1002/ptr.4873. Epub Oct 29, 2012.
68. Lin, T., Liu, Y., Shi, M., Liu, X., Li, L., Liu, Y., Zhao, G. (2012). "Promotive effect of ginsenoside Rd on proliferation of neural stem cells in vivo and in vitro." *Journal Ethnopharmacology.* Aug 1, 142(3):754–61. doi: 10.1016/j.jep.2012.05.057. Epub Jun 7, 2012.
69. Jiang, B., Xiong, Z., Yang, J., Wang, W., Wang, Y., Hu, Z. L., Wang, F., Chen, J. G. (2012). "Antidepressant-like effects of ginsenoside Rg1 are due to activation of the BDNF signalling pathway and neurogenesis in the hippocampus." *British Journal of Pharmacology.* July, 166(6):1872–87. doi: 10.1111/j.1476-5381.2012.01902.x.
70. Funakoshi, H., Kanai, M., and Nakamura, T. (2011). "Modulation of tryptophan metabolism, promotion of neurogenesis and alteration of anxiety-related behavior in tryptophan 2,3-dioxygenase-deficient mice." *International Journal of Tryptophan Research.* 4:7–18. Epub Apr 11, 2011. doi: 10.4137/IJTR.S5783. PMCID: PMC3195223.
71. Rivera, P., Pérez-Martín, M., Pavón, F. J., Serrano, A., Crespillo, A., Cifuentes, M., López-Ávalos, M. D., Grondona, J. M., Vida, M., Fernández-Llebrez, P., de Fonseca, F. R., Suárez, J. (2013). "Pharmacological administration of the isoflavone daidzein enhances cell proliferation and reduces high fat diet-induced

apoptosis and gliosis in the rat hippocampus." *PLoS One*. May 31, 8(5):e64750. doi: 10.1371/journal.pone.0064750.

72. Zheng, J., Zhang, P., Li, X., Lei, S., Li, W., He, X., Zhang, J., Wang, N., Qi, C., Chen, X., Lu, H., Liu, Y. (2013). "Post-stroke estradiol treatment enhances neurogenesis in the subventricular zone of rats after permanent focal cerebral ischemia." *Neuroscience*. Feb 12, 231:82–90. doi: 10.1016/j.neuroscience.2012.11.042. Epub Dec 2, 2012.
73. Bayer, J., Rune, G., Kutsche, K., Schwarze, U., Kalisch, R., Büchel, C., Sommer, T. (2013). "Estrogen and the male hippocampus: Genetic variation in the aromatase gene predicting serum estrogen is associated with hippocampal gray matter volume in men." *Hippocampus*. Feb, (2):117–21. doi: 10.1002/hipo.22059. Epub Aug 6, 2012.
74. Sarlak, G., Jenwitheesuk, A., Chetsawang, B., Govitrapong, P. (2013). "Effects of melatonin on nervous system aging: Neurogenesis and neurodegeneration." *Journal of Pharmacological Sciences*. Sep 20, 123(1):9–24. Epub Aug 27, 2013.
75. Ramírez-Rodríguez, G., Vega-Rivera, N. M., Benítez-King. G., Castro-García, M., Ortíz-López, L. (2012). "Melatonin supplementation delays the decline of adult hippocampal neurogenesis during normal aging of mice." *Neuroscience Letters*. Nov 14, 530(1):53–8. doi: 10.1016/j.neulet.2012.09.045. Epub Oct 6, 2012.
76. Chern, C. M., Liao, J. F., Wang, Y. H., Shen, Y. C. (2012). "Melatonin ameliorates neural function by promoting endogenous neurogenesis through the MT2 melatonin receptor in ischemic-stroke mice." *Free Radical Biology & Medicine*. May 1, 52(9):1634–47. doi: 10.1016/j.freeradbiomed.2012.01.030. Epub Feb 10, 2012.
77. Zhuang, P., Zhang, Y.,* Cui, G., Bian, Y., Zhang, M., Zhang, J., Liu, Y., Yang, X., Isaiah, A. O., Lin, Y., and Jiang, Y. (2012). "Direct stimulation of adult neural stem/progenitor cells in vitro and neurogenesis in vivo by salvianolic acid B." *PLoS One*. 7(4):e35636. doi: 10.1371/journal.pone.0035636 PMCID: PMC3335811. Epub Apr 24, 2012.
78. Kumar, S., Mondal, A. C. (2016). "Neuroprotective, neurotrophic and antioxidant role of Bacopa monnieri on CSU induced model of depression in rat." *Neurochem Res*. Nov, 41(11):3083–3094.
79. Lau, B. W., Lee, J. C., Li, Y., Fung, S. M., Sang, Y. H., Shen, J., Chang, R. C., So, K. F. (2012). "Polysaccharides from wolfberry prevents corticosterone-induced inhibition of sexual behavior and increases neurogenesis." *PLoS One*. 7(4):e33374. doi: 10.1371/journal.pone.0033374. Epub Apr 16, 2012.
80. Yoo, D. Y., Kim, W., Yoo, K. Y., Lee, C. H., Choi, J. H., Yoon, Y. S., Kim, D. W., Won, M. H., Hwang, I. K. (2011). "Grape seed extract enhances neurogenesis in the hippocampal dentate gyrus in C57BL/6 mice." *Phytotherapy Research*. May, 25(5):668–74. doi: 10.1002/ptr.3319. Epub Oct 29, 2010.
81. Crupi, R., Mazzon, E., Marino, A., La Spada, G., Bramanti, P., Battaglia, F., Cuzzocrea, S., and Spina, E. (2011). "Hypericum perforatum treatment: Effect on behaviour and neurogenesis in a chronic stress model in mice." *BMC Complementary and Alternative Medicine*. 11:7. doi: 10.1186/1472-6882-11-7. PMCID: PMC3041724. Epub Jan 27, 2011.
82. M. L.,* Bus, B. A. A., Spinhoven, P., Penninx, B. W. J. H., Prickaerts, J., Oude Voshaar, R. C., and Elzinga, B. M. (2011). "Serum levels of brain-derived neurotrophic factor in major depressive disorder: State–trait issues, clinical features and pharmacological treatment." *Molecular Psychiatry*. Nov, 16(11):1088–1095. doi: 10.1038/mp.2010.98. PMCID: PMC3220395. Epub Sep 21, 2010.
83. Abumaria, N., Yin, B., Zhang, L., Li, X. Y., Chen, T., Descalzi, G., Zhao, L., Ahn, M., Luo, L., Ran, C., Zhuo, M., and Liu, G. (2011). "Effects of elevation of brain magnesium on fear conditioning, fear extinction, and synaptic plasticity in the infralimbic prefrontal cortex and lateral amygdala." *Journal of Neuroscience*. Oct 19, 31(42):14871–14881. doi: 10.1523/JNEUROSCI.3782-11.2011.
84. Liu, G. (2012). (1):L24. doi: 10.1186/1750-1326-7-S1-L24. Epub Feb 7, 2012. Corona, C., et al. (2011). "Effects of dietary supplementation of carnosine on mitochondrial dysfunction, amyloid pathology, and cognitive deficits in 3xTg-AD mice" *PLOS One*. Mar 15.
85. Li, L. F., Lu, J., Li, X. M., Xu, C. L., Deng, J. M., Qu, R., Ma, S. P. (2012). "Antidepressant-like effect of magnolol on BDNF up-regulation and serotonergic system activity in unpredictable chronic mild stress treated rats." *Phytotherapy Research*. Aug, 26(8):1189–94. doi: 10.1002/ptr.3706. Epub Jan 5, 2012.
86. Mercola, J. (2018). "For optimal health, make sure you have a vitamin D level of 60ng/mL." Mercola.com. July 4.
87. Ma, T., et al. (2013). "Huperzine A promotes hippocampal neurogenesis in vitro and in vivo." *Brain Res*. April 19, 1506:35–43.
88. Manchanda, S., Kaur, G. (2017). "Withania somnifera leaf alleviates cognitive dysfunction by enhancing hippocampal plasticity in high fat diet induced obesity model." *BMC Complementary Alternative Medicine*. 17:136.
89. Cimini, A., Gentile, R., D'Angelo, B., Benedetti, E., Cristiano, L., Avantaggiati, M. L., Giordano, A., Ferri, C., Desideri, G. (2013). "Cocoa powder triggers neuroprotective and preventive effects in a human Alzheimer's disease model by modulating BDNF signaling pathway." *Journal of Cellular Biochemistry*. Oct, 114(10):2209–20. doi: 10.1002/jcb.24548.
90. Scholey, A., Owen, L. (2013). "Effects of chocolate on cognitive function and mood: A systematic review." *Nutrition Review*. Oct, 71(10):665–81. doi: 10.1111/nure.12065.

91. Sokolov, A. N., Pavlova, M. A., Klosterhalfen, S., Enck, P. (2013). "Chocolate and the brain: Neurobiological impact of cocoa flavanols on cognition and behavior." *Neuroscience & Biobehavioral Reviews*. June 26, pii: S0149-7634(13)00168-1. doi: 10.1016/j.neubiorev.2013.06.013.
92. Kittur, S., Wilasrusmee, S., Pedersen, W. A., Mattson, M. P., Straube-West, K., Wilasrusmee, C., Lubelt, B., Kittur, D. S. (2002). "Neurotrophic and neuroprotective effects of milk thistle (Silybum marianum) on neurons in culture." *Journal of Molecular Neuroscience*. June, 18(3):265–9.
93. Tsai, S. J. (2006). "Cysteamine-related agents could be potential antidepressants through increasing central BDNF levels." *Medical Hypotheses*. 67(5):1185–8. Epub Jun 22, 2006.
94. Park, H. J., Shim, H. S., Kim, K. S., Han, J. J., Kim, J. S., Ram Yu, A., Shim, I. (2013). "Enhanced learning and memory of normal young rats by repeated oral administration of krill phosphatidylserine." *Nutritional Neuroscience*. Mar, 16(2):47–53. doi: 10.1179/1476830512Y.0000000029. Epub Aug 8, 2012.
95. Maggioni, M., Picotti, G. B., Bondiolotti, G. P., Panerai, A., Cenacchi, T., Nobile, P., Brambilla, F. (1990). "Effects of phosphatidylserine therapy in geriatric patients with depressive disorders." *Acta Psychiatrica Scandinavica*. Mar, 81(3):265–70.
96. Jana, A., Modi, K. K., Roy, A., Anderson, J. A., van Breemen, R. B., Pahan, K. (2013). "Up-regulation of neurotrophic factors by cinnamon and its metabolite sodium benzoate: Therapeutic implications for neurodegenerative disorders." *Journal of Neuroimmune Pharmacology*. June, 8(3):739–55. doi: 10.1007/s11481-013-9447-7. Epub Mar 9, 2013.
97. Hyman, M. (2016). *Eat fat, get thin*. New York: Little, Brown and Company.
98. Elias, P., et al. (2005). "Serum cholesterol and cognitive performance in the Framingham heart study." *Psychosomatic Medicine*. 67(1):24–30.
99. Iowa State University. (2009). "Cholesterol-reducing drugs may lessen brain function, says researcher." *ScienceDaily*. Feb 26.
100. Mielke, M. M. (2005). "High total cholesterol levels in late life associated with a reduced risk of dementia." *Neurology*. May 24, Vol 64, No 10:1689–1695.
101. Senoff, S. (2009). "APOE: the clue to why low fat diet and statins may cause Alzheimer's." MIT webpage for Stephanie Senoff, Ph.D. Dec. 15.
102. Mann, G. (1993). *Coronary heart disease*. Austin, TX: Harry Ransom Humanities Research Center.
103. Kummerow, F., Kummerow, J. (2014). *Cholesterol is not the culprit*. Summerfield, FL: Spacedoc Media, LLC.
104. Steprans, I., et al. (2005). "The role of oxidized cholesterol and oxidized fatty acids in the development of atherosclerosis." *Mol Nutr Food Res*. Nov, 49(11):1075–1082.
105. Perlmutter, D. (2013). *Grain brain*. New York: Little, Brown and Co.
106. Uribarri, J., et al. (2010). "Advanced glycation end products in foods and a practical guide to their reduction in the diet." *J Am Diet Assoc*. Jun, 110(6):911–16 e12.
107. Choi, J., et al. (2017). "Long-term consumption of sugar-sweetened beverage during the growth period promotes social aggression in mice with proinflammatory responses in the brain." *Scientific Reports*. No 7, Article 45693.
108. Laplante, M., Sabatini, D. (2012). "mTOR signaling in growth control and disease." *Cell*. Apr 13, Vol 149, Issue 2:274–293.
109. Berg, J. M., et al. (2002). *Biochemistry*, 5th Edition. New York: F H Freeman.
110. Volek, J. & Phinney, S. (2011). *The art and science of low carbohydrate living*. Miami, FL: Beyond Obesity, LLC.
111. Asprey, D. (2017). *Head strong*. New York: Harper Wave.
112. Volek, J., & Phinney, S. (2012). *The art and science of low carbohydrate performance*. Miami, FL: Beyond Obesity, LLC.
113. Nokia, M., et al. (2016). "Physical exercise increases neurogenesis in male rats provided it is aerobic and sustained". *The Journal of Physiology*. Feb 24.
114. Sleiman, S. F., et al. (2016). "Exercise promotes the expression of brain derived neurotrophic factor (BDNF) through the action of the ketone body beta-hydroxybuterate." *eLife*. Jan 2.
115. Csilla, A., et al. (2017). "Exogenous ketone supplements reduce anxiety-related behavior in Sprague-Dawley and Wistar Albino Glaxo-Rijswijk rats." *Front. Mol. Neuroscience*. Feb 13.
116. Maneer, A., et al. (2016). "Bipolar disorder: Role of inflammation and the development of disease biomarkers." *Psychiatry Investigation*. Jan 13(1):18–33.
117. Salim, S., et al. (2012). "Inflammation in anxiety." *Adv Protein Chem Struct Biol*. 88–125.
118. Underwood, E. (2017). "The polluted brain." Science. Jan 26.
119. Biswas, K. S. (2016). "Does the interdependence between oxidative stress and inflammation explain the antioxidant paradox?" *Oxidative Medicine and Cellular Longevity*. Vol 2016, Article ID 5698931.
120. Sender, R., et al. (2016). "Revised estimates for the number of human and bacteria cells in the body." *BioRxiv*. Jan 6.
121. Carpenter, S. (2012). "That gut feeling." *APA Monitor*. Sep, Vol 43, No 8.
122. Messaoudi, M., et al. (2011). "Assessment of psychotropic-like properties of a probiotic formulation (Lactobacillus helveticus R0052 and Bifidobacterium longum R0175) in rats and human subjects." *Br J Nutr*. 105(5):755–64.

123. Messaoudi, M., Violle, N., Bisson, J. F., et al. (2011). "Beneficial psychological effects of a probiotic formulation (Lactobacillus helveticus R0052 and Bifidobacterium longum R0175) in healthy human volunteers." *Gut Microbes*. 2(4):256–61.
124. Sarkar, A., et al. (2016). "Psychobiotics and the manipulation of bacteria-gut-brain signals." *Trends in Neurosciences*. Nov, Vol 39, Issue 11:763–781.
125. Novkovic, B. (2018). "20 causes of leaky gut syndrome and 15 healing treatments." Selfhacked.com. Nov 27.
126. Ahrne, S., & Hagslat, M. J. (2011). "Effect of lactobacilli on paracellular permeability in the gut." *Nutrients*. Jan, 3(1):104–117.
127. Gong, Y., et al. (2016). "Effects of bacillus subtilis on epithelial tight junctions of mice with inflammatory bowel disease." *J Interferon Cytokine Res*. Feb, 36(2):75–85.
128. Ulluwishewa, D., et al. (2011). "Regulation of tight junction permeability by intestinal bacteria and dietary components." *Journal of Nutrition*. May, Vol 141, Issue 5:769–776.
129. Sonnenburg, E., et al. (2016). "Diet-induced extinctions in the gut microbiota compound over generations." *Nature*. Jan 14, 529:212–215.
130. Teunissen, C. E., et al. (2003). "Homocysteine: A marker for cognitive performance? A longitudinal follow-up study." *J Nutr Health Aging*. 7(3):153–9.
131. Adami, R., et al. (2018). "Reduction of movement in neurological diseases: Effects on neural stem cells characteristics." *Frontiers in Neuroscience*. May 23.
132. Duncan, E. (2018). "Leg exercise critical to brain and nervous system health." *EurekAlert*. May 23 Public Release.
133. Ahrne, S., & Hagslat, M. J. (2011). "Effect of lactobacilli on paracellular permeability in the gut." *Nutrients*. Jan, 3(1):104–117.
134. Gong, Y., et al. (2016). "Effects of bacillus subtilis on epithelial tight junctions of mice with inflammatory bowel disease." *J Interferon Cytokine Res*. Feb, 36(2):75–85.
135. Hairston, I. L., et al. (2005). "Sleep restriction suppresses neurogenesis induced by hippocampus-dependent learning." *American Journal of Psychiatry: Journal of Neurophysiology*. 94(6):4224–4233.
136. World Health Organization. (2016). Sep.

Chapter 3: Holistic Healing of Anxiety

1. National Institute of Mental Health (2018). "Prevalence of any anxiety disorder among adults." Data from National Comorbidity Study Replication 2017. August 21.
2. Gray, P. (2010). "The decline of play and rise in children's mental disorders." *Psychology Today*. Jan 26.
3. Twenge, J., et al. (2010). "Birth cohort increases in psychopathology among young Americans, 1938–2007: A cross-temporal meta-analysis of the MMPI." *Clinical Psychology Review*. 30:145–154.
4. Melville, N. A. (2017). "Most children with anxiety relapse, regardless of treatment." *Medscape*. April 18.
5. Mercola, J. (2017). "Anxiety overtakes depression as no. 1 mental health problem." Mercola.com. June, 29.
6. Fredrikson, M., et al. (1997). "Cerebral blood flow during anxiety provocation." *Journal of Clinical Psychiatry*. 58 Suppl 16:16–21.
7. Salim, S., et al. (2012). "Inflammation and anxiety." *Adv Protein Chem Struct Biol*. 88:1–25.
8. Sapolsky, R. (1999). "Stress and your shrinking brain" *Discover*. Vol 20, No 3:116–122.
9. Felleti, V. J., et al. (1998). "Relationship of childhood abuse and household dysfunction to many of the leading causes of death in adulthood: The adverse childhood experiences study." *American Journal of Preventive Medicine*. May, Vol 14, Issue 4:245–258.
10. Laing, R. D. (1987). Talk at Evolution of Psychotherapy conference. Phoenix, AZ.
11. Bernard, R., et al. (2010). "Altered expression of glutamate signaling, growth factor, and glia genes in the locus coeruleus of patients with major depression." *Molecular Psychiatry*. 16:634–646.
12. Friedman, R. (2018). "How to be more resilient." *New York Times*. Dec 16, front page.
13. Herman, J. (1992). *Trauma and recovery*. New York: HarperCollins.
14. Ogden, P. (2015). *Sensorimotor psychotherapy: Interventions for trauma and attachment*. New York: W. W. Norton & Co.
15. Freud, S. (1926). *Inhibitions, symptoms and anxiety*. New York: Vintage Classics.
16. Timulak, L., & McElvaney, J. (2018). *Transforming generalized anxiety*. New York: Routledge.
17. Wachtel. P. (2011). *Therapeutic communication*. New York: Guilford Press.
18. Kohut, H. (1977). *The restoration of the self*. Madison, CT: International Universities Press.
19. Kohut, H. (1971). *The analysis of the self*. Madison, CT: International Universities Press.
20. Bowlby J. (1988). *A secure base*. New York: Basic Books.
21. Sapolsky, R. (1994). *Why zebras don't get ulcers*. New York: W. H. Freeman and Company.
22. Cacioppo, S., et al. (2014). "Toward a neurology of loneliness." *Psychological Bulletin*. Vol 140, No 6:1464–1504.
23. Russek, L. G., et al. (1994). "Interpersonal heart-brain registration and the perception of parental love." *Subtle Energies*. Vol 5, No. 3.
24. Brisch, K. H. (2012). *Treating attachment disorders*. New York: Guilford Press.

25. May, R. (1994). *Existence*. New York: Jason Aronson.
26. Yalom, I. (1980). *Existential Psychotherapy*. New York: Basic Books.
27. Jacka, F. N. , et al. (2012). "Red meat consumption and mood and anxiety disorders." *Psychotherapy and Psychosomatics*. 81:196–198.
28. Reynolds, G. (2009). "Why exercise makes you less anxious." *New York Times*. Nov 18.
29. Gerlach, L. B., et al. (2018). "Factors associated with long-term benzodiazepine use among older adults." *JAMA Internal Med*. 178(11):1560–1562.
30. Barnes, E. M. (1996). "Use-dependent regulation of GABAA receptors." *Int Rev Neurobiology*. 39:53–76.
31. Mahtre, M. C., & Ticku, M.K. (1994). "Chronic GABA treatment downregulates the GABAA receptor a2 and a3 subunit mRNAS as well as polypeptide expression in primary cultured cerebral cortical neurons." *Molecular Brain Research*. July, 159–165.

Chapter 4: Holistic Healing of Depression

1. Abi-Habib, R., Luyten, P. (2013). "The role of dependency and self-criticism in the relationship between anger and depression." *Personality and Individual Differences*. Nov, Vol 55, Issue 6:921–925.
2. Blue Cross Blue Shield. May 10, 2018.
3. Butters, M. A., et al. (2008). "Pathways linking late-life depression to persistent cognitive impairment and dementia." *Dialogues Clin Neurosci*. Sept, 10(3):345–357.
4. May, R., et al. (1958). Existence. New York: Basic Books.
5. Lowen, A. (1972). *Depression and the body*. New York: Coward, McCann & Geoghegan.
6. Yalom, I. (1980). *Existential psychotherapy*. New York: Basic Books.
7. Kohut, H. (1971). *The analysis of the self.* New York: International Universities Press.
8. Masterson, J. (1981). *The narcissistic and borderline disorders*. Oxfordshire: Routledge.
9. Masterson, J. (1993). *Search for the real self.* Oxfordshire: Routledge.
10. Maslow, A. (1976). *The farther reaches of human nature*. New York: Penguin Books.
11. Sapolsky, R. (1998). *Why zebras don't get ulcers*. New York: W. H. Freeman & Co.
12. Greenberg, L., & Watson, J. C. (2005). *Emotion-focused therapy for depression*. Washington, D.C.: American Psychological Association.
13. Kohut, H. (1977). *The restoration of the self.* New York: International Universities Press, Inc.
14. Ristevska-Dimitrovska, G., et al. (2013). "Different serum BDNF levels in depression." *Psychiatr Danub*. Jun, 25(2):123–7.
15. Greenberg, L. S., & Paivio, S. C. (1997). *Working with emotions in psychotherapy*. New York: Guildford.
16. Seligman, M. (1975). *Learned helplessness*. San Francisco: W. H. Freeman.
17. Seligman, M. (1972). "Learned helplessness." *Annual Review of Medicine*. 23(1):407–412.
18. Greenberg. L. S., & Watson, J. C. (1994). *Emotion-focused therapy for depression*. Washington, D.C.: American Psychological Association.
19. Donovan, N. J. (2017). "Loneliness, depression and cognitive decline in older adults." *Int J Geriatric Psychiatry*. May, 32(5):564–573.
20. Majoribanks, D., & Bradley, A. D. (2017). "You're not alone: The quality of the UK's social relationships." *Relate*. Mar.
21. Beck, A. T., et al. (1987). *Cognitive therapy of depression*. New York: Guilford Press.
22. Beck, A. T., Alford, B. A., (2009). *Depression: causes and treatment*, 2nd edition. Philadelphia: University of Pennsylvania Press.
23. St. John of the Cross, translated by Kavanaugh, K., & Rodriguez, O. (1979). *The collected works of St. John of the Cross*. Washington, D.C.: ICS Publications.
24. Stein, M. (2014). *In midlife: A Jungian perspective. Asheville*, North Carolina: Chiron Publications.
25. Moore, T. (2005). *Dark nights of the soul*. New York: Avery.
26. Washburn, M. (1994). *Transpersonal psychology in psychoanalytic perspective*. Albany, New York: State University of New York Press.
27. World Health Organization. Sep.
28. Cortright, B. (2015). *The neurogenesis diet and lifestyle*. Mill Valley, CA: Psyche Media.
29. Santarelli, L. (2003). "Requirement of hippocampal neurogenesis for the behavioral effects of antidepressants." *Science*. 301(5634):805–809. Doi:10.1126/science.1083328.
30. Sahay, A. & Hen, R. (2008). "Hippocampal neurogenesis and depression." Novartis Foundation Symposium. 289:152–60; discussion 160–4, 193–5.
31. Breggin, P. (2019). "What does the evidence say about antidepressants?" Mercola.com. Apr 4; interview with Peter Breggin by Joe Mercola.
32. Klerman, G. L., et al. (1994). *Interpersonal psychotherapy of depression*. New York: Jason Aronson, Inc.
33. Bernard, R., et al. (2010). "Altered expression of glutamate signaling, growth factor, and glia genes in the locus coeruleus of patients with major depression." *Molecular Psychiatry*. 16:634–646.
34. Friedman, R. (2018). "How to be more resilient." *New York Times*. Dec 16, front page.

35. Colle, R., et al. (2017). "Plasma BDNF level in major depression." *Neuropsychobiology*,75(1):39–45.
36. Guo, L., et al. (2018). "Relationship between depression and inflammatory factors and brain-derived neurotrophic factor in patients with perimenopause syndrome." *Experimental and Therapeutic Medicine. May,* 15(5):44236–40.
37. Zonis, S., et al. "Chronic intestinal inflammation alters hippocampal neurogenesis." *Journal of Inflammation.* 12(65).

Chapter 5: Holistic Healing for Cognitive Decline

1. Beeri, M. S. & Sonnen, J. (2016). "Brain BDNF expression as a biomarker for cognitive reserve against Alzheimer disease progression." *Neurology.* 86:702–703.
2. Kennedy, R. E., et al. (2018). "Association of concomitant cholinesterase inhibitors or memantine with cognitive decline in Alzheimer's trials: A meta-analysis." *JAMA Network Open.* Nov 2, 1(7):e184080.
3. Peterson, R. (2009). "Early diagnosis of Alzheimer's disease: Is MCI too late?" Current Alzheimer Research. 6(4):324–330.
4. Kozareva, D. A., et al. (2019). "Born this way: Hippocampal neurogenesis across the lifespan." *Aging Cell.* July 12.
5. Parmet, S. (2019). "New neurons form in the brain into the tenth decade of life, even in people with Alzheimer's." *UIC Today.* May 24.
6. Tobin, M. K., et al. (2019) "Human hippocampal neurogenesis persists in aged adults and Alzheimer's disease patients." *Cell Stem Cell.* May 23.
7. Pascoal, T. A., et al. (2017). "Synergistic interaction between amyloid and tau predicts the progression to dementia." *Alzheimer's Dement.* Jun, 13(6):644–653.
8. Brion, J. P. (1998). "Neurofibrillary tangles and Alzheimer's disease." *Eur Neurol.* Oct, 40(3):130–40.
9. Bushche, M. A., et al. (2019). "Tau impairs neural circuits, dominating amyloid-beta effects, in Alzheimer's models in vivo." *Nature Neuroscience.* 22, 57–64.
10. Simen, A. A., et al. (2011). "Cognitive dysfunction with aging and the role of inflammation." *Ther Adv Chronc Dis.* 2(3):175–195.
11. Zonis, S., et al. (2015) "Chronic intestinal inflammation alters hippocampal neurogenesis." *Journal of Inflammation.* 12(65).
12. Kim, B., Feldman, E. L. (2015). "Insulin resistance as a key link for the increased risk of cognitive impairment in the metabolic syndrome." *Experimental and Molecular Medicine.* 47 e149.
13. Kerti, L., et al. (2013). "Higher glucose levels associated with lower memory and reduced hippocampal microstructures." *Neurology.* 81:1746–1752.
14. Ortega-Martinez, S., et al. (2019). "Deficits in enrichment-dependent neurogenesis and enhanced anxiety behaviors mediated by expression of Alzheimer's disease-linked Ps1 variants are rescued by microglial depletion." *Journal of Neuroscience.* August 21, 39(34):6766–6780.
15. Yuen, E. Y., et al. (2011). "Repeated stress causes cognitive impairment by suppressing glutamate receptor expression and function in prefrontal cortex." *Neuron.* Mar 8, 73(5): 962–977.
16. Tessman, R. (2018). "Stressed out? Study suggests it may affect memory, brain size in middle age." *EurkAlert.* Oct 24 public release.
17. Pietrzak, R. H., et al. (2015). "Amyloid-B, anxiety, and cognitive decline in preclinical Alzheimer's disease." *JAMA Psychiatry.* 72(3):284–291.
18. Mah, L., et al. (2014). "Anxiety symptoms in amnestic mild cognitive impairment are associated with medial temporal atrophy and predict conversion to Alzheime's disease" *American Journal of Geriatric Psychiatry.* Oct 29. ajgponline.org
19. Sutin, A. R., et al. (2018). "Loneliness and risk of dementia." Journal of Gerontology: Series B. Oct 26, gby112.
20. Donovan, N. J., (2017). "Loneliness, depression and cognitive decline in older adults." *Int J Geriatric Psychiatry.* May, 32(5):564–573.
21. Wilson, R., et al. (2007). "Loneliness and risk of Alzheimer's disease." *Arch Gen Psychiatry.* 64(2):234–240.
22. Giles, L. C., et al. (2012). "Social networks and memory over 15 years of followup in a cohort of older Australians." *Journal of Aging Research.* Aug 29, 2012:856048.
23. Holwerda, T. J., et al. (2014). "Feelings of loneliness, but not social isolation, predict dementia onset." *J Neurol Neurosurg Psychiatry.* Feb, 85(2):135–42.
24. Leuner, B., et al. (2012). "Oxytocin stimulates adult neurogenesis even under condition of stress and elevated glucocorticoids." *Hippocampus.* 22:861–868.
25. Murman, D. (2015). "The impact of age on cognition." *Seminars in Hearing.* Aug, 36(3):111–121.
26. Wang, J. Y., et al. (2006). "Leisure activity and risk of cognitive impairment." *Neurology.* Mar 28, 66(6): 911–3.
27. Hoang, T., et al. (2016). "Effect of early adult patterns of physical activity and television viewing on midlife cognitive function." *JAMA Psychiatry.* Jan 1, 73(1):73–79.

28. Wang, H. X., et al. (2013). "Late life leisure activities and risk of cognitive decline." *J Gerontol A Biol Sci Med Sci*. Feb, 68(2):205–13.
29. Hanson, R., & Mendius, R. (2009). *Buddha's brain*. Oakland, CA: New Harbinger Publications.
30. Goleman, D., & Davidson, R. J. (2017). *Altered Traits*. New York: Avery
31. Cortright, B. (2015). The neurogenesis diet and lifestyle. Mill Valley, CA: Psyche Media.

Appendix A

1. Ahrne, S., & Hagslat, M. J. (2011). "Effect of lactobacilli on paracellular permeability in the gut." *Nutrients*. Jan, 3(1):104–117.
2. Gong, Y., et al. (2016). "Effects of bacillus subtilis on epithelial tight junctions of mice with inflammatory bowel disease." *J Interferon Cytokine Res*. Feb, 36(2):75–85.
3. Novkovic, B. (2018). "20 causes of leaky gut syndrome and 15 healing treatments." Selfhacked.com. Nov 27.
4. Ulluwishewa, D., et al. (2011). "Regulation of tight junction permeability by intestinal bacteria and dietary components." Journal of Nutrition. May, Vol 141, Issue 5:769–776.

Appendix C

1. Chandrasekhar, K., et al. (2012). "A prospective, randomized double-blind, placebo-controlled study of safety and efficacy of a high-concentration full-spectrum extract of ashwagandha root in reducing stress and anxiety in adults." *Indian J Psychol Med*. Jul–Sep, 34(3):255–262.
2. Candalerio, M., et al. (2015). "Direct evidence for GABAergic activity of withania somnifera on mammalian ionotropic GABAAA and GABAp receptors." *J Ethnopharmacol*. Aug 2, 171:264–72.
3. Peng, W. H., et al. (2004). "Anxiolytic effect of berberine on exploratory activity of the mouse in two experimental anxiety models: Interaction with drugs acting as 5-HT receptors." *Life Sciences*. Oct 1, Vol 75, Issue 20:2451–2462.
4. Su, K. P., et al. (2018). "Association of use of omega-3 polyunsaturated fatty acids with changes in severity of anxiety symptoms: A systematic review and meta-analysis." *JAMA Network Open*. 1(5):e182327.
5. Kumar, S., Mondal, A. C. (2016). "Neuroprotective, neurotrophic and antioxidant role of Bacopa monnieri on CSU induced model of depression in rat." *Neurochem Res*. Nov, 41(11):3083–3094.
6. Calabrese, C., et al. (2008). "Effects of standardized bacopa monnieri extract on cognitive performance, anxiety and depression in the elderly: A randomized, double-blind, placebo-controlled trial." *Journal of Alternative and Complementary Medicine*. Jul 14, (6):707–713.
7. Li, S., et al. (2012). "Anti-depressant like effect of magnolol on BDNF up-regulation and serotonergic system activity in unpredictable mild stress treated mice and its possible mechanisms." *Life Science*. Aug 26, (8):1189–94.
8. Zhu, X., et al. (2019). "The antidepressant and anxiolytic effects of resveratrol." *Neuropharmacology*. July 15, 20–31.
9. Sowndhararajan, K., et al. (2018). "Neuroprotective and cognitive enhancement potentials of baicalin: A review." *Brain Sciences*. Jun, 8(6):104.
10. Hui, K. M., et al. (2000). "Interaction of flavones from the roots of scutellaria baicalensis with the benzodiazepine site." *Planta Med*. 66(1):91–93.
11. Lee, B., & Lee, H. (2018). "Systemic administration of curcumin affects anxiety-related behaviors in a rat model of posttraumatic stress disorder via activation of serotonergic systems." *Evid Based Complement Alternat Med*. Jun, 19:9041309.
12. Esmaily, H., et al. (2012). "An investigation of the effects of curcumin on anxiety and depression in obese individuals: A randomized, controlled trial." *Chin J Integr Med*. Sept 28. doi: 10.107/s11655-015-2160-z
13. Vignes, M., et al. (2016). "Anxiolytic properties of green tea polyphenol epigallocatechin gallate\ (EGCG)." *Science Direct Brain Research*. July 21. www.sciencedirect.com
14. Murakami, T., Furuse, M. (2010). "The impact of taurine and beta-alanine-supplemented diets on behavioral and neurochemical parameters in mice: Antidepressant versus anxiolytic-like effects." *Amino Acids*. Jul, 39(2):427–34.
15. Dolu, N., et al. (2014). "Investigation of dose-related effects of carnosine on anxiety with sympathetic skin response and T-maze." *Acta Medica*. 57(3):112–8.
16. Kanai, M., et al. (2009). "Tryptophan 2,3-dioxygenase is a key modulator of physiological neurogenesis and anxiety-related behavior in mice." *Molecular Brain*. March 27; 2:8.
17. Csilla, A., et al. (2016). "Exogenous ketone supplements reduce anxiety-related behavior in Sprague-Dawley and Wistar albino Glaxo/Rijswijk rats." *Front Mol Neurosci*. 9:137.
18. Gros, D. F., et al. (2009). "Frequency and severity of the symptoms of irritable bowel syndrome across the anxiety disorders and depression." *J Anxiety Disord*. Mar, 23(2):290–296.

19. Cohen, S., et al. (2012). "Chronic stress, glucocorticoid receptor resistance, inflammation and disease risk." *Proceedings of the National Academy of Sciences*. Apr 2.
20. Duivis, H. E., et al. (2013). "Differential association of somatic and cognitive symptoms of depression and anxiety with inflammation: Findings from the Netherlands study of depression and anxiety (NESDA)." *Psychoneuroendocrinology*. Sept, Vol 38, Issue 9:1573–1585.
21. Pitsavos, C., et al. (2006). "Anxiety in relation to coagulation markers among health adults: The ATTICA study." *Atherosclerosis*. Apr, Vol 185, Issue 2:320–326.
22. Hoban, A. E., et al. (2017). "Microbial regulation of microRNA expression in the amygdala and prefrontal cortex." *Microbiome*. 5:102.
23. Mohammadi, A. A., et al. (2016). "The effects of probiotics on mental health and hypothalamic-pituitary-adrenal axis: A randomized, double-blind, placebo-controlled trial in petrochemical workers." *Nutr Neuroscience*. Nov, 19(9):387–395.
24. Bravo, J. A., et al. (2011). "Ingestion of lactobacillus strain regulates emotional behavior and central GABA receptor expression in a mouse via the vagus nerve." *Proc Natl Acad Sci USA*. Sep 20, 108(38):16050–16055.
25. Bercik, P., et al. (2011). "The intestinal microbiota affect central levels of brain-derived neurotrophic factor and behavior in mice" *Gastroenterology*. Aug, 141(2):599–609.
26. Savignac, H. M., et al. (2014). "Bifidobacteria exert strain-specific effects on stress-related behavior and physiology in BALB mice." *Neurogastroenterol Motil*. Nov, 26(11):1615–27.
27. Messaoudi, M., et al. (2011). "Assessment of psychotropic-like properties of a probiotic formulation in rats and human subjects." *Br J Nutr*. Mar, 105(5):755–64.
28. Tavemiti, V., Guglielmetti, S. (2012). "Health-promoting properties of lactobacillus helveticus." *Front Microbiol*. Nov 19, 3:392.
29. Liu, Y. W., et al. (2016). "Psychotropic effects of lactobacillus plantarum PS128 in early life-stressed and naïve adult mice." *Brain Res*. Jan 15, 1631:1–12.
30. Buffington, S.A., et al. (2016). "Microbial reconstitution reverses maternal diet-induced social and synaptic deficits in offspring." *Cell*. June 16, Vol 165, Issue 7:1762–1775.
31. Cryan, J. F., O'Mahony, M. (2011). "The microbiome-gut-brain axis: From bowel to behavior." *Neurogastroenterology and Motility*. Feb 8, Vol 23, Issue 3:187–192.
32. Kimball, S. M., et al. (2018). "Database analysis of depression and anxiety in a community sample-response to a micronutrient intervention." *Nutrients*. Jan 30, 10(2).
33. Russo, A. J. (2011). "Decreased zinc and increased copper in individuals with anxiety." *Nutr Metab Insights*. 4:1–5.
34. Cope, E. C., Levenson, C. W. (2010). "Role of zinc in the development and treatment of mood disorders." *Curr Opin Clin Nutr Metab Care*. Nov, 13(6):685–9.
35. Brody, S., et al. (2002). "A randomized controlled trial of high dose ascorbic acid for reduction of blood pressure, cortisol, and subjective responses to psychological stress." *Psychopharmacology (Berl)*. Jan, 159(3):319–24.
36. Bjelland, I., et al. (2009). "*Choline in anxiety and depression*." Am J Clin Nutr. Oct, 90(4):1056–60.
37. Schiavin, A. P., et al. (2016). "Influence of single and repeated cannabidiol administration on emotional behavior and markers of cell proliferation and neurogenesis in non-stressed mice." *Prog Neuropsychopharmacol Biol Psychiatry*. Jan 4, 64:27–34.
38. Kuribara, H., et al. (2000). "The anxiolytic effect of two oriental herbal drugs in Japan attributed to honokiol from magnolia bark." *J Pharm Pharmacol*. Nov, 52(11):1425–9.
39. Reynolds, G. (2009). "Why exercise makes you less anxious." *New York Times*. Nov 18.
40. Sanders, L. (2018). "Poor sleep can be the cause of anxiety, study finds." *Washington Post* . Nov 10.
41. Walker, M. (2018). *Why we sleep*. New York: Scribner.
42. Pall, M. L. (2015). "Microwave frequency electromagnetic fields (EMFs) produce widespread neuropsychiatric effects including depression." *Journal of Chemical Neuroanatomy*. Sept, Vol 75, Part B:43–51.

Appendix D

1. Lopresti, A., et al. (2014). "Curcumin for the treatment of major depression: A randomized, double-blind, placebo controlled study." *Journal of Affective Disorders*. June 11.
2. Xu, Y., et al. (2005). "Antidepressant effects of curcumin in the forced swim test and olfactory bulbectomy models of depression in rats." *Pharmacology Biochemistry and Behavior*. Sep, Vol 82, Issue 1:200–206.
3. Ng, Q. X., et al. (2017). Clinical uses of curcumin in depression: A meta-analysis." *J Am Med Dir Assoc*. Jun 1, 18(6):503–509.
4. Lopresti, A., Drummond, P. (2017). "Efficacy of curcumin, and a saffron/curcumin combination for the treatment of major depression: A randomized, double-blind, placebo-controlled study." *Journal of Affective Disorders*. Oct 1, 207:188–196.
5. Hibbeln, J. R. (1995). "Dietary fatty acids and depression: When cholesterol does not satisfy." *Am J Clin Nutr*. 62:1–9.

6. Hibbeln, J. (2001). Interview with *Life Extension magazine October Report*
7. Osher, Y., Belmaker, R. H. (2009). "Omega-3 fatty acids in depression: A review of three studies." *CNS Neuroscience & Therapeutics*. 15(2):128–33.
8. Bonaterra, C. A., et al. (2018). "Neurotrophic, cytoprotective and anti-inflammatory effects of St. John's wort extract on differentiated mouse hippocampal HT-22 neurons." *Front Pharmacol.* Jan 18, 8:955. Doi: 10.33889/fphar.2017.00955.
9. Kimball, S. M., et al. (2018). "Database analysis of depression and anxiety in a community sample-response to a micronutrient intervention." *Nutrients*. Jan 30, 10(2).
10. Mercola, J. (2018). "For optimal health, make sure you have a vitamin D level of 60ng/mL." Mercola.com. July 4.
11. Murakami, T., Furuse, M. (2010). "The impact of taurine and beta-alanine-supplemented diets on behavioral and neurochemical parameters in mice: Antidepressant versus anxiolytic-like effects." *Amino Acids*. Jul, 39(2):427–34.
12. Shen, J., et al. (2016). "Berberine upregulates the BDNF expression in hippocampus and attenuates corticosterone-induced depressive-like behavior in mice." *Neuroscience Letters*. Feb 12, Vol 614:77–82.
13. Kulkami, S. K., Dhir, A. (2008). "On the mechanism of antidepressant-like action of berberine chloride." *Eur J Pharmacol.* Jul 28, 589(1–3):163–72.
14. Kumar, S., Mondal, A. C. (2016). "Neuroprotective, neurotrophic and antioxidant role of Bacopa monnieri on CSU induced model of depression in rat." *Neurochem Res.* Nov, 41(11):3083–3094.
15. Tomonaga, S., & Furuse, M. (2008). "Carnosine-induced antidepressant-like activity in rats." *Pharmacology, Biochemistry and Behavior* .June, Vol 89, Issue 4: 627–632.
16. Gangwisch, J. E., et al. (2015). "High glycemic index diet as a risk factor for depression: Analysis from the women's health initiative." *American Journal of Clinical Nutrition*. Aug, Vol 102, Issue 2:454–463.
17. Knuppel, A., et al. (2017). "Sugar intake from sweet food and beverages, common mental disorder and depression: Prospective findings from the Whitehall II study." *Scientific Reports*. July 27, Article 6287.
18. Murphy, P., Likhodii, S., Nylen, K., Burnham, W. (2004). "The antidepressant properties of the ketogenic diet." *Biol Psychiatry*. 56(12):981–3.10.1016/j.biopsych.2004.09.019.
19. Sussman, D., Germann, J., Henkelman, M. (2015). "Gestational ketogenic diet programs brain structure and susceptibility to depression & anxiety in the adult mouse offspring." *Brain Behav*. 5(2):e00300.10.1002/brb3.300
20. Hibbelin, J., et al. (2018). "Vegetarian diets and depressive symptoms among men." *Journal of Affective Disorders*. Jan, Vol 225:13–17.
21. Jacka, F. N., et al. (2012). "Red meat consumption and mood and anxiety disorders." *Psychother. Psychosom.* 81:196–198.
22. McAfoose, J., & Baune, B.T. (2009). "Evidence for a cytokine model of cognitive function." *Neurosci Biobehav Rev*. Mar, 33(3):355–66.
23. Felger, J. C., & Lotrich, F. E. (2013). "Inflammatory cytokines in depression: Neurobiological mechanisms and therapeutic implications." *Neuroscience*. Aug 29, 246:199–229.
24. Forsythe, C. E., Phinney, S. D., et al. (2008). "Comparisons of low fat and low carbohydrate on circulating fatty acid composition and markers of inflammation." *Lipids*. Jan, 43(1)65–77.
25. Kulkami, S. K., Dhir, A. (2008). "On the mechanism of antidepressant-like action of berberine chloride." *Eur J Pharmacol.* Jul 28, 589(1–3):163–72.
26. Yary, T., et al. (2017). "Serum dihomo-y-linolenic acid level inversely associated with the risk of depression." *J Affect Disord.* Apr 15, 213:151–156.
27. Valles-Colomer, M. V., et al. (2019). "The neuroactive potential of the human gut microbiota in quality of life and depression." *Nature Microbiology*. 4:623–632.
28. Wallace, C. J. K., Milev, R. (2017). "The effects of probiotics on depressive symptoms in humans: A systemic review." *Am Gen Psychiatry*. March 7, 16:18.
29. Kazemi, A. et al. (2018). "Effect of probiotic and prebiotic vs placebo on psychological outcomes in patients with major depressive disorder: A randomized clinical trial." *Clinical Nutrition*. Apr 24, pii: S0261-5614(18)30161-4.
30. Ait-Belgnaoui, A., et al. (2014). "Probiotic gut effect prevents the chronic stress-induced brain activity abnormality in mice." *Neurogastroenterol Motil.* 26(4):510–20.
31. Pinto-Sanchez, M. I., et al. (2017). "Probiotic Bifidobacterium longum reduces depression scores and alters brain activity." *Gastroenterology*. Aug, 153(2):448–459.
32. Mercola, J. (2017). "Depression is now the no. 1 cause of illness and disability worldwide." Mercola.com. Apr 13.
33. Mikkelsen, K., et al. (2016). "The effects of vitamin B on the immune/cytokine network and their involvement in depression." *Maturitas*. Nov 6, 2016 online pub: https://doi.org/10.1016/j.maturitas.2016.11.012
34. Petrilli, M. A., et al. (2017). "The emerging role for zinc in depression and psychosis." *Frontiers in Pharmacology*. 8:414.
35. Richarson, A. C., et al. (2015). "Higher body iron is associated with greater depression symptoms among young adult men but not women: Observational data from the daily life study." *Nutrients*. Aug, 7(8):6055–6072.

36. Juvenon Health Journal. (2018). "4 ways to ditch depression ... naturally." Juvenon.com.
37. Wang, S. M., et al. (2014). "A review of current evidence for acetyl-l-carnitine in the treatment of depression." *J Psychiatr Res.* Jun, 53:30–7.
38. Maes, M., et al. (2009). "Lower plasma coenzyme Q10 in depression." *Neuro Endocrinol Lett.* 30(4):462–9.
39. Wang, S., & Pan, J. (2016). "Irisin ameliorates depressive-like behaviors in rats by regulating metabolism." *Biochem Biophys Res Commun.* May 20, 474(1):22–28.
40. Huang, L., et al. (2019). "Irisin regulates the expression of BDNF and glycometabolism in diabetic rats." *Mol Med Rep.* Feb, 19(2):1074–1082.
41. Tarleton, E. K., et al. (2017). "Role of magnesium supplementation in the treatment of depression: A randomized clinical trial." *PLOS/One.* June 27. https://doi.org/10.1371/journal.pone.0180067
42. Tarleton, E. K., Littenberg, B. (2015). "Magnesium intake and depression in adults." *Journal of the American Board of Family Medicine.* Mar–Apr, 28(2):249–56.
43. Lin, T. W. & Kuo, Y. M. (2013). "Exercise benefits brain function: The monoamine connection." *Brain Sci.* 3:39–53.
44. Gordon, B. R., et al. (2018). "Association of efficacy of resistance exercise training with depressive symptoms." *JAMA Psychiatry.* 75(6):566–5756.
45. O'Connor, P. J., et al. (2010). "Mental health benefits of strength training." *American Journal of Lifestyle Medicine.* May 7, Vol 4, Issue 5.
46. Ahrne, S., et al. (2011). "Effect of lactobacilli on paracellular permeability in the gut." *Nutrients,* 3:104–117.
47. Pall, M. L. (2015). "Microwave frequency electromagnetic fields (EMFs) produce widespread neuropsychiatric effects including depression." *Journal of Chemical Neuroanatomy.* Sept, Vol 75, Part B:43–51.
48. Qato, D. M., et al. (2018). "Prevalence of prescription medications with depression as a potential adverse effect among adults in the United States." *JAMA.* 319(22):2289–2298.
49. You, H., et al. (2013). "The relationship between statins and depression: A review of the literature." *Expert Opin Pharmacother.* 14(11):1467–1476.

Appendix E

1. Jiao, S. S., et al. (2016). "Brain-derived neurotrophic factor protects against tau-related neurodegeneration of Alzheimer's disease." *Translational Psychiatry.* Oct 4, 6.
2. Beeri, M. S. & Sonnen, J. (2016). "Brain BDNF expression as a biomarker for cognitive reserve against Alzheimer disease progression." *Neurology.* 86:702–703.
3. Rezai-Zedah, K., et al. (2008). "Green tea epigallocatechin-3-gallate (EGCG) reduces beta-amyloid mediated cognitive impairment and modulates tau pathology in Alzheimer's transgenic mice." *Brain Research.* July, 1214(C):177–187.
4. Tang, M., Taghibiglou, C. (2017). "The mechanisms of action of curcumin in Alzheimer's disease." *J Alzheimer's Dis.* 58(4):1003–1016.
5. Cai, Z., et al. (2016). "Role of berberine in Alzheimer's disease." *Neuropsychiatr Dis Treatment.* 12:2509–2520.
6. Williams, P., et al. (2011). "Natural products as a source of Alzheimer's drug leads." *Nat Prod Rep.* Jan, 28(1);48–77.
7. Daiello, L. A., et al. (2015). "Association of fish oil supplement use with preservation of brain volume and cognitive function." *Alzheimer's Dement.* Feb,15(2):226–235.
8. Pottala, J.V., et al. (2015). "Higher RBC EPA & DHA corresponds with larger total brain and hippocampal volumes." *Neurology.* Feb 4, 82(5):435–442.
9. Tan, Z. S., et al. (2012). "Red blood cell omega-3 fatty acid levels and markers of accelerated brain aging." *Neurology.* Feb 28, 78(9):658–654.
10. Ren, H., et al. (2017). "Omega-3 polyunsaturated fatty acids promote amyloid beta clearance from the brain through mediating the function of the glymphatic system." *FASEB J.* Jan, 31(1):282–293.
11. Zhang, Y. P., et al. (2017). "Effects of DHA supplementation on hippocampal volume and cognitive function in older adults with mild cognitive impairment." *J Alzheimer's Dis.* 55(2):497–507.
12. Sehgal, N., et al. (2012). "Withania somnifera reverses Alzheimer's disease pathology by enhancing low-density lipoprotein receptor-related protein in liver." *Proc Natl Acad Sci USA.* Feb 28, 109(9): 3510–3515.
13. Wu, B., et al. (2012). "Icariin improves cognitive deficits and activates quiescent neural stem cells in aging rats." *J Ethnopharmacol.* Aug 1, 142(3):746–53.
14. Paula-Lima, A. C., et al. (2005). "Activation of GABA(A) receptors by taurine and muscimol blocks the neurotoxicity of beta-amyloid in rat hippocampal and cortical neurons." *Neuropharmacology.* Dec, 49(8):1140–8.
15. Jiao, S. S., et al. (2016). "Brain-derived neurotrophic factor protects against tau-related neurodegeneration of Alzheimer's disease." *Translational Psychiatry.* Oct 4, 6, e907.
16. Krikorian, R., et al. (2013). "Dietary ketosis enhances memory in mild cognitive impairment." *Neurobiol Aging.* 33(2):425.e27.

17. Jx, Y., et al. (2016). "Ketones block amyloid entry and improve cognition in an Alzheimer's model." *Neurobiol Aging*. 39:25–37.
18. Reger, M. A., et al. (2004). "Effects of beta-hydroxybutyrate on cognition in memory-impaired adults." *Neurobiol Aging*. 25(3):311–114.
19. Zheng, F., et al. (2018). "HbA1c, diabetes and cognitive decline: The English longitudinal study of ageing." *Diabetologia*. April, Vol 61, Issue 4:839–848.
20. Enzinger, C., et al. (2005). "Risk factors for progression of brain atrophy in aging." *Neurology*. May 24, 64(10):1704–11.
21. Kerti, L., et al. (2013). "Higher glucose levels associated with lower memory and reduced hippocampal microstructure." *Neurology*. Oct 13, 81:1746–1752.
22. Roberts, R. O., et al. (2012). "Relative intake of macronutrients impacts risk of mild cognitive impairment or dementia." *Journal of Alzheimer's Disease*. Jan 1: 32(2): 329-339
23. LaMotte, S., (2019). "Alzheimer's risk may be 75% higher for people who eat trans fats." CNN Health online Oct 24
24. Bredesen, D. (2017). *The end of Alzheimer's*. New York: Avery.
25. Brandt, J., et al. (2019). "Preliminary report on the feasibility and efficacy of the modified Atkins diet for treatment of mild cognitive impairment and early Alzheimer's disease." *Journal of Alzheimer's Disease*. Vol 68, No 3:969–981.
26. Parbo, P., et al. (2017). "Brain inflammation accompanies amyloid in the majority of mild cognitive impairment cases due to Alzheimer's disease." *Brain*. July, Vol 140, Issue 7:2002–2011.
27. Ozawa, M., et al. (2017). "Dietary pattern, inflammation and cognitive decline." *Clin Nutrition*. Apr, 36(2):506–512.
28. Walker, K., et al. (2017). "Midlife systemic inflammatory markers are associated with late-life brain volume." *Neurology*. Nov 28, 2262–2270.
29. Zonis, S., et al. (2015) "Chronic intestinal inflammation alters hippocampal neurogenesis." *Journal of Inflammation*. 12(65).
30. Akbari, E., et al. (2016). "Effect of probiotic supplementation on cognitive function and metabolic status in Alzheimer's disease." *Frontiers in Aging Neuroscience*. Nov 10. frontiersin.org
31. Nation, D. A., et al. (2019). "Blood-brain barrier breakdown is an early biomarker of human cognitive dysfunction." *Nature Medicine*. Jan 14, 25:270–276.
32. Novkovic, B. (2018). "20 causes of leaky gut syndrome and 15 healing treatments." Selfhacked.com. Nov 27.
33. Bushche, M. A., et al. (2019). "Tau impairs neural circuits, dominating amyloid-beta effects, in Alzheimer's models in vivo." *Nature Neuroscience*. 22, 57–64.
34. Sehgal, N., et al. (2012). "Withania somnifera reverses Alzheimer's disease pathology by enhancing low-density lipoprotein receptor-related protein in liver." *Proc Natl Acad Sci USA*. Jan 30, v.109(9):3510–3515.
35. Mancuso, C., et al. (2012). "Natural substances and Alzheimer's disease: From preclinical studies to evidence based medicine." *Biochimica et Biophysica Acta: Molecular Basis of Disease*. May, Vol 1822, Issue 5:616–624.
36. Comejo, A., et al. (2011). "Fulvic acid inhibits aggregation and promotes disassembly of tau fibrils associated with Alzheimer's disease." *J Alzheimers Dis*. 27(1):143–53.
37. Morello, M., et al. (2018). "Vitamin D improves neurogenesis and cognition in a mouse model of Alzheimer's disease." *Mol Neurobiol*. Aug, 55(8):64643–79.
38. Annweiler, C., et al. (2011). "Vitamin D-mentia" *Neuroepidemiology*. 37(3–4):117–41.
39. Goodwill, A. M., et al. (2018). "Vitamin D status is associated with executive function a decade later." *Maturitas*. Jan, 107:56–62.
40. Llewellyn, D. J., et al. (2010). "Vitamin D and risk of cognitive decline in elderly persons." *Arch Intern Med*. Jul 12, 170(13):1135–1141.
41. Mercola, J. (2019). "Top 4 reasons to check your iron level, not your cholesterol." Mercola.com. Jan 9.
42. Stough, C., et al. (2001). "The chronic effects of an extract of bacopa monnieri (Brahmi) on cognitive function in healthy human subjects." *Psychopharmacology (Berl)*. Aug, 156(4):481–4.
43. Stough, C., et al. (2008). "Examining the nootropic effects of a special extract of bacopa mannieri on human cognitive functioning." *Phytother Res*. Dec, 22(12):1629–34.
44. Cohut, M. (2018). "Can beets tackle Alzheimer's at its root?" *Medical News Today*. March 22.
45. Parnetti, L., et al. (2001). "Choline alphoscerate in cognitive decline and in acute cerebrovascular disease: An analysis of published clinical data." *Mech Ageing Dev*. Nov, 122(16):2041–55.
46. Dysken, M. W., et al. (2014). "Effect of vitamin E and memantine on functional decline in Alzheimer's disease." *JAMA*. Jan 1, 311(1):33–44.
47. Hoder, H., et al. (2018). "Midlife cardiovascular fitness and dementia." *Neurology*. Mar 14.
48. Blumenthal, J. A., et al. (2018). "Lifestyle and neurocogntion in older adults with cognitive impairments." *Neurology*. Dec 19. n.neurology.org
49. Colcombe, S. J., et al. (2006). "Aerobic fitness training increases brain volume in aging humans." *Journal of Gerontology: Series A*. Nov 1, Vol 61, Issue 11:1166–1170.
50. Kennelly, S. P., et al. (2009). "Blood pressure and dementia." *Ther Adv Neurol Dosord*. Jul, 2(4): 241–260.

51. Arvanatakis, Z., et al. (2018). "Late-life blood pressure association with cerebrovascular and Alzheimer's disease pathology." *Neurology*. July 12. n.neurology.org
52. Cortright, B. (2015). *The neurogenesis diet and lifestyle*. Mill Valley, CA: Psyche Media.
53. Erikson, K. I., et al. (2011). "Exercise training increases size of hippocampus and improves memory." *Proceedings of the National Academy of Sciences*. Feb 15, 108(7):3017–3022.
54. Lourenco, M. V., et al. (2019). "Exercise-linked FNDC5/irisin rescues synaptic plasticity and memory defects in Alzheimer's models." *Nature Medicine*. Jan 07, 25, 163–175.
55. Shokri-Kojori, E., et al. (2018). "Beta-amyloid accumulation in the human brain after one night of sleep deprivation." *Proceedings of the National Academy of Sciences*. April 24, 115(7):4483–4488.
56. Walker, M. (2018). *Why we sleep*. New York: Scribner
57. Ren, H., et al. (2016). "Omega-3 polyunsaturated fatty acids promote amyloid beta clearance from the brain through mediating the function of the glymphatic system." *FASEB Journal*. Oct 7 online.
58. Nevado-Holgado, A. J., et al. (2016). "Commonly prescribed drugs associate with cognitive function." *BMJ Open*. Nov 30. bmjopen.bmj.com
59. Moore, A. R. & O'Keeffe, S. T. (1999). "Drug-induced cognitive impairment in the elderly." *Drugs Aging*. Jul, 15(1):15–28.
60. Coupland, C. A. C., et al. (2019). "Anticholinergic drug exposure and the risk of dementia." *JAMA Internal Medicine*. 179(8):1084–1093.

ACKNOWLEDGMENTS

My patients over the decades have been the greatest source of inspiration for this book. I am grateful to be in a profession that allows me to be with people in a deeply vulnerable, authentic way in their journey of healing. This book is a direct result of what I have learned from them.

Several friends and colleagues have provided invaluable feedback to the manuscript. Philip Brooks and Mark Fromm read the entire work and gave very specific, helpful comments. Bill Melton provided big picture feedback that was enormously constructive in shaping the final form. Devon Cortright and Ron Moshontz provided sensitive advice on the tone of the book. Rachael Vaughn read an early version of the first two chapters and pointed out some important gaps and missing links.

A sabbatical from my university gave me extra time to write, and a grant from the Green Earth Foundation gave material support to this work which was very much appreciated.

My editor, Madeline Hopkins, was a godsend. She has been tireless and meticulous in bringing greater clarity and order to its final form.

Thank you all.

ABOUT THE AUTHOR

Brant Cortright, Ph.D., is *professor emeritus* in psychology with the California Institute of Integral Studies. He maintains a private psychotherapy pratice in San Francisco and works as a consultant and coach with individuals around the globe. The author of four books, he speaks and gives workshops in the U.S., Europe, and Asia. Visit him on the web at: brantcortright.com

Made in the USA
Las Vegas, NV
20 March 2021

19854346R00208